EPIDEMIOLOGY AND CONTROL OF NEMATODIASIS IN CATTLE

CURRENT TOPICS IN VETERINARY MEDICINE AND ANIMAL SCIENCE

VOLUME 9

EPIDEMIOLOGY AND CONTROL OF NEMATODIASIS IN CATTLE

Other titles in this series

Series ISBN: 90-247-2429-5

EPIDEMIOLOGY AND CONTROL OF NEMATODIASIS IN CATTLE

An Animal Pathology in the CEC Programme of
Coordination of Agricultural Research, held at the
Royal Veterinary and Agricultural University, Copenhagen,
Denmark, February 4-6, 1980

Sponsored by the Commission of the European Communities,
Directorate-General for Agriculture, Coordination of
Agricultural Research

Edited by

P. Nansen

Royal Veterinary and Agricultural University,
Copenhagen, Denmark

R. Jess Jørgensen

Royal Veterinary and Agricultural University,
Copenhagen, Denmark

E.J.L. Soulsby

Veterinary School,
Cambridge, United Kingdom

1981
MARTINUS NIJHOFF PUBLISHERS
THE HAGUE / BOSTON / LONDON

for

THE COMMISSION OF THE EUROPEAN COMMUNITIES

Distributors

for the United States and Canada
Kluwer Boston, Inc.
190 Old Derby Street
Hingham, MA 02043
USA

for all other countries
Kluwer Academic Publishers Group
Distribution Center
P.O. Box 322
3300 AH Dordrecht
The Netherlands

ISBN 90-247-2502-X (this volume)
ISBN 90-247-2429-5 (series)

SF
967
P3
EC
1981

Publication arranged by
Commission of the European Communities,
Directorate-General Information Market and Innovation

EUR 6901 EN

Manuscript Preparation by
Janssen Services, 33a High Street, Chislehurst, Kent BR7 5AE, UK

PRINTED IN THE NETHERLANDS

PREFACE

This publication is the Proceedings of a workshop held at the Royal
Veterinary and Agricultural University in Copenhagen, Denmark on 4th –
6th February, 1980, sponsored by the Commission of the European
Communities (CEC) as a part of the programme of coordination of
agricultural research in the field of animal pathology. The CEC wishes
to thank those who took responsibility for the organisation of the
workshop, those who presented the papers, and all participants.

CONTENTS

X

SESSION I

METHODOLOGY I
Chairman: D. Düwel

MONITORING PASTURE INFECTIVITY AND PASTURE CONTAMINATION WITH INFECTIVE STAGES OF *Dictyocaulus viviparus*

R.J. Jørgensen

Institute of Veterinary Microbiology and Hygiene,
Royal Veterinary and Agricultural University,
Bülowsvej 13, DK-1870 Copenhagen V. Denmark

ABSTRACT

The technique for the estimation of pasture larval contamination by the examination of herbage is presented. Samples are taken near to faecal pats where the larvae are expected to be concentrated; a second sample taken at least 100 cm from the faecal pat provides information on the horizontal distribution of the pasture contamination.

The bile-agar technique for herbage samples is compared with results obtained with tracer calves. It is concluded that the two parameters are not directly comparable, nevertheless they both provide useful information on the presence of infective stages in the pasture.

P. Nansen, R.J. Jørgensen, E.J.L. Soulsby (eds), Epidemiology and Control of Nematodiasis in Cattle.
Copyright © 1981 ECSC, EEC, EAEC, Brussels – Luxembourg. All rights reserved.

INTRODUCTION

The purpose of monitoring the number of lungworm larvae
on a grazing area may be to determine whether the infection has
over-wintered or not or it may be to follow fluctuations
during the grazing season. In addition, the demonstration of
infective larvae in the pasture before clinical disease has
developed may be used in the surveillance of parasitic
bronchitis.

Two methods are available; the use of tracer calves and
the examination of pasture samples for infective stages. These
methods express the pasture infectivity and the pasture larval
contamination, respectively.

The methods and experiences with these techniques will be
presented and discussed.

METHODS

Pasture larval contamination

Sampling

When sampling for over-wintered larvae, an important
problem is that such larvae are present in extremely low numbers
at the time of the turning out of animals to pasture. Under
Danish conditions the contamination may be lower than 1 larva
per kg of herbage. Therefore the collection of fairly large
samples may be necessary. The disappearance rate of over-
wintered larvae seems to follow a logarithmic course (Jørgensen,
1980a). Hence sampling in early spring may permit extrapolation
of the contamination later on. The highest contamination of
over-wintered larvae is found in the herbage around faecal
deposits.

During the grazing season maximum larval counts are obtained similarly from the herbage sampled close to faecal pats (Figure 1). For this a pooled sample of herbage is collected within a distance of 5 cm around 40 - 50 randomly selected pats, avoiding newly deposited and very old ones. A second sample may be picked at a distance of at least 100 cm from any faecal droppings. Though the collection of this sample is more tedious and it will contain comparatively few larvae, nevertheless it will give an indication of the horizontal distribution of the pasture contamination when related to the results of the first sample (Jørgensen, 1980a, b, c).

In general, the time of sampling is not critical. In very dry periods, maximum numbers are recovered 4 - 6 hours after sunrise (Jørgensen, 1980b). Relatively high counts may be obtained by separate sampling of wet areas of the field (e.g. around water holes and drinking troughs). Due to the rapidity with which the larvae appear and disappear, sampling at weekly intervals may be essential in order to disclose shortlived peaks.

Storage of herbage samples

Herbage samples contained in plastic bags may be stored in the refrigerator for one or two weeks without any significant loss of viable *D. viviparus* larvae.

Washing

Thorough washing is essential. A modified cement mixer or household washing machine will allow easy processing of large samples and easy handling of large volumes of water. A comparison between the efficiency of the cement mixer and a Colworth Stomacher Lab. Blender[*] has shown that they are

[*] Model 3500, Seward Laboratory, UAC House, Blackfriars Rd., London SE1 9UG, England.

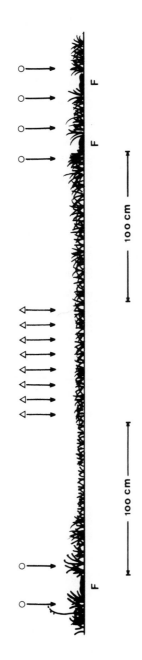

Fig. 1. Sampling for the recovery of *D. viviparus* larvae. F = faecal pats; O = sample taken 5 cm from faecal pats; Δ = sample taken at least 100 cm from pats.

equally efficient in recovering larvae from samples of 250 g of herbage. The stomacher apparatus is quicker to operate, but is not recommended for samples of more than 300 g.

Laboratory technique

The experience of this laboratory with the agar-bile technique (Jørgensen, 1975) may be summarised as follows: laboratory capacity; a maximum of 50 samples/week/2 persons (including washing and microscopical examination) can be dealt with; sensitivity (i.e. ability to detect low numbers of *D. viviparus* larvae) and specificity (i.e. efficient separation of larvae and debris) is satisfactory; laboratory variation may reach 100% when few larvae are present but this is greatly reduced if sediments are split into two sub-samples which are processed separately; for relative efficiency (recovery rate and comparison with traditional techniques): see Jørgensen (1975) and Duncan et al. (1979); technicians favour the work with agar; specially made glass cylinders and racks involve extra expenses; the recovery rate of trichostrongyle larvae is satisfactory (Mwegoha and Jørgensen, 1977) however differential counting of trichostrongyle larvae is complicated by the ex-sheathment of a certain proportion of these larvae during incubation.

Identification of lungworm larvae

D. viviparus larvae may be identified under the microscope according to Iskander and Jørgensen (1980).

Pasture infectivity (tracer calves)

The number of worms present in the lungs of susceptible calves grazed for maximum two weeks and stabled for 2 - 3 weeks is often used for a parameter in experimental work. However, the clinical signs, including larval excretion, may also be monitored. The individual variation is considerable, possibly due to variations in uptake of larvae and variations in the explusion of immature worms (Michel, 1969).

COMPARISON BETWEEN PASTURE LARVAL CONTAMINATION AND PASTURE
INFECTIVITY

The difference between these two parameters in the field
is reflected in the data presented in Table 1. It is concluded
however, that the two parameters are not directly comparable,
but that they both provide valuable information on the presence
of *D. viviparus* infective stages on the pasture.

TABLE 1

HERBAGE INFECTIVITY, EXPRESSED AS MEAN LUNGWORM COUNTS OF SUSCEPTIBLE PAIRS
OF CALVES (TRACERS), AND HERBAGE CONTAMINATION, EXPRESSED AS MEAN *Dictyocaulus*
LARVAL COUNTS OF 3 WEEKLY HERBAGE SAMPLES TAKEN DURING THE SAME 2 WEEK
PERIODS GRAZED BY THE RESPECTIVE TRACER PAIRS. THE FIELD WAS GRAZED
PERMANENTLY (MAY – SEPTEMBER) BY CALVES DURING BOTH SEASONS.

Grazing period	Mean worm counts of tracers	Mean herbage contamination (L_3/kg)	
		Away from faeces	Close to faeces
1974			
30th April – 14th May	0	1.3	1.3
28th May – 11th June	110	4	21
25th June – 9th July	904	8	12
23rd July – 6th Aug.	2 400	54	171
20th Aug. – 3rd Sept.	1 427	13	71
17th Sept. – 30th Sept.	964	1.0	7
1975			
29th July – 12th Aug.	155	16	18
12th Aug. – 26th Aug.	37	0	5
26th Aug. – 9th Sept.	231	2	48
9th Sept. – 23rd Sept.	143	2	170
23rd Sept. – 7th Oct.	413	1	166

(The figures are extracts of data published by Jørgensen, 1980b).

Several factors, some of them interacting, are likely to complicate such a comparison. These include the stocking rate, climate, grass growth and individual variation between calves, including variations in grazing behaviour. From a cost-benefit viewpoint the author has found that examination of the herbage contamination close to faecal pats is easy to perform, is inexpensive and sensitive.

REFERENCES

Duncan, J.L., Armour, J., Bairden, K., Urquhart, G.M. and Jørgensen, R.J., 1979. Studies on the epidemiology of bovine parasitic bronchitis. Vet. Rec. 104, 274-278.

Iskander, A.R. and Jørgensen, R.J., 1980. Identification of infective *Dictyocaulus viviparus* larvae isolated from herbage by the bile-agar technique. Acta vet. Scand. 21 (in press)

Jørgensen, R.J., 1975. Isolation of infective *Dictyocaulus* larvae from herbage. Vet. Parasitol. 1, 61-67.

Jørgensen, R.J., 1980a. Recent Danish studies on the epidemiology of bovine parasitic bronchitis. Proceedings of a CEC Workshop meeting on 'The epidemiology and control of nematodiasis in cattle', Copenhagen, 4th to 6th February, 1980 (in press).

Jørgensen, R.J., 1980b. Epidemiology of dictyocaulosis in Denmark. Vet. Parasitol. 7, 153-167.

Jørgensen, R.J., 1980c. An experimental study on the epidemiology and prevention of naturally acquired verminous bronchitis. Acta vet. Scand. (In press).

Michel, J.F., 1969. Experiments on the loss of *Dictyocaulus filaria* from the lungs of infected sheep. V. Some general conclusions. Folia Parasitologica (Praha) 16, 361-363.

Mwegoha, W.M. and Jørgensen, R.J., 1977. Recovery of infective 3rd stage larvae of *Haemonchus contortus* and *Ostertagia ostertagi* by migration in agar gel. Acta vet. Scand. 18, 293-299.

THE CORRECT HANDLING OF FAECAL SAMPLES USED FOR EXAMINATION OF *Dictyocaulus viviparus* LARVAE

H.J.W.M. Cremers[*]

Institute of Veterinary Parasitology and Parasitic Diseases,
State University, Utrecht, The Netherlands

ABSTRACT

Faecal samples for examination for larvae of Dictyocaulus viviparus *were stored in plastic bags at room temperature and at 4 - 6°C. Larvae were collected by the Baermann method at varying times after collection and storage. After one day of storage at room temperature there was a marked decrease in the number of larvae recovered by the Baermann method. However, many larvae were found on the wall of the plastic bag and not in the faeces.*

It is concluded that the faeces to be used for examination for Dictyocaulus *larvae should be stored in a refrigerator when storage for more than one day is necessary.*

* Presented by Professor J. Jansen

P. Nansen, R.J. Jørgensen, E.J.L. Soulsby (eds), Epidemiology and Control of Nematodiasis in Cattle.

INTRODUCTION

Many of the faecal samples of calves and yearlings, which are sent from veterinary practices to our Institute for examination for lungworm larvae, fail to show larvae although the clinical signs, grazing history and time of the year would suggest that a positive result might be expected. Most of these samples do not reach the laboratory on the same day they are collected, but one, or a few, days later. This is especially so when they are sent by mail. Since it is known that larvae of *Dictyocaulus viviparus* can only survive for a short time in dry faeces (Rose, 1956), an experiment was done to compare the survival of larvae following storage of faecal samples at room temperature or in the refrigerator.

MATERIALS AND METHODS

Faeces were collected from the rectum of yearling arrivals (Experiment 1) or calves (Experiment 2) suffering from parasitic bronchitis on two farms in the neighbourhood of Utrecht. After transport to the Institute, the faeces were well mixed by hand and samples of 20 g were prepared. In each experiment four samples were placed immediately in a modified Baermann apparatus, as used in our Institute. The remaining samples were put in small plastic bags and divided in two groups: Group 1 was placed in a refrigerator (4 - 6°) and Group 2 was held at room temperature (20 - 23°C) in the daylight. At varying times, two samples of each group were placed in a Baermann apparatus for 24 h at room temperature and the larvae were collected and counted. In Experiment 2, after scraping the faeces from the plastic bag, the bag was washed onto the screen of another Baermann apparatus, which was then handled as mentioned above.

RESULTS

The results are given in Table 1. The average number of larvae from the two samples, stored at the same temperature during the same time, is expressed in the percentage of the average

number of larvae found in four samples, which were placed
directly in the Baermann apparatus. The average number of these
four samples was 52 (= 100% in the Table) in Experiment 1 and
133 (= 100% in the Table) in Experiment 2.

TABLE 1

RECOVERY OF LARVAE OF *D. viviparus* IN SAMPLES OF 20 g FAECES AFTER STORAGE
AT 4 - 6°C AND 20 - 23°C.

Time after collection from the animal	Percentage of recovered larvae			
	4 - 6°C		20 - 23°C	
(Hours)	Faeces	Faeces + plastic bag	Faeces	Faeces + plastic bag
Exp. 1 2			100	
13	60		12	
24	60		15	
48	37		4	
73	29		0	
Exp. 2 4			100	
20	111	158	59	113
28	92	159	22	75
52	111	168	0.8	2.8
76	92	153	0	0.8
166	42	120	0	0

DISCUSSION

As can be seen in Table 1, there is a rapid decrease in
the recovery of larvae from faeces stored at room temperature
after one day. There is no obvious explanation for the marked
decrease in Experiments 1 and 2. In Experiment 2 it is evident
that, because of condensation of water on the wall of the plastic
bag, larvae soon migrated from faeces to the plastic. More
larvae were found in faeces plus washings from the plastic bag
after storage at low temperatures than with fresh faeces so
treated. This can possibly be explained by an increased motility

of the larvae when they are placed at the higher temperature
of the water in the Baermann apparatus after storage at low
temperatures. Because of the almost complete absence of faecal
debris in the plastic bag-Baermann, the migration of the living
larvae is much easier than from faeces.

The conclusions of these experiments are that faecal samples
for examination on *D. viviparus* larvae should be examined directly
or, if storage is necessary before examination, the material
should be stored in a refrigerator. When faeces are kept for
one day at room temperature (e.g. in a car or in the post) it
is very useful to examine the plastic bag as well as the faeces.
Storage of faeces for a longer time renders them unfit for
examination with the Baermann method.

REFERENCE

Rose, J.H. 1956. The bionomics of the free-living larvae of *Dictyocaulus*
    viviparus. J. Comp. Path. 66, 228-240.

DISCUSSION

H.-J. Bürger *(FRG)*

Is the time given in the table that when the examination procedure was begun, or was it the time when the larvae were examined? How long did these samples stay in the Baermann apparatus?

J. Jansen *(The Netherlands)*

The time stated in the table is the number of hours of storage at a given temperature. The examination occupied about 24 h.

J.F. Michel *(UK)*

I would like to comment on Dr. Jørgensen's finding that the largest concentrations of larvae are to be found on the herbage at noon, or thereabouts. This is similar to observations by Crofton about 30 years ago. I wonder whether this is due to the fact that at mid-day a given bulk of herbage probably weighs less because it is drier. In other words, it is an artefact.

R.J. Jørgensen *(Denmark)*

The drying up of the herbage in the field took place before the increase in the herbage larval contamination.

J-P. Raynaud *(France)*

In your results you detect more *Dictyocaulus* by the use of tracer animals than by the herbage estimates. The ideal system of detection could be the tracers for *Dictyocaulus*?

R.J. Jørgensen

This is very difficult to answer. I have often found the situation where larvae are found on the pasture close to faeces and while tracers may be on the pasture they would not reflect

pasture burdens in such a case. I think that was the case in
the table, but this also could be due to technical problems in
recovering small numbers of parasites from lungs.

J-P. Raynaud

So you are not concluding there is a relationship between
the tracer animals and the larvae on herbage?

R.J. Jørgensen

No, I do not think they are directly comparable. In the
tracer animals one runs into problems of very large individual
variations between calves. One may find one animal negative
whereas another may be almost dying from parasitic infection.

J. Eckert   *(Switzerland)*

Do you have any recommendations for the practitioners,
Dr. Jansen? You said that you examined the faecal samples on
the spot. What practical recommendations do you have?

J. Jansen

I think that an examination, even with a simple Baermann
apparatus, is easy enough for the practitioner to do for himself.

J. Eckert

But do they accept this?

J. Jansen

I don't think so. Even with the ordinary faecal examinations for eggs, we often do these ourselves. But I think a
practitioner should do it himself, especially in the case of
Dictyocaulus. There may be a delay which could compromise the
results. For example, if he sends the sample by rail, first it
may be in his car for some hours, then it may take a couple of
days to reach the animal health station. I advise him to do it
himself.

SOME EFFECTS OF STORAGE ON THE RECOVERY OF
Dictyocaulus viviparus LARVAE FROM FAECES

M.T. Fox[*]

Department of Microbiology and Parasitology,
Royal Veterinary College,
University of London, UK.

ABSTRACT

Storage of faeces at +8°C for 1 - 2 weeks improved the numbers of Dictyocaulus viviparus *larvae that could be recovered with the Baermann technique.*

[*] Presented by D.E. Jacobs.

P. Nansen, R.J. Jørgensen, E.J.L. Soulsby (eds), Epidemiology and Control of Nematodiasis in Cattle.

INTRODUCTION

The rate of collection of faecal samples from cattle during a large scale field epidemiology study exceeded the capacity of this laboratory to process the material, thus creating a severe storage problem. A cold chamber kept at +8°C was available for storage but the suitability of this temperature for keeping faeces intended for the diagnosis of lungworm infection was unknown. The investigations described below were therefore instituted.

MATERIAL AND METHODS

Faeces from lungworm infected calves were kindly supplied by Glaxo Research Laboratories, Ware. Sixty 25 g faecal samples were taken from a single bulk collection, after thorough mixing, and placed in 1 oz polypots with tightly fitting lids. Thirty of the prepared pots were stored in the cold chamber at +8°C, the remainder were kept at room temperature. At approximately weekly intervals, lungworm larvae were recovered from the contents of each of six pots (of which three had been stored at +8°C), using the Baermann technique and counted.

This procedure was repeated on three occasions using faeces from different donor animals.

RESULTS

Larval recoveries are displayed in Figure 1.

Storage at room temperature resulted in a rapid decline in the numbers of larvae recovered by the Baermann technique. By two weeks, larval counts had fallen by more than 80%. In contrast, storage at +8°C resulted in the detection of increasing numbers of larvae over the first 6 - 15 days, maximum numbers exceeding Day 0 values by factors of between

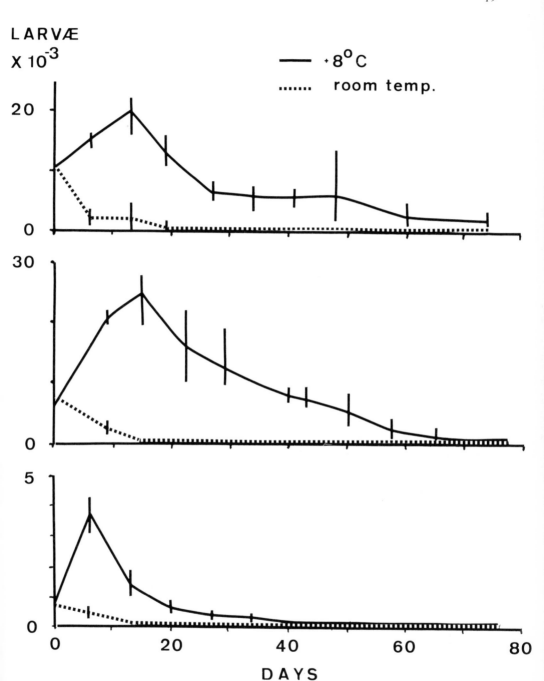

Fig. 1. The numbers of *D. viviparus* larvae recovered from 25 g faecal samples by the Baermann technique after storage at +8°C or room temperature. Vertical lines display range of counts on each occasion.

1.9 and 5.6. Numbers were reduced thereafter but substantial recoveries (more than 50% of the Day 0 value) were achieved for 35 - 55 days after collection of the sample. A few larvae could still be found after 70 - 80 days.

At Day 0, all recovered nematodes were in the first larval stage. After storage at +8°C for 6 - 9 days a variable proportion of the larvae were observed to be ensheathed. One week later the majority of larvae were ensheathed.

DISCUSSION

D. viviparus larvae are known to be only sluggishly motile. This characteristic hinders the recovery of larvae by procedures, such as the Baermann technique, which depend upon the active migration of the nematodes. Although direct experimental evidence has not been sought it is assumed that the higher counts obtained after storage at +8°C for 1 - 2 weeks are associated with the observed development of larvae at that temperature. It is possible that the ensheathed larvae are more actively motile than the first stage larvae allowing a greater proportion to migrate from the faecal mass in the Baermann apparatus.

The three bulk faecal collections used for this work all contained relatively high numbers of larvae but it is presumed that the same phenomenon would occur if numbers were sparse. If this is the case, storage at +8°C for 10 days would be expected to increase the sensitivity of the Baermann technique thereby increasing its reliability as a diagnostic tool.

ACKNOWLEDGEMENTS

This work was made possible by a research grant awarded by Imperial Chemical Industries Ltd. Mr. W. Mazhowu provided the technical assistance.

DISCUSSION

G. Urquhart *(UK)*

Did you eventually find more larvae than you started with?
Were these first stage larvae in fresh faeces?

D.E. Jacobs *(UK)*

Yes, that is so. The larvae were not reproducing during
the course of the experiment, and I think the results
demonstrate the inefficiency of the Baermann technique.

G. Urquhart

You calculated the number of larvae in fresh faeces by
using a Baermann technique?

D.E. Jacobs

Yes.

G. Urquhart

You started with about 500 and ten days later you estimate
about 2 000?

D.E. Jacobs

Yes. We get substantially more.

G. Urquhart

That is very odd, but it is consistent.

D.E. Jacobs

It is consistent, yes. The same thing happened three
times over. We feel that, when we have the first stage larvae,
our technique as we apply it is very inefficient, yet after ten
days storage the technique becomes more efficient; we recover a
greater proportion of the larvae.

G. Urquhart

You do not do any parallel examinations by using, e.g. a salt flotation?

D.E. Jacobs

No. We have not done this yet.

J. Armour *(UK)*

Are you absolutely sure that in faeces stored at room temperature the larvae are dead? It could be that they remain inactivated and when you alter the temperature they then migrate into the Baermann.

D.E. Jacobs

Possibly. All I know is that when we process the two sets of samples, side by side, using exactly the same technique, we get a lot of larvae when they are stored at $8^{\circ}C$, and very few larvae when stored at room temperature.

J. Armour

How do you relate this to what goes on in the summer in the fields? Supposing you get a warm wet day, are you suggesting that the larvae are dying in the faeces all that time?

D.E. Jacobs

I really would not like to comment. There are so many people in this room who have more experience in the field situation than I have.

J. Eckert *(Switzerland)*

Did you carry out the Baermann examinations always at the same temperature? There is an American paper which demonstrates that the yield of larvae at $20^{\circ}C$ is maximum, and if you have higher temperatures, about $25 - 30^{\circ}C$, the number

of larvae which can be recovered decreases. This is of
relevance for examinations occurring in summer time. It was
our experience in one case, that during summer time, samples
sent to the laboratory were negative although the animals
are infected with *Dictyocaulus*.   I think these higher
temperatures are very critical. Therefore, I am asking you
if you carried out these experiments at a constant temperature?

D.E. Jacobs

No, not at a constant temperature. They were carried out
at room temperature, and the room temperature at our laboratory
never rises above 20°C.

R.J. Jørgensen *(Denmark)*

How quickly, after the samples were taken, did you
Baermannise them?

D.E. Jacobs

The first Baermann examination was done between 24 and
48 hours after the faeces had been produced.

R.J. Jørgensen

So during the time lapse the samples were kept at room
temperature before they were put out for Baermannisation?

J.F. Michel *(UK)*

I was wondering whether your results demonstrate that at
8°C larvae are developing, so that your results reflect the
differences in activity between different developmental stages.
Further, your results might suggest that the Baermann funnel is
not to be regarded as a quantitative method. Perhaps you would
be better off with some sort of flotation technique?

D.E. Jacobs

I certainly accept this.

EXPERIENCES WITH OUR TECHNIQUES FOR THE RECOVERY OF NEMATODE LARVAE FROM HERBAGE

H.-J. Bürger

Institute of Parasitology,
Hannover School of Veterinary Medicine, Bünteweg 17,
D 3000 Hannover 71, Federal Republic of Germany.

ABSTRACT

The technique of Sievers Prekehr (1973) for the recovery of larvae from herbage samples included six basic steps:

1. *Washing a representative sample of herbage in a commercial washing-machine.*

2. *Collecting larvae on a 25 μm sieve.*

3. *Concentrating larvae in a saturated magnesium sulfate solution.*

4. *Counting and differentiating larvae microscopically.*

5. *Drying the herbage to a constant weight at $70^{o}C$.*

6. *Calculating the number of larvae/kg dry herbage.*

We have used this technique routinely since 1973. Twentyfour to 30 samples were usually processed for microscopic examination by one person during a working day of eight hours. The microscopic examination took another 10 to 25 minutes per sample, mainly depending on the number of larvae to be differentiated. The rate of recovery was approximately 60%. No significant differences between replicate samples processed and counted by different individuals could be traced.

There was a close correlation between the arithmetic mean of two duplicate larval counts of a pasture and the total worm burdens of the gastrointestinal tract of 28 tracer calves. Duplicate herbage samples had been taken on the days on which a tracer calf was put on, or taken from, a pasture used by first season stock. The calves had been reared wormfree from one week to three months of age before being turned out, and for 16 or 17 days after housing when they were autopsied and examined quantitatively for their gastrointestinal worm burdens.

P. Nansen, R.J. Jørgensen, E.J.L. Soulsby (eds), Epidemiology and Control of Nematodiasis in Cattle.
Copyright © 1981 ECSC, EEC, EAEC, Brussels – Luxembourg. All rights reserved.

INTRODUCTION

The technique used for the recovery of nematode larvae from herbage samples is a modification of Lancaster's (1970) technique, worked out in our laboratory by Sievers Prekehr (1973).

METHODS

Two herbage samples are taken from each pasture by pinching 100 small samples of herbage on a W-shaped walk across the pasture and collecting them in a bag made from curtain cloth and closed by a zipper. Each sample is handled separately. The procedure for the evaluation of the number of larvae includes six basic steps:

The bag with the herbage is washed three times in a commercial washing-machine equipped with a siphon at the outlet.

The larvae are collected on a 25 μm screen after removal of grass blades and coarse debris by a 250 μm sieve.

The larvae are concentrated by three centrifugations (250 x g, 5.5 and 3 minutes) in a saturated solution of magnesium sulfate (s.ç = 1.28). The supernatant is resuspended in tap water to reduce the concentration of salt and reconcentrated on a 25 μm sieve and stored until examination.

Microscopic examination is carried out in a counting chamber adapted to the microscope.

The herbage in the bag is dried to constant weight at $70^{\circ}C$.

The number of larvae/kg dry herbage is calculated for each sample. The arithmetic mean of the two counts is designated the 'infestation of the pasture'.

The technique is illustrated diagrammatically in Figure 1.

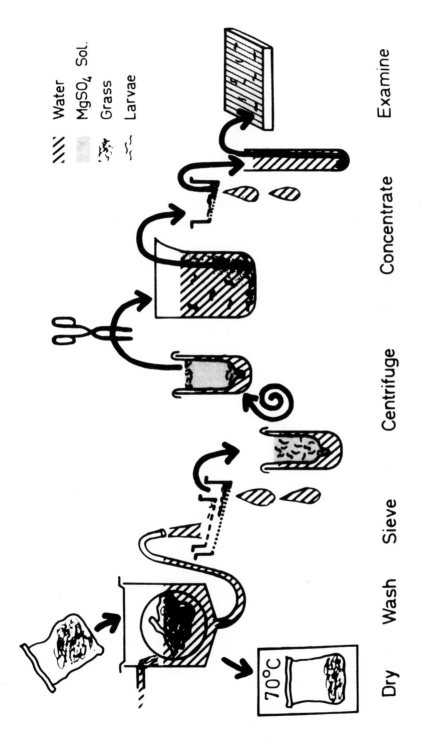

Fig. 1. Technique for the recovery of nematode larvae from herbage samples.

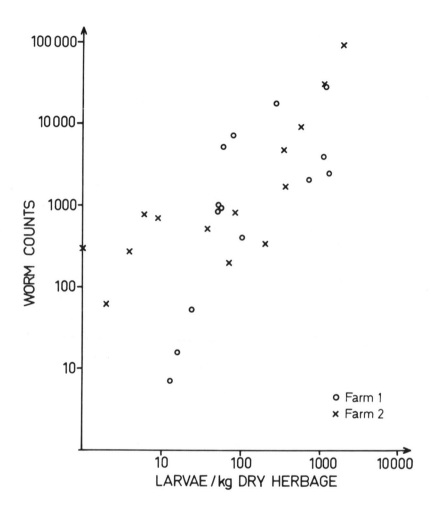

Fig. 2. Correlation of worm burdens of tracer calves and larval counts in herbage samples.

Two points of technique should be pointed out:

> Our sieves are all equipped with prominent corners.
> This enables us to concentrate the debris on the sieves
> to very small volumes which can be easily transferred to
> small tubes.

> A rubber condom is put into the centrifuge tube when
> contrifuging the sample in the saturated salt solution.
> By using a long clamp the supernatant can easily be
> separated from the sediment.

Merits of the technique

Twentyfour to 30 samples are usually processed through
steps 1 - 3 by one person during a normal working day of eight
hours. Microscopic examination takes 10 - 25 minutes per sample,
mainly depending on the number of larvae to be differentiated.
We use long-distance objectives (Zeiss, Oberkochem, Fed. Rep. of
Germany) in our microscopes which enable us to cover the
counting chambers by a relatively thick slide. The whole
procedure in the laborabory takes approximately 40 minutes per
sample. The samples can be stored in the refrigerator for
microscopic examination. The rate of larval detection is
approximately 60%. Results from replicate samples, either
processed by one person or by different sets of two individuals,
did not differ significantly. The technique has been used
routinely since 1973.

Correlation between larval counts and worm burdens of tracer calves.

In order to compare our sampling technique and our
laboratory procedure with the actual risk of infection for
grazing animals, duplicate herbage samples were taken from
pastures on the day individual tracer calves were put on or
taken from a given pasture. A total of 28 worm-free tracer
calves grazed one of two pastures for a fortnight covering a
whole grazing season. The animals were necropsied 16 or 17
days after removal from pasture, being kept under conditions

which excluded further infection. There was a good correlation
between the average of the four larval counts and the total
worm burdens of the tracer calves (Figure 2). Ranking these
two parameters and comparing the rans by means of the U-test
did not show any significant differences. This indicates
that larval counts do reflect the actual risk for grazing
calves.

CONCLUSION

The results of the comparison show that our technique
can well be used for larval counts in some epidemiological work
thus saving costs and efforts due to the use of tracer animals.

REFERENCES

Lancaster, M.B., 1970. The recovery of infective nematode larvae from
herbage samples. J. Helminth. **44**, 219-230.

Sievers Prekehr, G.H., 1973. Methode zur Gewinnung III. Strongyliden-
larven aus dem Wiedegras. Vet. med. Dissert., Hannover, p59.

DISCUSSION

H.J. Over *(The Netherlands)*

I did not quite get the point when you described the
correlation between the larval count on the herbage and the
worm burden in the tracer animals. Worm counts are no problem,
but what measure did you take for your larval count in the
herbage? For a period of weeks?

H.-J. Bürger *(FRG)*

We put the tracer calves on a pasture for 2 weeks and
we took two samples at the start, and two samples at the end
of this period, and averaged them.

A TECHNIQUE FOR THE RECOVERY OF INFECTIVE TRICHOSTRONGYLE LARVAE FROM SOIL

K. Bairden, J.L. Duncan and J. Armour

Wellcome Laboratory for Experimental Parasitology,
University of Glasgow, Veterinary School,
Bearsden Road, Bearsden, Glasgow, G61 IQH, UK.

The recovery of infective trichostrongyle larvae from soil was achieved by a technique similar to that developed by Jørgensen (1975) to isolate *Dictyocaulus viviparus* larvae from herbage. Thus a process of sedimentation and filtration followed by extraction using a Baermann apparatus resulted in a clean and easily read preparation.

The technique may be summarised as follows:

Core samples of 28 cm^2 are removed to a depth of 10 cm and divided into four layers namely:

1) Herbage

2) Root-mat layer (ca 0.5 cm)

3) Upper 5 cm of soil

4) Lower 5 cm of soil.

Aggregated samples of each layer are then soaked in 20 litres of water for a minimum of 12 hours in a large bin.

After thorough mixing, the soil suspension is allowed to stand for 30 seconds during which time the heavier soil particles etc. settle to the bottom of the container leaving the larvae in suspension.

The supernatant is then passed through a 27 micron aperture nylon sieve (Figure 1) and the process of mixing the soil suspension and washing through the sieve is repeated four times. The larvae retained in the nylon sieve are then washed into a bucket.

P. Nansen, R.J. Jørgensen, E.J.L. Soulsby (eds), Epidemiology and Control of Nematodiasis in Cattle.

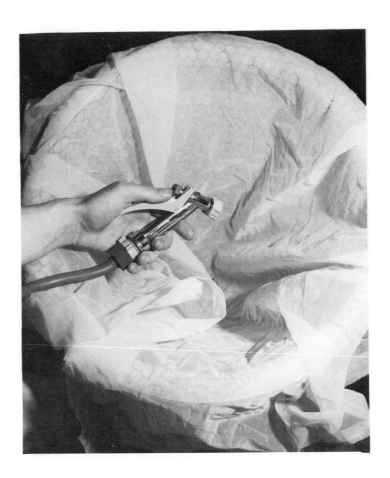

Fig. 1.

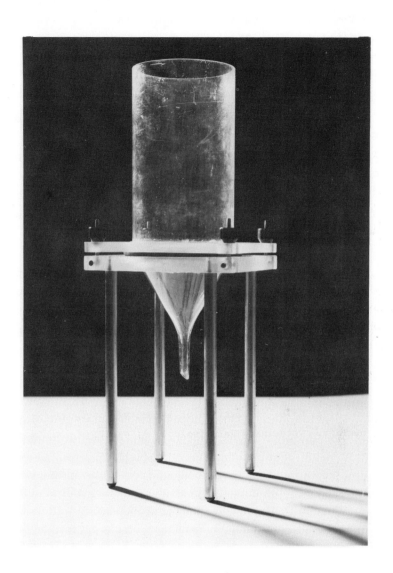

Fig. 2.

The above process removes most of the soil debris and the relatively clean larval suspension is then further concentrated by filtration through a 15 cm. circle of nylon gauze (aperture size 27 microns) using the apparatus illustrated in Figure 2. The larvae retained by this filter are recovered using the Baermann technique.

After 12 hours the larvae present in the neck of the Baermann apparatus are run off and concentrated to a volume of 10 ml. to which a drop of Lugol's iodine is added. Prior to microscopic examination of the 10 ml. a few drops of 5% sodium hypochlorite are added; this facilitates the examination since any free living larvae are decolourised whereas the trichostrongyle larvae retain the stain.

The numbers of larvae present in each area of the sample can then be calculated and expressed as L_3 per acre or hectare. We have found that it is necessary to examine 125 cores of soil per unit area studied to obtain a statistically acceptable result.

REFERENCE

Jørgensen, R.J., 1975. Isolations of infective *Dictyocaulus* larvae from herbage. Veterinary Parasitology, 1, 61-67.

DISCUSSION

T. O'Nuallain *(Ireland)*

Have you had an opportunity to observe variations in soil types?

J. Armour *(UK)*

All sampling has been done within ten miles of Glasgow and I don't think that there has been a variation in the soil. The site is the university farm and the experimental plots are our own. However, work in the USA has shown that *Ostertagia* larvae, buried at 15 cm, will migrate vertically. Perhaps we are not going deep enough, though we have some difficulty in going deeper than 10 cm.

H.J. Over *(The Netherlands)*

Your description of the herbage sample suggested that the roots did not go deeper into the soil than 1 cm.

J. Armour

I called it the 'root/mat layer' to give it a name.

H.J. Over

You described it as being about 1 cm or 0.5 cm deep.

J. Armour

Yes, 0.5 cm.

H.J. Over

This suggests that you are working on soil that is rather heavy, or that is very, very sandy. One or the other?

J. Armour

I would not have said that we are on a sandy soil. No.

H.J. Over

Well then it is very heavy. If so it is very interesting since larvae are moving very deep into the soil when the amount of free space between particles is very limited.

J. Armour

That is the geologist coming out in you, Hans!

G. Urquhart *(UK)*

Have you attempted to calibrate the efficiency of your system by taking known negative samples of soil then, adding a known number of larvae, by syringe, and ascertaining the recovery rate?

J. Armour

Yes. There was a 60% recovery.

J.F. Michel *(UK)*

I am reminded of some observations made by my colleague, Mr. Everett, some six or seven years ago. He buried Nematodirus larvae at a depth of two feet and found they very promptly returned to the surface. They could in fact be buried several times and would do this. However, Weybridge has an atypical soil type and therefore, I regard all results done locally as entirely suspect.

J. Armour

What time of year did he do this?

J.F. Michel

I think it was during the summer.

J-P. Raynaud *(France)*

Do you have a chance to work in the winter time as well?

J. Armour

Yes, but it is rather difficult. We should be taking
samples this week but the snow cover will make it rather
difficult.

E.J.L. Soulsby *(UK)*

Since you have divided your samples up into four parts,
is there any differential location of larvae in these different
parts?

J. Armour

We are looking for movement of larvae in the soil. The
trend so far suggests that larvae disappear rapidly from the
herbage and the root/mat layer. There is an increase in deeper
layers though we may have not gone down far enough with our
samples. It remains to be seen whether there is a reverse
migration to the surface in the spring.

H.-J. Bürger *(FRG)*

What is the diameter of your samples?

J. Armour

The total surface area is 28 cm^2. An interesting point
is that we have examined some sheep pastures by this technique.
These were contaminated with *Ostertagia, Trichostrongylus, Chabertia*
and *Haemonchus* species and we were unable to recover any larvae
from the soil. Also we are interested in looking for lungworm
larvae (as will be mentioned in a later paper), and we have
found a few lungworm larvae in the soil, but the number is much
smaller than with *Ostertagia* and *Cooperia* that it is almost like
looking for a needle in a haystack.

R.J. Thomas *(UK)*

I would like to support Professor Armour's argument that
the soil is an important reservoir of larvae. We injected
larvae to various depths in the soil and then observed recoveries

on the grass. Initially no larvae were found on the surface, but over a period of time we did recover increasing numbers from the herbage. This was from larvae injected to a depth of 5 cm. Therefore, this evidence indicates that larvae are not lost when they enter the soil. Our experience would suggest that the soil could be an important reservoir of infective larvae for the grazing animal.

J. Armour

Using the 'Weybridge technique' for estimating numbers of larvae/kg herbage, we find that on pasture not grazed in the spring, we get up to 4 000 - 5 000 larvae/kg by the middle of the summer. Pasture burdens are at zero from the third week in May to the third week in June, which is a period when traditionally we all have difficulty in finding larvae.

J-P. Raynaud

How did you work out the numbers in the samples?

J. Armour

The numbers are worked out on a unit area. We have worked it out per 28 cm^2, per 280 cm^2, and per hectare. The per hectare calculation seems, in the end, to be the best, because we are trying to express the numbers of larvae available - or potentially available - to the grazing animal. This estimates at several million, based on a 60% recovery. It is likely this is an underestimation, but whether such larvae detected in the soil return to the herbage, and how many do so, remains to be determined.

N. Downey *(Ireland)*

Did you consider using the mist chamber? This is suitable for recovering nematodes from soil.

J. Armour

This is the apparatus used by workers with root nematodes. Yes, we did look at these and we decided to use the present method. Rolf Jørgensen has been our mentor. He has helped Ken Bairden who has been in Copenhagen to discuss this. We are hoping to combine it with the *D. viviparus* agar-bile sampling technique, to find out more about lungworm larvae. Details of the root nematode techniques are available from the Commonwealth Institute of Helminthology, St Albans, England.

R.J. Jørgensen *(Denmark)*

I would like to comment on the Cramer paper and the Fox paper presented by Jacobs dealing with the recovery of lungworm larvae from faeces by the Baermann techniques.

I would like to show details from a study of the motility of lungworm larvae, which coincides with data presented today. Fluctuations are seen in motility during the development of larvae in the culture and this supports the explanation advanced by Dr. Jacobs. The period of inactivity, observed in my experiment, took place when the larvae were in their second lethargus, that is, when they developed from the second to the third stage. (See Figure).

H.J. Over

What was the room temperature in Dennis' experiments?

D.E. Jacobs *(UK)*

About 18°C.

R.J. Jørgensen

I was interested in the refrigerator graph.

H.J. Over

The phase was ten hours?

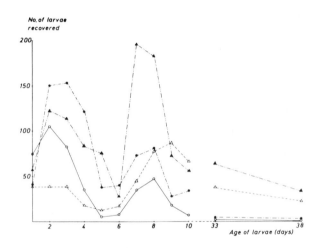

Fig. 1: The response of larvae towards CO_2 and bile during their cult-
ivation in water at $16°C$:

(o) non-exposed larvae,

(Δ) bile exposure,

(●) CO_2 exposure,

(▲) bile plus CO_2 exposure.

Each determination is the mean larval count of 6 plates in Petri
dishes.

D.E. Jacobs
<u>D.E. Jacobs</u>

No, in ten days!

<u>R.J. Jørgensen</u>

That is another interesting thing. I have only observed one period of inactivity, or low activity, in larval cultures which, in fact, is in contrast to the description of the free-living stages as described by Daubney in 1920. He described two periods of inactivity, so he had all the three stages to look at but he started his cultures from the eggs from the female. So I don't know if they are more or less 2nd stage at the time they are excreted. But that is a different matter. I just wanted to show you the similarities between the two graphs.

<u>J. Armour</u>

Dr. Jacobs, when you take your samples out of the container - the ones kept at room temperature - do you do as Dr. Cremers does, and wash the surface of the container?

<u>D.E. Jacobs</u>

No, I must admit I don't. But when I get home I will try it.

<u>J. Armour</u>

I saw a technique at Rahway which was used for culturing *D. viviparus*, in which they are washed clear of the faeces and then left at room temperature in shallow water. They get very good yields of infective larvae using this technique. The temperature used might be as high as or even higher than 20°C.

<u>E.J.L. Soulsby</u>

Dr. Jacobs, do you have any information as to whether 8°C is critical for this development of *D. viviparus*?

D.E. Jacobs

I do not have that information. The objective of our
study was a purely practical one: how long could we keep these
samples before we examined them. We obtained the answer to
our practical problem and we have not investigated other
possibilities.

SESSION I

METHODOLOGY II
Chairman: R.J. Jørgensen

A MODIFIED AND SIMPLE MCMASTER TECHNIQUE

Sv. Aa. Henriksen

State Veterinary Serum Laboratory,
Copenhagen, Denmark

ABSTRACT

A modified McMaster technique is described. The technique involves the use of inexpensive disposable materials (polystyrene cups and gauze). Comparative testing showed it to be sufficiently reliable for routine diagnostic examinations of bovine faecal samples for trichostrongyle eggs.

INTRODUCTION

Modifications of the McMaster technique have been described by Levine et al.(1960), Van den Brink (1971), Mines (1977) and Raynaud et al.(1979). The following modification (Henriksen and Aagaard, 1976) was developed to use disposable materials in routine diagnostic examinations.

DISPOSABLE EQUIPMENT

Two polystyrene cups (Figure 1 (I & II)) were used for each faecal sample. The bottom of Cup II had been cut off and slits were made in the side. Gauze (cloth) with a mesh size of 200 - 450 µm x 200 - 450 µm and synthetic fabric, mesh size 350 x 800 µm were assessed. Wire mesh with a mesh size of 400 x 400 µm was used in the conventional McMaster technique.

TECHNIQUE

A 4 g sample of faeces is weighed into Cup I and mixed thoroughly with 56 ml of the flotation solution. The gauze is placed over the cup and pressed down by means of Cup II whereby a filtrate of the faecal suspension is obtained in the inner cup. The appropriate amount of filtrate is immediately transferred to a McMaster slide by means of a pipette. The preparation is allowed to stand for a few minutes before counting. The cups as well as the remaining filtrate are discarded.

P. Nansen, R.J. Jørgensen, E.J.L. Soulsby (eds), Epidemiology and Control of Nematodiasis in Cattle.

COMPARATIVE TESTS

The efficiency of the technique was tested on subsamples,
each of 4 g and it was compared with a conventional McMaster
technique in which the faecal suspension was sieved through a
400 μm wire mesh. The results of the egg counts are summarised
in Table 1. The number of eggs counted when gauze and synthetic
fabric were used averaged approximately 80% and 100%, respectively, of those counted with the conventional method. The lower
rate obtained with gauze should probably be ascribed to struct-
ural features of that material such as the inconstant mesh width
and the end of microfibres projecting into most of the meshes.

It is concluded that egg counting by the described modification of the McMaster technique is sufficiently reliable for
routine diagnostic examinations.

TABLE 1

FAECAL EGG COUNTS AND RELATIVE EFFICIENCY (%) OF THE MODIFIED McMASTER
TECHNIQUE COMPARED WITH CONVENTIONAL TECHNIQUE

| Test No. | Modified McMaster | | Conventional McMaster |
	Gauze	Synthetic fabric	(Wire net)
1	40	38	44
2	32	44	39
3	30	46	41
4	35	57	50
5	41	57	49
6	35	40	52
7	32	39	26
8	24	32	38
9	24	34	32
10	25	30	30
Average	31.8	41.7	40.1
%	79	102	100

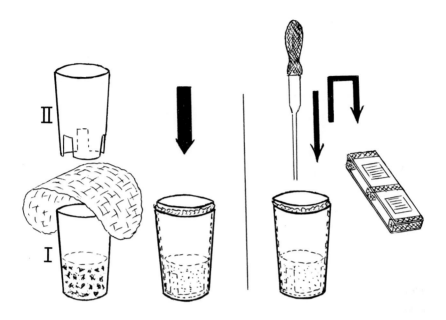

Fig. 1.   Diagrammatic illustration of the modified McMaster technique.

REFERENCES

Brink, R. van den 1971. Een eenvoudige McMastermethode voor het tellen van
     Trichostrongyliden eieren in runder-faeces. (A simple McMaster egg
     counting procedure for strongylid eggs in cow's faeces). Tijdschr.
     Diergeneesk. 96, 859-862

Henriksen, Sv. Aa. and Aagaard, K. 1976. En enkel flotations- og McMaster-
     metode. (A simple flotation and McMaster method). Nord. Vet.-Med., 28,
     392-397

Levine, N.D., Krishna, N.M., Clark, D.T. and Aves, I.J. 1960. A comparison
     of nematode egg counting techniques for cattle and sheep faeces. Am.
     J. Vet. Res., 21, 511-515

Mines, J.J. 1977. Modifications of the McMaster worm egg counting method.
     Austr. Vet. J., 53, 342-343

Raynaud, J.-P., Leroy, J.-C., Virat, M. and Nicolas, J.-A. 1979. Une tech-
     nique de coproscopie quantitative polyvalente par dilution et sediment-
     ation en eau. Flottaison et solution dense (D.S.F.) et numeration en
     lame de Mac Master. I. (A polyvalent egg count technique by dilution
     and sedimentation in water. Flotation in a high s.d. solution (D.S.F.)
     and counting in Mac Master slide. I.). Rev. Méd. Vét., 130, 377-404

DISCUSSION

R.J. Jørgensen *(Denmark)*

Thank you Dr. Henriksen for this very useful modification of the McMaster technique.

F.H.M. Borgsteede *(The Netherlands)*

How do you deal with sheep faeces?

Sv. Aa. Henriksen *(Denmark)*

That is a problem. This technique is primarily for cattle faeces. Perhaps one could let sheep faeces soak in water for about an hour.

A. Kloosterman *(The Netherlands)*

When you press down the plastic cup, the faecal particles will tend to block the gauze. This would suggest that with the last half of the suspension the sieve will work as much finer gauze. Does this make a difference to your recovery?

Sv. Aa. Henriksen

Yes. As far as we can see from comparative experiments on subsamples from the same faecal sample, we have found an average recovery of 80% with the modified technique, sieving through gauze. However, I don't think this is of any importance for routine diagnostic examinations.

G. Urquhart *(UK)*

Have you ever tried this technique for *Dictyocaulus* larvae?

Sv. Aa. Henriksen

No.

G. Urquhart

I have never used this technique but I remember in the old days doing a McMaster in the orthodox way by mixing faeces in water and then spinning and adding in salt later. I seemed to get much better results than if the faeces were mixed directly with salt. Yours is an even further simplification. Do you have any comparative data?

Sv. Aa. Henriksen

No.

COMPARISON OF TECHNIQUES FOR ASSESSMENT OF THE CONTAMINATION OF PASTURE HERBAGE WITH INFECTIVE NEMATODE LARVAE

J.-P. Raynaud[1] and L. Gruner[2]

[1]Agricultural R & D Station, Pfizer International,
37400 Amboise, France.

[2]INRA, Station de Pathologie Aviaire et de
Parasitologie, Unité d'Ecologie Parasitaire,
37380 Monnaie, France.

ABSTRACT

Comparison of various sampling and laboratory techniques to evaluate the concentration of infective nematode larvae on pasture herbage for cattle and to estimate the workload in the laboratory has been undertaken. We recommend for routine use (a) for pasture sampling procedures to take separately and at random a large number of sub-samples near the dung pats (near DP) and far from the dung pats (far DP); (b) for laboratory procedures the herbage sample can be processed either with one-day soaking or with washing in a cement mixer and sieved on a specially designed funnel. The larvae are collected on a 20 μm sieve and recovered on mercuric and potassium iodide solution (sg = 1.44).

P. Nansen, R.J. Jørgensen, E.J.L. Soulsby (eds), Epidemiology and Control of Nematodiasis in Cattle.
Copyright © 1981 ECSC, EEC, EAEC, Brussels – Luxembourg. All rights reserved.

INTRODUCTION

To determine which techniques should be applied for future work in our laboratories we have compared various sampling and laboratory methods for the estimation of nematode larvae on pasture.

The efficacy of the techniques was evaluated by performing total and differential counts of larvae of gastro-intestinal nematodes and lungworm larvae. The investigation was carried out mainly using pasture herbage samples from pastures grazed by calves, but cores of soil were also examined.

The sampling technique ("W"-shaped pattern) described by Taylor (1939) was compared with the sampling of strips (10 areas of 100 x 10 cm each), with the sampling near dung pats (Jørgensen, 1980) and with the sampling of cores of soil plus herbage (Gruner et al., 1980). In addition, the soaking versus washing of herbage samples followed by sieving, were compared and these two procedures also were compared to Baermannization.

MATERIALS AND METHODS

Pastures

Pastures in western France (Departments of Mayenne, Sarthe and Eure), grazed by calves at a stocking rate of 10 per hectare, were used.

Sampling

Samples were taken either before the calves were turned out (February - March) or during the grazing season (April - November). Pastures were sampled according to Taylor's technique by following the proscribed W-shaped route and the grass was cut at ground level with shears. A total of 300 to 400 cuts was taken. In an initial experiment, 2 "W" patterns were compared in the same field. Sampling of herbage on 10 randomly selected strips (total area: 1 sq. metre) was carried out by means of a battery operated automatic shearer. Sampling around faecal pats was done by hand: four sub-samples were picked around each of 50 randomly selected pats within a distance of 10 centimetres from the pat. Soil cores, plus the herbage growing on them, were collected with a cylinder-like garden tool for planting flower bulbs. It had a diameter of 5 cm and a height of 7 cm. A total of 60 cores were sampled at random, representing an area of 0.12 m^2.

Laboratory procedures

Soaking was carried out in buckets containing water and detergent. The grass was removed at the end of the first day and the contents were sieved through a 200 μm and then a 20 μm screen. A second soaking was performed on some occasions on the same grass samples. The material retained on the 20 μm screen was examined for larvae.

Washing was performed in a washing machine or a cement mixer modified according to Jørgensen (Personal communication). The contents were poured over a large screen with an aperture of 200 μm and the larvae collected underneath in a specially designed stainless steel funnel with holes fitted with a nylon mesh inside with an aperture size of 20 μm. This allowed efficient washing and rinsing by the use of a shower head fitted to the water hose.

Baermannization of soil plus herbage was carried out with the cores upside down over a large screen in a bucket filled with water.

Diagrammatic drawings of the three laboratory procedures are shown in Figure 1.

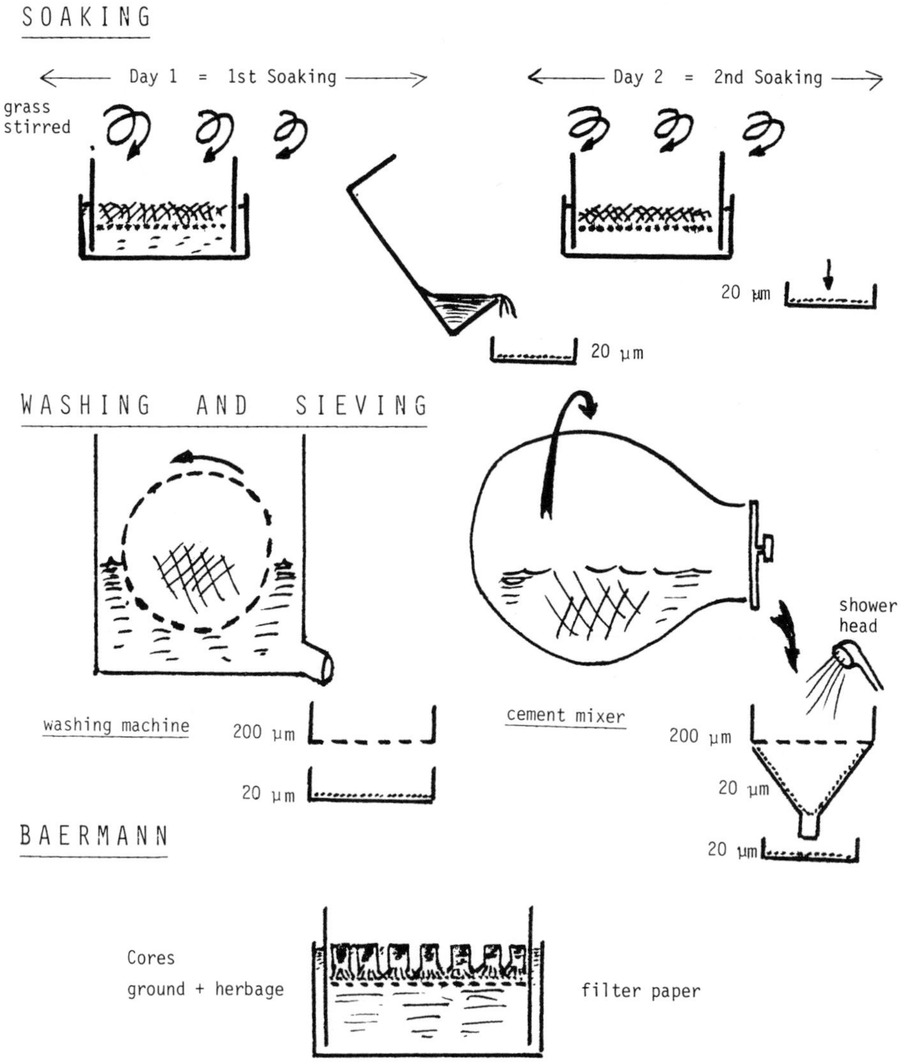

54

SOAKING

Fig. 1. Diagrammatic drawings of the three laboratory procedures: soaking, washing and Baermannization

RESULTS

Sampling techniques

Comparison between two W's

The weight and quality (dry matter) of the herbage
collected in two opposite W-shaped routes on the same paddock
were similar. The results from examination of pairs of samples
are shown in Table 1. In February and March the differences
between the counts of the two samples are less important than
during the other months both for the total larval counts (the
ratio of the highest/lowest is 1.5 on average) and for the
different species. August to October was the period when heterogeneity of the two parts of the same paddock is the highest.

TABLE 1

COMPARISON BETWEEN TWO OPPOSITE W's TAKEN ON THE SAME PADDOCK

	Period of sampling		
	April to July 1978	August to October 1978	February to March 1979
Number of pairs of W's	10	11	12
L3/kg dry herbage			
Ratio highest/ lowest counts; mean (range)	1.8 (1.1-3.4)	2.3 (1.1-5.3)	1.5 (1.0-2.8)
Difference in the percentage of the species			
mean (range)			
Ostertagia	14 (5-24)	9 (0-26)	8 (1-30)
Cooperia	15 (6-25)	11 (0-26)	9 (1-33)
Trichostrongylus	2 (6-25)	1 (0-1)	2 (1-4)
Bunostomum	-	17 (0-67)	-
Nematodirus	16 (8-24)	-	-

Comparison between "W" and "strip" sampling

The number of strips of one tenth of a square metre was fixed at 10 so as to have nearly the same weight of herbage as with the W sampling. It appears that the quality (dry matter) of the two samples was the same, but as shown in Table 2, the number of L3 per kg dry herbage is higher for the W than for the square metre strips.

TABLE 2

COMPARISON BETWEEN "W" AND STRIP SAMPLING. A TOTAL OF 13 COMPARISONS WERE PERFORMED

	2 W's/paddock	10 strips (= 1 m^2)/paddock
L3/kg dry herbage		
mean	305	39
range	0 to 31,247	0 to 8,833

In Table 3 the results of samplings on two paddocks using two W-shaped routes processed by soaking or washing, and 4 to 6 strips also processed by the same two techniques, are presented. It appears that 10 samples of 1/10th square metre are not enough to be representative of pasture contamination. It is estimated that 40 sub-samples of 1/10th square metre each would be better to compare with the results of the W technique; however, the amount of laboratory work involved would be quadrupled.

Comparison between "W" and "near dung pat" samples

From May 29th to September 25th, 117 comparisons of the two sampling techniques were done on the same paddock. The results are summarised in Table 4. On average, with samples taken in all periods tested, the "near the dung pat" samples carry more L3 than the W for *Dictyocaulus* (large difference), *Ostertagia* and *Cooperia*; the W counts are higher for *Nematodirus*. However, a variation appears if the samples collected before

July 1st are compared with those collected after this date.
Before July 1st the counts were higher for the W with *Ostertagia*
and significantly higher for *Cooperia* and *Nematodirus*.   After
July 1st the counts are higher for the "pats" with *Ostertagia*
and *Cooperia*.   W-counts were always significantly higher for
Nematodirus.

TABLE 3

COMPARISON BETWEEN "W" AND STRIP SAMPLING PROCESSED BY 2 SOAKINGS OR BY
WASHING   (L3/KG DRY HERBAGE)

| | 2 W's/paddock | | x times 1 m^2/paddock | |
	2 soakings	washing	2 soakings	washing
Paddock No.1	2 354	1 110	4 times/m^2 individual values 0; 64; 385; 7564 Average = 2003	
Paddock No.2	14 901	1 008	6 times/m^2 individual values 787; 1102; 2362; 4409; 9055; 16378 Average = 5289	6 times/m^2 individual values 189; 472; 583; 2402; 3402; 5157 Average = 2034

Comparison between cores and strip samplings

The results are shown in Table 5. The comparisons between
60 cores and 10 strips of 1/10th square metre show higher
counts for *Ostertagia* and *Cooperia* with the core technique, but
the difference was not significant and this is reflected in the
heterogeneity of the results of the samples taken throughout the
year. The comparisons between 5 times 60 cores and 4 times
1 m^2 give better results for core sampling (significantly for
Cooperia). *Ostertagia* appear to be more frequently present on
strip samples.

TABLE 4

IN THE "W"s, OR IN "HERBAGE NEAR THE PATS" ("PATS") SAMPLES TAKEN AT THE SAME TIME, ON THE SAME PADDOCKS
- NUMBER OF L3 RECOVERED IN L3/KG DRY HERBAGE BEFORE OR AFTER JULY 1ST
- FREQUENCY OF POSITIVE SAMPLES DURING THE WHOLE SEASON

Parasites		*Ostertagia*		*Cooperia*		*Nematodirus*		*Dictyocaulus*	
Samples		No. (Sig.)	Ave	No. (Sig.)	Ave	No. (Sig.)	Ave	No. (Sig.)	Ave
Before July 1st	"Pats"	15	79	17	47	13	65		
	"W"	(NS)	241	(S)	348	(S)	225		
After July 1st	"Pats"	84	2 364	63	3 097	41	311	5	3 290
	"W"	(NS)	1 958	(NS)	2 601	(HS)	459		616
Whole season									
% positive samples	"Pats"	80%		79%		87%		80%	
	"W"	75%		78%		52%		100%	

No. = number of samples

(Sig.) = significance: HS, S or NS

Ave = average values

TABLE 5

COMPARISON OF CORES OF SOIL $+_2$HERBAGE AND m^2 FROM STRIPS
FOR 1 SERIES (60 CORES OR 1 m^2 = 10 TIMES 1 x 0.1 m) OR MULTIPLE SERIES IN
THE SAME PADDOCK = 5 x 60 CORES OR 4 x 1 m^2
RESULTS IN $L3/m^2$

	No. of samplings	*Ostertagia*	*Cooperia*
No. $L3/m^2$ for each paddock			
1. 60 cores	59	133	122
1 m^2 herbage	46	77	45
significance		NS	NS
2. 5 x 60 cores	12	208	142
4 x 1 m^2	12	90	43
significance		NS	S
Frequency of presence of L3			
60 cores	59	25%	42%
1 m^2	46	52%	48%

Different laboratory procedures

Comparison of 1 soaking (1 day) with 2 soakings on 2 successive days

One hundred and four (104) samples of herbage collected
on different paddocks during the pasture period were soaked on
two successive days, the larvae being counted after each day.
The proportion of larvae collected after one soaking was
compared with the total number after two soakings (Table 6).
The results indicate that 77 to 99 percent of larvae are collected with only one soaking; the results are most consistent
with *Dictyocaulus* and least consistent with *Nematodirus*, where
there was high variability.

TABLE 6

COMPARISON OF THE PERCENTAGE OF LARVAE (FOR THE DIFFERENT SPECIES) COLLECTED
AFTER 1 SOAKING WITH THE TOTAL COUNTS OF 2 SOAKINGS ON 2 SUCCESSIVE DAYS

	Ostertagia	*Cooperia*	*Nematodirus*	*Dictyocaulus*
No. of comparisons	93	81	32	8
Average % L3 1 soaking / L3 2 soakings	82.1	85.8	77.5	99.4
Standard error	4.5	3.9	15.9	1.2

TABLE 7

COMPARISONS BETWEEN LARVAL COUNTS AFTER 2 SOAKINGS AND AFTER WASHING

	Ostertagia	*Cooperia*	*Nematodirus*	*Trichostr.*
No. of comparisons	43	34	24	8
% comparisons L3 2 soakings > L3 washing	63%	65%	79%	87%
Significance of difference	NS	NS	HS	S

Comparison of soakings and washings

Herbage was collected 52 times all through the grazing
season along two parallel W-shaped routes, on different
paddocks. One sample was processed by soaking and the other by
washing.

The results of the comparisons of the larval counts are
presented in Table 7. This table shows that two soakings improve significantly the recovery of *Nematodirus* and *Trichostrongylus* species, and slightly that of *Ostertagia* and *Cooperia*
species.

DISCUSSION

The estimation of the number of infective larvae present
on the pasture is an essential part of epidemiological studies
of nematodiasis in calves (Michel and Parfitt, 1956; Michel,
1966; Kloosterman, 1971; Downey, 1973). The main purpose is
to determine the seasonal variations of the larval content of
herbage (Henriksen et al., 1976; Borgsteede and Kloosterman,
1977), the sampling work being done every two weeks or even
every week for lungworm studies. The necessity of collecting
and processing a large number of samples makes it desirable to
have an economic and rapid laboratory technique, which at the
same time yields reliable results.

With respect to sampling techniques, grass generally is
collected and the contamination is expressed as the number
of larvae per kilo of dry herbage. However, the efficacy of
the technique is rarely assessed because of the necessity of
conducting many replicates. For example, Kloosterman (1971)
takes 8 samples each time in the same paddock to calculate the
confidence limits. In our work, we compared two W-shaped
routes; this was not sufficient to determine the confidence
limits, but it gave some idea of the heterogeneity of the
larval distribution in the pasture. For example, at the
beginning of the year, when the overwintering larvae had had
time to spread out, and a lot of pats were disintegrated, the
counts of the two samples were equivalent. Later, when calves
had been turned out, the heterogeneity increased with the
appearance of new generations of larvae from the new pats.
Such information was useful to understand the efficacy of the
different sampling techniques under comparison.

The comparison of the W and strip sampling shows that
the former gave better results because the sub-samples are more
numerous and better distributed on the paddock. The collecting
of the grass along the strips is mechanical and less dependent on the operator, but 10 strips are not sufficient to allow
for the heterogeneity of larval distribution. With 40 strips

the larval counts are similar to those from the W technique, but the amount of grass to be processed is much too great.

A major drawback of grass sampling techniques is that results depend on climatic conditions and these could differ markedly during the day (Gevrey, 1970). Additionally, the sampling of the herbage is not representative enough when the grass is more than 15 cm tall. For these reasons we try to collect simultaneously, herbage, litter and 5 cm of ground by the core technique. However, the results showed that 60 cores were not enough, but rather 5 times 60 cores (i.e. 300 cores) per paddock gave the best results.

In comparison of the W technique and the "near the pat" sampling, differences were found for samples collected before or after July 1st. The counts from samples near the pats were higher after this date, and this increase in larval numbers was evident earlier in these samples than in others (i.e. the new generation of larvae derived from Spring infection of calves was initiated at this date). In practice, when collecting along the W-shaped route, when a stop occurs near a pat, the operator walks one metre away and cuts the grass "away from the pats", thereby making this sampling comparable to the sampling "far from the pats" used by Henriksen et al. (1976) and Jørgensen (1980). Our results confirmed those of the authors who work on *Dictyocaulus* larvae and gastro-intestinal nematodes, mainly *Ostertagia*. Particular attention must be paid to *Nematodirus*: during the year the counts are higher in the W samples. This may be due to the fact that larvae are very active and migrate very rapidly far from the pat, but the main reason may be the particular epidemiology of this genus, as Boag and Thomas (1975) and Rose (1975) explain for the different species in Great Britain. For example, the eggs deposited one year developed to free living larvae the following year.

In regard to laboratory procedures, one soaking gives good results in comparison to two soakings for the different species, the lowest and most heterogenous results being for

Nematodirus (77.5%). In practice, one soaking is sufficient, since more than 80% of the larvae are recovered by this technique.

The comparisons between soaking and washing were mainly done with two soakings. The results are slightly higher in this case, so we can consider that one soaking gives similar results to washing for *Ostertagia* and *Cooperia*. Soaking is slightly better for *Nematodirus* larval detection. Lancaster (1970) found better results with washing, mainly for *Nematodirus*, but he did sedimentation after soaking. In practice, soaking is the simplest technique, giving cleaner samples that are easier to count, but washing remains an interesting and useful technique if results are needed rapidly after the collection of the herbage.

We have extended the sampling technique used by Jørgensen (1980) for lungworms to the other nematode species of parasites of cattle: one sample of grass collected "near the pats" (up to 10 cm) and one sample of grass collected "far from the pats" (more than 1 metre), the two counts being presented separately. The main interest of the W-shaped route is that the number of sub-samples is high. Using the same number of sub-samples, we can distribute them randomly on the paddock. In the laboratory, soaking one day or washing for 10 minutes, before sieving and counting by flotation on mercuric and potassium iodide, gave satisfactory results.

CONCLUSIONS

The homogeneity of the sub-samples taken on the same paddock is good when collection is done at the beginning or at the end of the grazing season, when the counts in L3 are high or average. It is poor in mid-season when the counts are low.

For pasture sampling procedures, a large number of sub-samples should be taken. The "strips of herbage" technique can be discarded, and for the assessment of concentration of L3 in pasture herbage we recommend sampling separately at random

near the dung pats and far from the dung pats. This seems more
appropriate for the determination of parasite risk and a better
understanding of nematodiasis, as the samples cover the lowest
and the highest counts on the paddock. The cores of soil plus
herbage have a different objective, i.e., to reflect all the
L3 available on and in the ground, but the procedure requires
improvement to become a feasible procedure in the laboratory.

For laboratory procedures, the reference technique is
soaking the same herbage sample in a bucket for two successive
days. For routine work, the easiest and fastest technique is
the washing with a washing machine or a cement mixer. We have
developed, in collaboration with R.J. Jørgensen, a specially
designed funnel which allows very easy handling of a large
number of individual samples.

REFERENCES

Boag, B. and Thomas, R.J., 1975. Epidemiological studies on *Nematodirus* species in sheep. Res. Vet. Sci. 19, 263-268.

Borgsteede, M. and Kloosterman, A., 1977. Epidemiology and prevention of Trichostrongylid infections in cattle. Tijdsch. Diergeneesk 102, (24) 1428.

Downey, N.E., 1973. Nematode parasite infections of calf pasture in relation to the health and performance of grazing calves. Vet. Rec. 93, 505-514.

Gevrey, J., 1970. Etude du peuplement d'une prairie naturelle par les larves infestantes de "Strongles" parasites du tractus digestif des ovins. II. Déplacements larvaires verticaux. Ann. Rech. Vet. 1 (2), 233-252.

Gruner, L., Mauleon, H., Hubert, J. and Sauve, D., 1980. Study of gastro-intestinal strongylosis in a flock on permanent pasture. II Pasture infestation in 1977 and epidemiological discussion. Ann. Rech. Vet. 11 (2)(in press).

Henriksen, S.R., Bentholm, B.R. and Neilsen-Englyst, A., 1976. Investigations on bovine gastro-intestinal strongylidae. II Seasonal variations in infestation of herbage with infective larvae. Nord. Vet. Med. 28, (415), 201-209.

Jørgensen, R.J., 1980. Epidemiology of bovine dictyocaulosis in Denmark. Vet. Parasitol. 7, (2), 153-167.

Kloosterman, A., 1971. Observations on the epidemiology of Trichostrongylosis of calves. Medel. Land. Wageningen No. 71-70, 114p.

Lancaster, M.B., 1970. The recovery of infective Nematode larvae from herbage samples. J. Helminth. 44, (2), 219-230.

Michel, J.F., 1966. The epidemiology and control of parasitic gastro-enteritis in calves. Proc. 4th int. Meet. Wld. Ass. Buiatrics 272-288.

Michel, J.F. and Parfitt, J.W., 1956. An experimental study of the epidemiology of parasitic bronchitis in calves. Vet. rec. 68, 706-710.

Rose, J.H., 1975. The significance of *Nematodirus helvetianus* eggs which have survived on a pasture throughout the winter in the transmission of infection to calves. Res. vet. Sci. 18, 175-177.

Taylor, E.L., 1939. Technique for estimation of pasture infestation by strongyle larvae. Parasitology 31, 473-478.

DISCUSSION

R.J. Thomas *(UK)*

Do you have an explanation for the fact that the recovery by the "W" technique is higher up until July, and then the recovery around the pats is higher from July onwards?

J.-P. Raynaud *(France)*

We have worked in the west part of France and last year the herbage was high early in the season. So even if we gave precise instructions to the collectors to pick around the pats, it is very difficult to do so early in the season, to isolate a pat which is not a fresh one and to really work around the pat.

R.J. Thomas

So it is partly a technical problem rather than one of epidemiology?

J.-P. Raynaud

Yes. It is due to the amount of the herbage.

J. Armour *(UK)*

How much soil did you collect in your core? Secondly, what do you think is the reason for the difference in the behaviour of *Nematodirus* compared to the *Ostertagia* and *Cooperia* species?

J.-P. Raynaud

It is interesting to note that the W system is better for *Nematodirus* than the technique of collecting around the pats. So the only conclusion is that the *Nematodirus* dislike the pats. The system our people use for cores is the approved system for gardeners which you use yourself.

F.H.M. Borgsteede *(The Netherlands)*

I have a question related to that of Dr. Thomas. Regarding the difference between the sampling before July and thereafter, have you looked at the age of the larvae? You can determine how their condition is and whether they have overwintered or not? One can see the intestinal cells of the larvae;' when they are filled up and very green, then you know that they are fresh larvae. When they are not so green and when they are rather empty then you can assume that they are overwintered larvae. Have you looked at these differences?

J.-P. Raynaud

Unfortunately, though we have determined the species in the samples, we did not examine the state of the intestinal cells.

J.F. Michel *(UK)*

I am puzzled about this question of pats before July and pats after July. Before July very few larvae will have emerged from the present season's faeces. Last season's faeces will have disintegrated, and will not be recognised as such.

J.-P. Raynaud

I would like to refer to one of the graphs shown by Dr. Jørgensen. Early in the season, on a permanent pasture, there are very few pats, but later they increase in number. A more practical aspect is to detect the pats and to collect correctly around them.

J.F. Michel

But with the pats of fresh faeces the larvae will not have emerged from them until July.

J.-P. Raynaud

That is probably true. This is a reason why, in the W system, random areas away from the pats are higher. Before July the pats represent nothing more than a reservoir for the future.

R.J. Thomas

I think a possible explanation why the W system is better for the *Nematodirus* is that larvae remain in the egg and only develops when it leaves the pat. We have found with sheep *Nematodirus* spp that the distribution on *Nematodirus* eggs is probably mostly by earthworm activity, which distributes the eggs from the pat. Therefore one might expect a much more random distribution than where the larvae develop to the 3rd stage within the pat and then come out of it.

J. Armour

Do you think it is the same with the cattle species?

R.J. Thomas

I would think it is probably the same with cattle. Until the pat is broken down you don't get the eggs developing unless they have been actively carried and disseminated by earthworms.

RECOVERY OF *Ostertagia* FROM THE BOVINE ABOMASAL
MUCOSA BY IMMERSION IN WARM NORMAL SALINE

N.E. Downey
The Agricultural Institute,
Dunsinea, Castleknock, Co. Dublin, Ireland.

INTRODUCTION

Theodorides and Actor (1967) reported that immature nematodes
could be successfully recovered at necropsy by allowing them to
migrate from segments of murine small intestine into a surrounding medium of normal saline. This is the principle underlying
the method described here for recovering mainly early fourth
stage larvae (EL_4) of *Ostertagia ostertagi* from the abomasal
mucosa of cattle. The adoption of a similar procedure for this
purpose was reported by Williams et al. (1977). Preliminary
estimations of recovery rates achieved by the method were carried
out.

METHOD

Having opened up the abomasum and collected its contents
in the usual way for worm count, the organ is placed in a 2
gallon (9 litre) plastic bucket and covered with normal saline
at 40°C. The saline containing the abomasum is held at 40°C for
4 - 5 hours. Immediately afterwards, the abomasum is dipped
several times in a second bucket containing 2 gallons of water
at 40°C and then discarded. The contents of both buckets are
poured over a sieve (aperture size, 38 micron) and the residue
on the sieve made up to a suitable volume for a dilution
count.

The abomasums of five naturally infected cows were
thoroughly washed preparatory to counting the mature worms in
the abomasal contents (Table 1). Each abomasum was then
processed in the manner already outlined. Afterwards, the
abomasums were subjected to pepsin/HCl digestion (Herlich, 1956)

P. Nansen, R.J. Jørgensen, E.J.L. Soulsby (eds), Epidemiology and Control of Nematodiasis in Cattle.
Copyright © 1981 ECSC, EEC, EAEC, Brussels – Luxembourg. All rights reserved.

and the results show that only a few worms remained to be recovered by this latter procedure (Table 1).

TABLE 1

Ostertagia BURDENS IN COWS - SPRING, 1979 - 'N. SALINE METHOD' FOLLOWED BY PEPSIN/CHl DIGESTION FOR MUCOSA

Cow No.	Abomasal contents		Abomasal mucosa			
			Mature	EL_4	LL_4	L_5
7 630	9 900	N. saline	800	2 180	–	3 760
		P. HCl	< 20	400		20
7 631	5 400	N. saline	320	< 20	4 320	< 20
		P. HCl	20	20	380	< 20
7 648	4 400	N. saline	1 700	25 220	< 20	< 20
		P. HCl	400	780	< 20	< 20
7 181	300	N. saline	200	79	< 20	< 20
		P. HCl	< 20	9	< 20	< 20
7 603	1 700	N. saline	3 200	5 500	–	–
		P. HCl	500	1 200	–	–

TABLE 2

PERCENTAGE OF WORMS IN MUCOSA RECOVERED BY 'N SALINE METHOD'

Animal No.	Mature	EL_4	LL_4	L_5
7 630	100	84	–	99
7 631	94	–	92	–
7 648	81	97	–	–
7 181	100	90	86	–
1 030	86.5	82.1	–	–
	92.3	88.3	89	–

Note (Tables 1 and 2): EL_4 = early 4th stage larvae; LL_4 = late 4th stage larvae; L_5 = 5th stage larvae.

Expressing the results as percentages (Table 2), it is apparent that 88.3 percent of EL_4 were recovered by the use, as described, of normal saline.

The abomasums of two cows were cut in half after the contents had been thoroughly washed out. One half of each organ was then processed by the 'saline/migration' method, the other by the digestion method. Table 3 shows that approximately the same number of EL_4 were recovered by both methods. Rather more mature worms were obtained by the use of normal saline. This presumably resulted from failure to recover these forms during preliminary washing, a failure also reflected in the high percentage values for mature worms shown in Table 2.

TABLE 3

PROCESSING HALF ABOMASUM BY EACH METHOD

Cow No.	Method	Worm numbers		
		Mature	EL_4	L_5
44	N. saline	120	270	0
	Pepsin/HCl	60	300	0
21	N. saline	210	1 980	60
	Pepsin/HCl	120	2 880	60

It may be concluded that this method is almost as efficient as the digestion method, compared with which it has certain advantages:

1. It is quicker.

2. The liquid fraction passes more readily through the sieve.

3. The residue is easier to examine (no fat or shreds of mucosa).

4. Worm specimens recovered are in excellent conditions.

5. It eliminates the cost of expensive pepsin.

A possible drawback is that the method may only be suitable for abomasums of freshly killed animals.

REFERENCES

Herlich, H., 1966. A digestion method for post-mortem recovery of nematodes
        for ruminants. Proceedings of the Helminthological Society of
        Washington, 23, 102-103.
Theodorides, V.J. and Actor, P., 1967. Simple method for the recovery and
        counting of helminths of mice. The Journal of Parasitology, 53, 210.
Williams, J.C., Knox, J.W., Sheehan, D. and Fuselier, R.H., 1977. Efficacy
        of albendazole against inhibited early fourth stage larvae of
        Ostertagia ostertagi. The Veterinary Record, 101, 484-486.

DISCUSSION

J.W. Hansen *(Denmark)*

You say that the contents of the abomasum were counted in
the usual way and you show figures indicating that the abomasal
contents have a certain number of worms in them. Is that only
adult worms or does it include larvae?

N. Downey *(Ireland)*

The figures for the abomasal contents are for the adult
worms in the lumen.

J.W. Hansen

So you are not considering larvae that might be in the
contents of the abomasum?

N. Downey

No!

J.W. Hansen

It is our impression that the number of larvae in the
content may vary in relation to the time between slaughter and
examination. The larvae seem to migrate out of the mucosa
within an hour or two. If one examined the mucosa ten minutes
after slaughter one would have a much higher count in the mucosa

than if one waited two or three hours. Then they would be
found in the contents. We believe it is very important to look
for the larvae in the content as well as in the mucosa.

N. Downey

   I agree.

R.M. Connan *(UK)*

   I would like to support that observation. My belief is
that as the techniques become more sophisticated it is necessary
to become less sophisticated.   We separate the parasites from
the abomasum in the same way as does Dr. Downey, we then put
them all together -- the washings and the contents. Then we
sample this, perhaps 10 or 20 times, and examine the whole sample,
in a petri dish, without sieving.

R.J. Jørgensen *(Denmark)*

   Thank you Dr. Downey. It is a very useful observation
to know that we can isolate the larval stages in warm saline.

CONTROLLED/CRITICAL TESTS IN THE EVALUATION
OF ANTHELMINTIC ACTIVITY

D. Düwel

Hoechst Aktiengesellschaft Helminthologie,
Postfach 80 03 20, D-6230 Frankfurt, M.80,
Federal Republic of Germany.

INTRODUCTION

Registration authorities and consumers are justified in demanding extensive information on veterinary drugs: this includes the spectrum of activity, pharmacological data, residues and tolerance/toxicity. These data can be obtained only in animal studies, and studies should be so designed that the minimum number is used. Thus, an internationally agreed standard for test methods could be a prerequisite for the registration authorities of various countries. The first symposium of the 'World Association for the Advancement of Veterinary Parasitology' was held in Hannover in 1963, under the title, 'Evaluation of Anthelmintics'. Since then, efforts to standardise the methods of laboratory and field evaluation of anthelmintics have continued.

Workers in the field of the evaluation of anthelmintics will be familiar with controlled or critical tests, which were described by Moskey and Harwood (1941), Gibson (1963), and Hall and Forster (1918). The critical test is applicable in laboratory studies. It is particularly suitable for studies of *Dictyocaulus viviparus* and *Fasciola hepatica*. The controlled test is applicable to studies of gastro-intestinal nematodes and to field studies. Technical details of these tests are presented as follows.

CRITICAL TEST

An animal, infected with helminths, is treated with the anthelmintic under test. The parasites expelled after treat-

ment in the faeces, sputum, tracheal exudate, etc., are counted
and identified. Five to seven days later, the animal is killed
and the remaining worm burden is counted and identified. The
time of autopsy can be decisive for the evaluation, as the duration of the time for the elimination of parasites is dependent
on the mechanism of action of the anthelmintic under test. The
efficacy is calculated according to the formula:

$$\frac{\text{number of parasites expelled}}{\text{number of parasites expelled} + \text{remaining parasites}} \times 100 = \text{percentage efficacy}$$

The advantage of this method is that each animal serves
as its own control, and individual variations in worm burdens
do not lead to erroneous calculations. This method can become
uncertain when the efficacy of a compound against nematodes of
the stomach and small intestine is under consideration. Thus,
digestion of worms may occur during passage through the intestine and this may lead to erroneous calculations. Results may
vary with vermicidal as opposed to vermifugal preparations
under test.

The critical test is of no value against immature stages.
In our experience, the critical test is of value in two circum-
stances: the evaluation of efficacy of drugs against lungworms
(D. viviparus) and against Fasciola hepatica.

The method used for lungworms is as follows: tracheotomy
is performed under local anaesthesia and a curved plastic tube
is inserted into the severed trachea and connected to a muslin
bag in which the lungworms are collected. The bag is held open
with the aid of a wire or plastic support.

Tracheotomised animals have been maintained for more than
two months, but the collection bag has to be changed every
4 - 6 hours.

In trials, a number of untreated animals are used as controls to assess the natural expulsion which may occur in severe infections.

CONTROLLED TEST

Matched groups, as regards weight, age, clinical findings, worm infestation, origin, etc., are established. One group is treated with the drug under test and the other is used as the untreated control. In this case, autopsy normally commences 5 - 7 days after treatment and the worm burden of both groups is compared.

With artificially infected animals the worm burden is approximately the same in all animals, so that a limited number of animals will be required for a controlled test. With naturally infected animals, where worm burden variation is to be expected, the number of experimental animals will need to be increased, in order to obtain statistically significant results.

Evaluation of the efficacy of compounds against immature stages is possible only by means of the controlled test. Similarly, field trials, undertaken to extend laboratory findings, are best evaluated by this technique.

In all tests there is need for uniform test methods. Thus, the times between infection, treatment and autopsy should be standardised so that the same developmental stages of a parasite are considered by different workers in different locations. By this, comparable data can be obtained for evaluation. Examples are given in Figures 1 and 2.

78

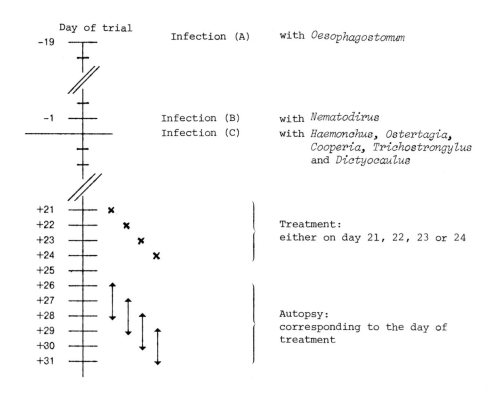

Fig. 1:   Scheme of testing anthelmintics in cattle.   Investigation of
adult nematodes.

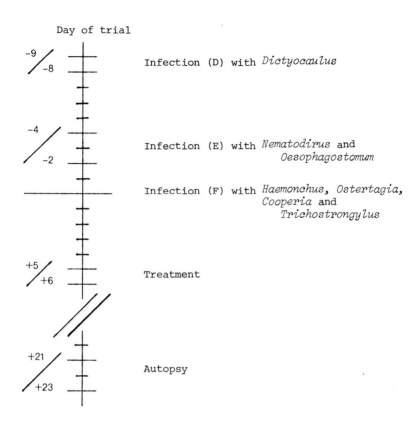

Day of trial

-9
-8   Infection (D) with *Dictyocaulus*

-4
-2   Infection (E) with *Nematodirus* and
                            Oesophagostomum

          Infection (F) with *Haemonchus, Ostertagia,*
                            Cooperia and
                            Trichostrongylus

+5
+6   Treatment

+21
+23   Autopsy

Fig. 2:   Scheme for testing anthelmintics in cattle.   Investigation of
           immature nematodes.

DISCUSSION

J. Eckert *(Switzerland)*

I would like to make some comments regarding Dr. Düwel's paper. He mentioned the standardisation of the techniques for anthelmintic testing and I would like to report that the World Association for the Advancement of Veterinary Parasitology has asked an international commission to prepare international guidelines for the evaluation of anthelmintics. Members of this group are Dr. Powers from the USA, Dr. Gibson from Great Britain, myself and some other colleagues. The proposal is to prepare international guidelines for the evaluation of anthelmintics so that national registration authorities could accept the results of anthelmintic testing which had been carried out in different countries according to these guidelines. In 1977/78 the American group started to prepare such guidelines and I attempted to contact this group to propose that European proposals should also be included in these guidelines. However, I was not successful with my proposal. Consequently, a small group met in Zürich; it was attended by representatives from various companies and we collected data and material as a basis for guidelines. I would propose now that we establish a sub-group of this group, which would finalise European proposals for such guidelines. When these guidelines are finalised, we should contact the American group and prepare international guidelines for the standardisation of techniques and the evaluation of efficacy.

J.W. Hansen *(Denmark)*

I hope that we will have further discussions on this and it could, perhaps, be included in the discussion on Wednesday afternoon.

GENERAL DISCUSSION

J. Armour *(UK)*

I would like to ask Dr. Jones, what were the numbers of tracer calves used, per acre or per hectare,

R.M. Jones *(UK)*

We used approximately one tracer calf per hectare in the studies.

A. Kloosterman *(The Netherlands)*

We have had interesting experiences with tracer calves. We place them two by two in a field where we have also done larval counts. We found a satisfactory correlation between herbage counts and wormburdens, but there may be big differences between the worm counts of the two calves grazing on one particular pasture. For example, a first calf had 100 worms and the second calf, grazing the same pasture simultaneously, had 81 000 worms! To minimise the variation between calves, these were calves that were all from one sire. Later, it was observed that some animals graze closer to the faecal pats than others, and hence grazing behaviour may play an important role in the acquisition of larvae.

J.-P. Raynaud *(France)*

I would like to refer to an experiement which was done on two paddocks. Each paddock was of one hectare and each had ten grazing animals, according to the normal system that we have in Normandy. On these two paddocks we put tracers every month. We calculated L_3/kg herbage and the total amount of the worm count, irrespective of developmental stage, for both *Ostertagia* and *Cooperia*. Also, we have calculated the herbage dry matter intake per day and have estimated the total hypothetical intake of L_3. There was a large discrepancy between the potential intake of larvae and the number of worms in the tracer animals when the numbers were very low. However, when the numbers were

high there was only a small discrepancy between the total
intake of larvae and the wormburden. Our conclusion is that,
in the second half of the grazing season, the tracer animal
reflects satisfactorily to the herbage count. However, in the
early part of grazing, the herbage probably shows more larvae
than the tracer acquires. On some occasions there was a good
correlation between the total possible intake and the real
intake of the calves.

N. Downey *(Ireland)*

The level of pasture contamination is important. At low
levels the pasture sampling techniques are not very good at
showing differences. Then it may be better to use egg counts
of susceptible animals.

R.M. Connan *(UK)*

I would like to refer to the difference in the correlation
between pasture larvae and wormburden in tracer animals in the
second half of the season, compared with the correlation in
the first half. This may be related to the amount of herbage
which is available. When the herbage is growing, and it is
reasonably plentiful and reasonably nutritious, animals can be
fairly selective. As the herbage becomes less nutritious and
less readily available, then they can be less selective in
their grazing. This is certainly my experience with sheep.

R.M. Jones

I would agree with Dr. Connan. Additionally, distinct
differences may occur in grazing behaviour when a strange animal
is placed in a herd. Even when the age and sex of the animal
are matched with the grazing herd, even then new arrivals may
be isolated and it may be a long time before they are accepted
into the grazing herd. Therefore, they do not necessarily
reflect the precise intake of the animals of the main herd.

J. Armour

On the other hand, if Dr. Michel's L_3 data in the 60s
is compared with our data on tracers, done at the same time in
a different part of Britain, there is a close relation to both
sets of data. Therefore, in view of what was presented this
morning, both methods are good indicators of parasitism.

J.F Michel *(UK)*

There was a great deal of talk about techniques this
morning but people were reluctant to relate these techniques
to specific purposes. Surely, what technique you choose does
depend very much on the specific purpose to which you wish to
put it?

I am also wondering whether one needs the degree of
precision that people seem to be aiming at. The outlines being
looked for are broad and does it matter if there is some
imprecision?

R.J. Jørgensen *(Denmark)*

I think precision is important in some circumstances.
I have presented some data on the horizontal distribution of
lungworm larvae. If the trichostrongyle larvae are counted in
the same samples, an equally uneven distribution of these
larvae is noted. In an experiment last year between two groups
of calves - one group was treated and the other untreated - we
found pasture larval counts which were the same both close to
the pat and away from the pat in one field, but on another
field, where there was a control group, there was a very high
concentration around the faecal pats and a very low concentration
away from faecal pats. I wonder what kind of counts we would
have got had we just taken random samples from these two fields.

E.J.L. Soulsby *(UK)*

We have heard papers on how to measure infective larvae
and other larvae in herbage and soil, and this has been correl-

ated with the numbers of worms found in tracer animals. Of course there is a large area of unknown between the situation in the soil or on the herbage and the occurrence of the adult worm in the animal. I wonder if any worker has thought of trying to assess the number of larvae ingested, for example, by an oesophageal fistula. How many larvae are taken in but never mature?

J. Armour

I think that Bill Southcott, and his colleagues at Armidale, used oesophageal fistulae. However, this raised problems in relation to appetite. They did not attach too much importance to the results they got using the technique of oesophageal fistulation.

R.J. Thomas *(UK)*

It is a question of how normal the animal is once it has been prepared for an oesophageal fistula.

P. Nansen *(Denmark)*

Last summer we tried to make a compromise between herbage larval counts and wormburdens in animals. The idea was to take samples by fistulae from the rumen of grazing animals.

There are differences between having an oesophageal fistulae and a rumen fistulae because grazing with a ruminal fistula does not seem to effect the animal very much.

However, we could not recover the larvae from the rumen for technical reasons. Nevertheless, it may be worthwhile to study this method further since it would be cheaper, probably, than tracer calves.

SESSION 2

ADULT CATTLE

Chairman: J. Armour

OBSERVATIONS ON THE EPIDEMIOLOGY AND PATHOGENICITY OF NEMATODE INFECTIONS IN ADULT DAIRY CATTLE IN GREAT BRITAIN

M.T. Fox and D.E. Jacobs

Department of Microbiology and Parasitology,
Royal Veterinary College, University of London, UK.

ABSTRACT

Preliminary results are presented from a continuing 3 year investigation of the effect of nematode infections on milk production in adult cows in 9 large dairy farms. Examination showed that 85.2% of 460 cows were passing nematode eggs or larvae in the faeces, thereby contaminating the pasture. The application of slurry to fields was observed to be an additional source of contamination. A new method is described for calculating the number of infective larvae ingested daily by dairy cattle and examples are given of estimated intake of infective larvae by cows kept under different management systems. Analysis of pooled milk production data from 5 farms in the first year of the study failed to show a response to treatment with levamisole although a significant increase in milk yield was noted on one farm.

P. Nansen, R.J. Jørgensen, E.J.L. Soulsby (eds), Epidemiology and Control of Nematodiasis in Cattle.

INTRODUCTION

Work in the USA (Bliss and Todd, 1973; 1976) and the
Benelux countries (Pouplard, 1978; Pluimers, 1979) suggests
that the treatment of dairy cows with a nematocidal drug at
the time of calving may increase milk yield significantly
during the ensuing lactation. This report gives interim
results from a continuing three year project designed to
measure the effect of a nematocidal treatment (levamisole) on
milk production under British conditions and to provide information on the epidemiology of nematode infections in adult
cattle.

MATERIAL AND METHODS

As many as possible of the cows on nine well-managed dairy
herds (Table 1) were allocated to pairs using the criteria
displayed in Table 2. On eight farms, one member of each pair
was given a placebo treatment (oxyclozanide) while the other
was treated with oxyclozanide plus the nematocide levamisole at
the recommended dose-rate of 2.3 - 5.5 mg/kg. No placebo was
used on the ninth farm. The remaining animals i.e. those that
could not be paired, were assigned to treatment groups
alternately according to their calving dates.

Milk production data were abstracted from Milk Marketing
Board computer printouts while health, nutrition and management
parameters were monitored by regular visits to the farms and
inspection of herd records. As there is no generally agreed
standard procedure for the comparison of milk yields, results
have been calculated by two alternative methods (Figure 1)
using data from a) the paired cows only and b) paired and
alternately treated animals. In each case calculations were
repeated i) with and ii) without inclusion of animals that
succumbed to disease during the period of observation (Table 3).

TABLE 1

HERD SELECTION

Geographical location: main drying areas (Somerset/Wiltshire .. 4 farms Oxfordshire .. .. .. 1 farm Staffordshire .. .. 4 farms) Breed: British Friesian .. .. 8 farms Canadian Holstein .. .. 1 farm Milk Marketing Board Milk Recording Scheme .. .. all farms Size: >200 cows .. 3 farms; >130 cows .. 4 farms; >80 cows .. 2 farms Calving pattern: Autumn calving .. 8 farms; Spring calving .. 1 farm Milk cell count: <500,000 .. .. 8 farms; <600,000 .. .. 1 farm Av. milk yield: range: .. .. .. 5 150 - 6 900 kg Health/management problems: .. .. minimal Reliability of data collection: .. good

TABLE 2

PAIR SELECTION CRITERIA

Calving dates .. .. within 14 days Lactation number .. .. same up to number 3 Latest complete lactation performance .. .. .. within 450 kg

TABLE 3

REASONS FOR REJECTION OF DATA

Disease	%
Mastitis	61.2
Endometritis/vaginal discharge	16.1
Milk fever	8.7
Retained placenta	5.8
Lameness	4.5
Others	3.7

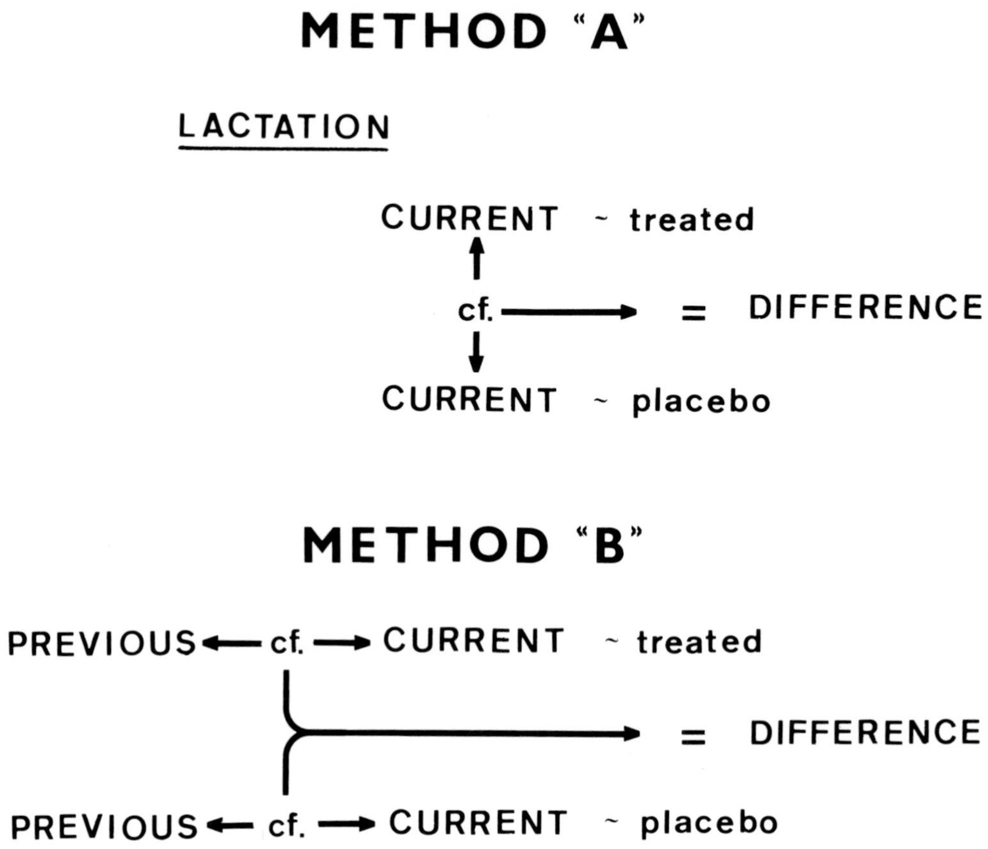

METHOD "A"

LACTATION

CURRENT ~ treated

cf. ⟶ = DIFFERENCE

CURRENT ~ placebo

METHOD "B"

PREVIOUS ← cf. → CURRENT ~ treated

= DIFFERENCE

PREVIOUS ← cf. → CURRENT ~ placebo

Fig. 1. Methods for the comparison of milk yields from treated cattle and control animals.

Faecal samples were taken from a proportion of the cows in the study and examined by the Baermann method and centrifugal flotation techniques using saturated MaCl and $ZnSO_4$ solutions. Herbage samples were taken from pastures used by the herds at the time of each visit and they were examined by the method of Lancaster (1970). Daily larval intakes for representative cows in two herds - one using traditional feeding methods, the other a complete feeding system - were calculated by multiplying the pasture larval count at each visit by the figure obtained by subtracting the dry matter content of the food fed to each animal at that time (i.e. concentrates hay, silage etc.) from its estimated total dry matter requirement (Figure 2).

$$L_3/day = L_3/KgDM \times DMI \text{ (grass)}$$

$$DMI \text{ (grass)} = DMI \text{ (total)} - DMI \text{ (fed)}$$

$$DMI \text{ (total)} = -4.14 + 0.43C + 0.015 \, LW - 0.095 \, WL$$

$$+ 4.04 \log_{10} WL + 0.208 \, MY + S$$

C = concentrate (Kg)   LW = liveweight (Kg)

WL = weeks post partum   MY = milk yield (Kg)

S = source effect

Fig. 2.   Method for calculating the daily intake of infective larvae
(L_3 per day) of dairy cows from the pasture larval count
(L_3 per kg DM) and the dry matter intake (DMI) of individual cows.

RESULTS

This study is not yet complete, and milk production data
are presented for only the first full lactations of cows on
the five farms in southern England. Whatever method of
calculation used (Table 4), no significant differences were
found when the pooled results from these herds were compared.
Examination of data from the individual herds, however,
revealed a significant response to treatment (+ 576 kg) on one
farm (Table 5).

Faecal examination demonstrated the presence of nematode
eggs and/or larvae in 85.2% of 460 pre-treatment samples. The
average egg-count was 4.8 epg. Larval culture revealed
Ostertagia and *Cooperia* to be the most common genera but
Trichostrongylus, *Oesophagostomum*, *Dictyocaulus*, *Fasciola*, *Trichuris*,
Capillaria, *Moniezia* and *Nematodirus* were found on occasion.

TABLE 4

EFFECT OF NEMATOCIDAL TREATMENT ON MILK YIELD - POOLED RESULTS FROM SOUTHERN FARMS, YEAR 1

	Yield (complete lactation)	
	kg extra milk	
	Paired cows only	Paired and non-paired cows
Method A*	(a)	(b)
Healthy and diseased cows (i)	+35	+165
Healthy cows only (ii)	- 3	+196
Method B*		
Healthy and diseased cows (i)	+17	+ 73
Healthy cows only (ii)	-211	+ 74
Total number cows:	170	351
Eliminated because of disease:	44.9%	
P > 0.05 in all cases		

*For explanation see Figure 1.

TABLE 5

EFFECT OF NEMATOCIDAL TREATMENT ON MILK YIELD - RESULTS FOR INDIVIDUAL SOUTHERN FARMS, YEAR 1

		Yield (complete lactation)		
Farm	Pasture larval counts (L_3/kg DM-range)	kg Extra		
		Milk	Butterfat	Protein
S1	0 - 510	+576*	+16.4*	+18.2*
S5	0 - 261	+466	+17.4	+ 3.8
S2	0 - 213	+ 98	- 5.5	- 3.5
S3	0 - 150	-170	+ 5.2	- 2.6
S4	0 - 135	- 69	-16.0	- 2.2

* P < 0.05

(Analysis: Method A - healthy cows only).

Pasture larval counts for the five southern herds are summarised in Table 5 and more detailed information on pasture larval counts and estimated daily larval intakes for two herds (one in the south of England, the other in the north) are given in Figure 3. The pasture larval count often increased, sometimes substantially, after the winter application of slurry (Table 6).

TABLE 6

PASTURE LARVAL COUNTS BEFORE AND AFTER SLURRY APPLICATION COMPARED WITH UNTREATED NEIGHBOURING FIELDS

Farm	Field	Slurry applied?	L_3/kg DM	
			Before	After
N_2	a	Yes	42	172
	b	No	20	0
	c	No	102	17
N_3	a	Yes	0	223
	b	No	0	0
	c	No	0	0

DISCUSSION

The effect of the nematocidal treatment on the overall milk production of five farms in the first year of the study appeared to vary from -211 kg to +196 kg depending on the method of calculation used (Table 4). This illustrates the care that must be taken when interpreting published data - especially where authors describe 'trends' without statistical validation. In studies of this kind, the method of calculation used should be defined and reasons for the choice given. Method A i b (Table 4) - i.e. a direct comparison of all animals in the trial, gives an estimate of the benefit of treatment to the farmer on that one occasion, but does not necessarily quantitate the deleterious effect of parasitism as this may be masked by the influence of a wide variety of extraneous factors.

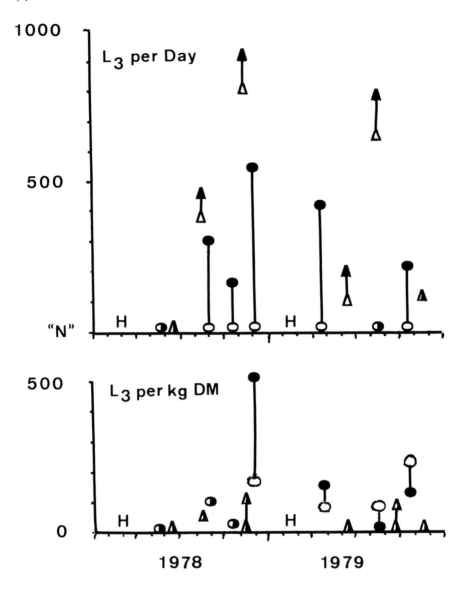

Fig. 3. Pasture larval counts (below) and the daily intake of infective larvae (above) for high yielding (closed shapes) and low yielding (open shapes) cows on a farm using traditional feeding methods (triangles) and one employing a complete feed system (circles).

'N' = larval intake associated with the 'Nibble effect' i.e. grass eaten in small quantities by animals whose appetite is theoretically satisfied by manger fed food - this effect is very difficult to quantify.

H = period of winter housing.

These complications can be minimised and a more meaningful result obtained by the meticulous pairing of cows on carefully selected farms, followed by the strict rejection of data should either member of a pair succumb to any disease that might affect milk production (i.e. Method A ii a in Table 4). However, this approach suffers from the disadvantage that only a small proportion of the cows in the herd can be used for the analysis. To overcome this problem Bliss and Todd (1976) have suggested the use of Method B (Figure 1) which reduces the need for pairing by exploiting the principle that future performance can be predicted with some accuracy from past lactation records. As successive lactations may be of different lengths a correction factor may also be applied to bring each to a standard 305 day figure. In the USA further correction factors are available to allow for differences in the age of animals by converting each milk yield to a 'mature equivalent'. Such figures are not yet available for British cattle. A comparison is then made of the relative improvements in milk yield between past and current lactations in treated and control animals. This gives a theoretical rather than a measured benefit attributable to worming but does have the great advantage that data from many more cows within each herd can be used for statistical evaluation.

In the present study, no method of analysis gave a statistically significant difference in milk yield (or quality) between treated and control groups i.e. there was no demonstrable effect that could be attributed to the nematocidal treatment. However, considerable farm to farm variation occurred (Table 5) with one herd giving a strongly positive response to treatment. As there is also the possibility of year to year variation, these preliminary results do not necessarily prejudge the final outcome of this investigation.

Inspection of the pasture larval counts recorded in Table 5 might suggest that the biggest responses to treatment were obtained on the farms with the highest pasture larval counts. However, as cows do not always derive the whole of their nutrition from grass but are fed concentrate rations, hay, silage, etc., pasture larval counts are not necessarily an indicator of parasitic challenge in this class of animal. The formula shown in Figure 2, derived from the work of Vadiveloo and Holmes (1979), accounts for 73% of the variability in dry matter intake of dairy cows and is therefore a most useful tool for the calculation of daily intakes of infective larvae from the pasture. The main source of error in the calculation is the failure of the pasture larval count technique to recover all larvae on the grass (Lancaster, 1970).

As expected, the daily larval intake of traditionally managed cows (i.e. supplementary feed restricted to 4 kg concentrate given for each 10 kg milk produced) was found to be considerably higher than that of cows kept on a complete feed system (i.e. separate ingredients of daily diet mixed into a homogenous blend designed as the main source of food) even when pasture larval counts were lower (Figure 3). More surprising was the finding that in every case high yielding animals were ingesting larger numbers of larvae than were the low yielders. In the case of the complete feeding farm, these differences were often substantial. These figures reflect the larger appetite of the high yielding animals and may explain the observation made by Bliss and Todd (1973) that the biggest responses to anthelmintic treatment ofen occur in the most productive dairy herds. Maximum daily larval intakes recorded for the traditional and complete feed systems were 927 and 541, respectively. By way of comparison, an intake of around 4,000 *Ostertagia* larvae per day is required to produce clinical signs in susceptible calves (Michel, 1969).

ACKNOWLEDGEMENTS

This work was supported by a research grant from Imperial Chemical Industries Ltd. The authors also wish to thank Mr. David Budget for the statistical analyses, the Veterinary Epidemiology Unit at Reading University, the Milk Marketing Board the the many others who have assisted in the compilation of the data presented in this report.

REFERENCES

Bliss, D.H. and Todd, A.C., 1973. 'Milk production by Wisconsin dairy
    cattle after deworming with Baymix^R'. Veterinary Medicine/Small
    Animal Clinician, 68, 1034-1038.

Bliss, D.H. and Todd, A.C., 1976. 'Milk production by Vermont dairy
    cattle after deworming (two dewormings during the first 90 days
    of lactation)'. Veterinary Medicine/Small Animal Clinician,
    71, 1251-1254.

Lancaster, M.B., 1970. 'The recovery of infective nematode larvae from
    herbage samples'. Journal of Helminthology, 44, 219-230.

Michel, J.F., 1969. 'Some observations on the worm burdens of calves
    infected daily with *Ostertagia ostertagi*'. Parasitology 59, 575-595.

Pouplard, L., 1978. 'Anthelmintic treatment of dairy cows'. Veterinary
    Record, 103, 434.

Pluimers, E.J., 1979. 'Milk production increase following treatment of
    Dutch dairy cattle with thiabendazole'. The Veterinary Quarterly
    1, 82-89.

Valdiveloo, J. and Holmes, W., 1979. 'The prediction of the voluntary
    feed intake of dairy cows'. Journal of Agricultural Science,
    Cambridge, 93, 553-562.

DISCUSSION

H.-J. Bürger *(West Germany)*

What was the system on the farm with the highest differences and the highest larval counts on pasture?

D.E. Jacobs *(UK)*

It was one of complete feeding. With the complete feeding system for high yielding cows the food is brought to the animals, and every component in the feed is carefully measured. The dry matter intake of the cow is closely monitored, and the nutritional content of the feed is 'tailor-made' to the industrial level of milk production.

H.-J. Bürger

Where and how do they get the larvae from the pasture?

D.E. Jacobs

This is from what we call a 'worm lot'. The food required for milk production is presented to the cows, but also they are put out onto a small paddock - not to graze but to get exercise and fresh air. These are the paddocks where we found the highest pasture larval counts. Also, we found that for high yielding cows the diets, although they fulfilled the milk production requirements, did not entirely satisfy the appetite of the cow. High yielding cows were acquiring more larvae because they made up the appetite difference by eating grass. There is also the 'nibble effect'. Thus cows like eating grass and, even if their appetite is satisfactory they nibble grass because they enjoy it. Unfortunately we have no way of quantifying that nibble.

G. Urquhart *(UK)*

I wish to clarify something. Were these cows dosed just the once at the time of calving or just after?

D.E. Jacobs

Yes! Once.

G. Urquhart

Were the cows in yards or byres or out of doors? How were they looked after?

D.E. Jacobs

We had nine farms with nine different management systems. In the complete feeding herd they were in yards.

G. Urquhart

And under the other systems?

D.E. Jacobs

Dry cows were on grazing and they are brought indoors for calving.

R.M. Connan *(UK)*

You said you used levamisole and then as a placebo you used an oxyclozanide. At the peak of feeding, do you not think that you were taking a risk of eliminating *Fasciola* in the one group, and *Ostertagia* in the other?

D.E. Jacobs

We considered that, the treatment group was levamisole and oxyclozanide and the placebo group was oxyclozanide alone. We included the oxyclozanide because some of our farms were on flukey ground and, because we thought we ought to give a placebo and it seemed to be as good a placebo as any to use.

AN EVALUATION OF ANTHELMINTIC TREATMENT IN A DAIRY HERD

R.J. Thomas and P. Rowlinson
Faculty of Agriculture,
The University of Newcastle upon Tyne, U.K.

ABSTRACT

Faecal egg count and milk production data are given for 48 pairs of cows from a single herd, paired on previous yield, parity and expected calving date, one of each pair being dosed at calving with 66 mg/kg Thiabendazole. Mean 305 day yields were 5 445 kg and 5 608 kg respectively in treated and control groups, and no significant differences in yield, milk fat or protein were recorded. Faecal egg counts were similar in both groups, a salt flotation method showing 25 - 29% infection and 3.7 - 3.9 epg at mid lactation, and flotation was shown to be more sensitive than a modified McMaster method. Data analysis showed a high degree of within group variation and a consideration of this and other reported data suggests that large groups of cows should be used for these trials in preference to smaller numbers of closely paired animals.

P. Nansen, R.J. Jørgensen, E.J.L. Soulsby (eds), Epidemiology and Control of Nematodiasis in Cattle.
Copyright © 1981 ECSC, EEC, EAEC, Brussels – Luxembourg. All rights reserved.

INTRODUCTION

Cox and Todd (1962) carried out a survey of parasitism in dairy cattle in Wisconsin, and found an overall infection rate of 78% with gastro-intestinal nematodes.   Surprisingly, the infection rate increased with age from 37% in young calves to 87.5% in milking cows, and this led to renewed interest in the possible effect of infection and response to anthelmintic treatment, in adult cattle as well as young stock.   Subsequently Todd et al. (1972) reported an increase in milk output in the 8 days following anthelmintic treatment of 1.0 kg/day compared with untreated controls in a trial involving over 1,000 cattle. These authors attributed earlier failure to recognise the widespread nature of parasitism in dairy cattle to the use of a McMaster egg count technique which they showed to be very inefficient in detecting the low levels of egg output which occurred compared with a sugar flotation system.   Following further work by Bliss and Todd (1973, 1974, 1976) the value of anthelmintic treatment was clearly demonstrated in several states in the USA, and a routine anthelmintic medication at calving has become accepted practice.

Studies in Europe have been reported by Plumiers (1977) in Holland and Pouplard (1977) in Belgium in which considerable improvement in milk yield following treatment was again recorded and a good deal of interest has been aroused in Britain, where the practice is being increasingly adopted.   However, no published evidence was available on the value of anthelmintic treatment of dairy cows in this country, and the trial reported in this paper was carried out to assess the effect of treatment in a single herd.   Virtually all the data reported in the literature is based on relatively large numbers of animals spread over a number of farms and therefore subject to considerable differences in management and nutrition, and in most cases the improvement in milk output has been assessed by comparison with previous lactation.   In this trial, facilities were not available to handle large numbers of animals, and so an alternative method aimed at reducing the variability between cows was employed, namely to work within a single herd, in which management and nutrition and breed were uniform, and to pair treated and control animals as far as possible.

MATERIALS AND METHODS

The trial was carried out at the University farm in south-east Northumberland which comprises 350 hectares, largely in arable crops and carrying a herd of approximately 200 Friesian milking cows together with replacement young stock. The cows are set-stocked at pasture from mid-April to early October and housed in winter in covered straw yards. During summer, grazing may be supplemented with parlour-fed concentrates and winter feeding is based on grass silage, barley and concentrates. Breeding policy is directed to winter milk production and calving mainly takes place between August and January. Cows were paired as closely as possible on the basis of parity, expected calving date and previous milk yield, thus excluding heifers, and as a result of pairing 124 cows were included in the trial, which commenced in August 1977. One of each pair was treated with 66 mg/kg thiabendazole within 24 hours of calving, the other being kept as an untreated control. Dosage was based on individual body weight, the animals being weighed after calving and again after the next calving. Fourteen animals were culled during the trial, and these and their pairs were excluded from the results, which are based on 96 cows.

PARASITOLOGICAL DATA

Faeces samples were taken on the day of calving and examined by a McMaster method modified to record a minimum count of 10 eggs per gram (epg). However, since a high proportion of zero counts were recorded, subsequent samples, taken at approximately mid-lactation and at the next calving, were examined by a salt flotation technique. In this technique, 1 g of faeces was centrifuged in 10 ml saturated salt solution under a cover-glass on which the eggs were deposited and subsequently counted under a microscope.

MILK YIELD

Milk production, milk fat and protein for each animal were recorded monthly using the Milk Marketing Board National Milk Recording Service. In order to compare output at different stages of lactation, yields were corrected to a 35 day, 100 day and 305 day basis, and the data analysed using a paired 't' test.

RESULTS

Using the McMaster technique, very low levels of infection were recorded (Table 1), only 8.8% of the treated and 15.1% of the controls giving positive counts pre-treatment. Mean counts were 18 epg in infected animals and 2.2 epg overall. At mid-lactation and next calving, considerably higher proportions of infected animals were recorded using the flotation technique and the increase is almost certainly attributable to the increased sensitivity of the latter technique. This was confirmed by carrying out comparative counts on 19 samples using the two methods, in which 1 positive count was detected by the McMaster technique and 17 positives by flotation.

TABLE 1

WORM EGG COUNTS

	At calving[1]		Mid lactation[2]		Subsequent Calving[2]	
	Treated	Controls	Treated	Controls	Treated	Controls
No. sampled	57	53	48	46	32	37
% positive	8.8	15.1	29.2	25.5	46.9	35.1
mean epg						
a) infected cows	18	18.8	3.9	3.7	4.4	4.3
b) overall	1.6	2.8	1.1	0.9	2.0	1.5

[1] McMaster technique

[2] Flotation technique

Milk production has been compared in two ways. The direct within-lactation comparison between treated and control animals on a paired basis is shown in Tables 2 - 4 for yield, fat and protein respectively. In all three cases output is similar in both groups, being slightly higher for the controls. The level of yield at 5400 - 5600 kg over a 305 day lactation is quite satisfactory for a herd of this nature, as is the fat level of 41 g/kg. Breakdown of these figures into three stages of lactation also show only very slight differences between the groups even in the first 35 days when any treatment effect might have been expected to be most marked, during the rise to peak output. The second comparison, between current and previous yield for each group and therefore in line with the comparative base used in most earlier trials, is shown in Table 5. Both groups show a considerable increase over the previous lactation, of +763 kg and +889 kg respectively for treated and control animals, but again very little difference between the two groups.

TABLE 2

MILK YIELD OF TREATED AND UNTREATED GROUPS

Stage of lactation (days) approx.	Cumulative mean yield (kg) Treated	Control	Overall SD	LSD
35	887.5	862.5	373.2	108.8
100	2 362.2	2 364.8	531.1	158.2
305	5 445.0	5 608.0	933.1	381.6

TABLE 3

CUMULATIVE MILK FAT YIELD (kg), TREATED AND UNTREATED GROUPS

Stage of lactation (days) approx.	Cumulative mean yield (kg) Treated	Control	Overall SD	LSD
35	34.42	35.29	14.42	4.13
100	89.93	93.43	23.53	7.00
305	219.40	229.02	40.21	16.92

TABLE 4

CUMULATIVE MILK PROTEIN YIELD (kg) , TREATED AND UNTREATED GROUPS

Stage of lactation (days) approx.	Cumulative mean yield (kg) Treated	Control	Overall SD	LSD
35	29.50	28.96	10.55	3.06
100	75.15	76.30	18.04	5.37
305	177.44	186.90	38.58	12.17

TABLE 5

COMPARISON OF SUCCESSIVE LACTATIONS

Total lactation yield		Treated	Control	Overall SD
Milk (kg)	Previous	4 682	4 719	956
	Current	5 445	5 608	925
	Difference	+ 763	+ 889	
Fat (kg)	Previous	191.3	198.1	31.8
	Current	219.4	229.0	40.2
	Difference	+ 28.1	+ 30.9	

Analysis of the milk production data reveals the very large within group differences which occurred, the overall standard deviation in yield at 305 days being 933 kg, with corresponding figures of 40 kg and 38 kg for fat and protein respectively.

Body weights of the two groups of cows were similar at calving, 597 kg in the treated group and 578 kg in the controls, and these increased respectively to 600 kg and 587 kg at the subsequent calving, again showing no influence associated with treatment.

DISCUSSION

There are perhaps three main features of interest in these results, namely the infection levels as indicated by egg counts, the failure to achieve any improvement in milk output, and the large within groups variations which occurred despite the pairing of control and treated animals.

FAECAL EGG COUNTS

The results of the faecal examinations confirm those of other workers in demonstrating the marked superiority of centrifugal flotation techniques over the McMaster technique for cattle nematode infections, in which egg output is usually low. Modifying the latter to increase sensitivity to a minimum of 10 epg was clearly not adequate, since a flotation technique showed that almost all the positive counts were in the range 1 - 8 epg.

This flotation technique used only 1 g of faeces in 10 ml of saturated salt solution, which is less than the normally recommended 5 g sample, but this allowed the use of one centrifuge tube per sample and made for a simple, rapid technique. If, as appears likely, the monitoring of egg output in adult cattle is to be a desirable routine, then further work on the flotation technique should be carried out to develop a simple, rapid method of known and repeatable accuracy.

The egg count data using the flotation method indicate infection rates of 25 - 40%, with counts up to a maximum of 20 epg, and these results are similar to those recorded by Plumiers (1977) who found an incidence of 16% and a range of 1 - 30 epg. Levels recorded in America by Todd and his co-workers (1962, 1972, 1973, 1976) generally show higher infection rates of 80 - 95%, but similar mean egg counts of 3.3 - 15 epg. In Canada, McGregor and Kingscote (1957) reported 36% positive in cattle of 1 - 2 years old and 16.5% in adults by a flotation technique, with corresponding mean egg counts of 11 epg and 29 epg by a McMaster method. A more recent report from England by McBeath et al. (1979) also records mean counts generally below 5 epg but does not indicate the rate of infection. In Europe, *Ostertagia* is likely to be the dominant genus, while in

the American work *Haemonchus* is more common, but the pattern of
low egg counts in adult animals appears to be common throughout.

Actual levels of infection from postmortem worm counts
were not available during the trial, but four abomasal recoveries
were made from animals subsequently culled from the herd and
these showed counts of 3 050, 3 300, 19 500 and 4 500 predominantly *Ostertagia ostertagi*, and this limited sample suggests
quite high levels of infection in the herd. Pouplard (1978) in
Belgium reports large numbers of cows with burdens in excess
of 10 000 in abattoir studies, but does not indicate related
egg counts. Few other reports of worm burden levels are
available, and since there is general agreement, which the above
observations support, that there is no close correlation between
worm burden and faecal egg count in adult cattle, more extensive
abattoir surveys to establish the general level of infection
are required.

MILK OUTPUT

The level of milk output in this trial of approximately
5 500 kg is similar to that recorded by McBeath et al. (1979) at
6 600 kg., Plumiers (1977) at 6 300 kg, and rather higher than
the 3 500 kg reported by Pouplard (1977). The Wisconsin herds
varied from 4 000 kg (Todd et al., 1972) to 6 300 kg (Bliss and
Todd, 1974), and in Vermont, 5 900 kg (Bliss and Todd, 1976).
Thus the production status of herds in the various trials, and
the infection levels indicated by faecal egg count, are quite
similar and comparable treatment results might have been
expected. However, in this trial no improvement in milk output
resulted following treatment, either by within-lactation or
between-lactation comparison. Correction of the data for weight
change, parity, season of calving (autumn or winter), or previous
yield still failed to show a significant treatment response. By
contrast, Pouplard (1977) obtained a within-lactation improvement
of 399 kg and between-lactation improvements ranging from 173 kg
in England (McBeath et al., 1979) to 230 kg in Holland (Plumiers,
1977) and up to 530 kg in America (Bliss and Todd, 1976) have
been reported.

When the differences between current and previous yield are considered, the increases seen in this trial of approximately 800 kg are similar to those recorded elsewhere. This may be regarded as a typical level of increase between successive lactations and it is due to two main factors. The first is associated with year and general management, and the Milk Marketing Board mean figures show an improvement of 341 kg from 1976 - 77 recording year to 1977 - 78. The second factor is associated with the increasing age of the animals involved in the trial, and for the University herd this is calculated to be + 394 kg when moving from first to second lactation, and + 530 kg when moving from second to third lactation. Thus non-treatment factors have a very considerable influence on between-lactation comparisons and must reduce their reliability.

The failure to obtain a positive response to treatment is difficult to explain, particularly since more detailed analysis of the milk records shows that no response occurred even in the 35 days following treatment. The fact that infection levels as indicated by flotation egg counts were similar in both treated and control animals at mid-lactation suggests that re-infection may have occurred, possibly from bedding, as suggested by Bliss and Todd (1976), but it seems unlikely that this would have been sufficiently rapid to prevent an initial response. Alternatively, the influence of parasitism may be modified by other factors such as the level of nutrition. However, there are brief reports in the literature of failure to demonstrate any improvement following treatment by Moore et al. (1974) and Harris and Wilcox (1976) in America, and Fox (1979) has recently given a preliminary report on a trial in England involving 900 cows in which no significant increase was recorded.

YIELD VARIATION

Statistical examination of the milk production data shows that a high level of yield variation occurred despite the careful pairing of treated and control cows, and a similar degree

of variation is apparent when the current yield is compared
with that in the previous lactation. Calculation of the least
significant difference indicates that due to this variability
an improvement of 382 kg in the yield of treated animals over
the controls was required to be of statistical significance
(P < 0.05). Similarly for statistical significance a yield
difference of over 100 kg in the 850 - 900 kg production to 35
days would have been necessary in the initial stage of lactation. These are large increases, and well above the response
which would be required to make treatment an economic proposition, which is, of course, the determining factor to the
dairy farmer.

Consideration of the published information shows that
only a limited amount of statistical data has been presented,
and it therefore seemed of interest to carry out a statistical
exercise on the published information to assess its significance. This was done by calculating the least significant
difference in yield required between treated and control cows
at each of 5 levels of coefficient of variation in yield from
10% to 30%. These coefficients were selected on the basis of
general milk production records which indicate that a variation
of 15% to 25% may normally be expected to occur, and the actual
variation in the present trial was 17%.

Results of such analysis are shown in Table 6 for a number
of reported trials, together with relevant comments. The results
indicate that the improvements in yield have generally reached
significance in the American work and that of Plumiers (1977)
assuming a coefficient of variation of around 20%, while the
results of Pouplard (1977), where a large improvement was
recorded, are significant even at the highest expected level of
variation. However, the trial carried out by McBeath et al.
(1979) would not seem to show statistically significant results
by this analysis, and the conclusions drawn by the authors must
be treated with a good deal of caution.

TABLE 6

ANALYSIS OF REPORTED TRIALS

111

TRIAL WORKERS	TRIAL DETAILS *	Compound	Number of animals Control (C)	Treatment (T)
1 Todd et al., 1972	USA: 34 farms: Unpaired: Various:	CuSO$_4$ Phenothiazine Thiabendazole	244	448 183 153
2 Bliss & Todd, 1973	USA: 22 farms: Unpaired: $\bar{X}$ Day 155 of Lactation:	Coumaphos	295	708
3 Bliss & Todd, 1974	USA: 12 farms: Alternate cows: Calving	Thiabendazole	244	244
4 Bliss & Todd, 1976	USA: 9 farms: Unpaired: Calving (i) + Day 60-90 of Lactation (ii):	Thiabendazole (i) Coumaphos (ii)	121	146
5 Pouplard, 1977	Belgium: 12 farms: Unpaired: Calving	Thiabendazole	84	106
6 Plumiers, 1977	Holland: 29 farms: Alternate cows: Calving	Thiabendazole	266	276
7 McBeath et al., 1979	UK: 9 farms: Unpaired: Dry period:	Fenbendazole	130	138
8 Fox, 1979	UK: 9 farms: Paired: Calving	Levamisole	900	
9 Thomas & Rowlinson, 1980	UK: 1 farm: Paired: Calving	Thiabendazole	48	48

* The four aspects of the trial given under TRIAL DETAILS are: country, number of farms, whether cows were paired and time of treatment

TABLE 6 (Continued)

TRIAL WORKERS	Response (T) v (C)[H] kg/day	Calculated Response (T) v (C) kg/lactation	Reqd. Least Significance Diff. (P < 0.05) in milk yield (kg/lactation) at 5 levels of Coefficient of Variation				
			10	15	20	25	30
1. Todd et al., 1972	+ .94 + 1.10 + 1.02 (overall **)	287 336 168	96	144	192	240	288
2. Bliss & Todd, 1973	+ 0.55 (+)	168	79	118	158	197	237
3. Bliss & Todd, 1974	+ 0.63 (+)	192	112	169	225	282	339
4. Bliss & Todd, 1976	+ 0.80 (*)	242	139	209	279	349	419
5. Pouplard, 1977	+ 1.31 (*)	400	99	149	198	248	298
6. Plumiers, 1977	+ 0.75 (**)	229	103	155	206	258	309
7. McBeath et al., 1979	+ 0.57 (+)	173	148	222	296	370	441
8. Fox, 1979	+ 0.11 (n.s.)	35	73	110	147	183	220
9. Thomas and Rowlinson, 1980	- 0.53 (n.s.)		382 (at a 17% C of V)				

[H] The statistical significance of response is stated as follows: ** P< 0.01; * P< 0.05: n.s. Not statistically significant (P< 0.05); + Significance not stated

Comments (Refer to the specific Trials in the above Table).

COMMENTS ON TRIALS IN TABLE 6

1. The statistical significance of the individual treatments is not stated, but all three are likely to be significant given coefficients of variation not in excess of 25%. Overall, treatment gave a significant (P < 0.01) milk response in the 8 day period in which response was assessed, but care must be exercised in extrapolating this response to a whole lactation.

2. Statistical significance is not stated. With a coefficient of variation below 21% significance would result, but should it be higher than 21%, which is possible with unpaired animals on a number of farms, then the recorded milk yield would not be significant. As with (1), there is the inherent danger of extrapolating results from in this case a 60 day post-treatment period, to a whole lactation.

3. Statistical significance is not stated. The recorded treatment difference of 192 kg in the lactation is very much on the borderline of statistical significance. With unpaired animals from 12 farms, if the coefficient of variation was above 17% (the level in the present trial (9), with paired animals on a single farm), then this apparently large difference would not be statistically significant.

4. The double dosing of treated animals in this trial gave a significant increase in lactation milk yield (+ 242 kg, P < 0.05). The coefficient of variation may be expected to be about 17% despite animals not being paired.

5. In this trial, although only one individual herd (out of 12) gave a significant response and the coefficient of variation would probably be high, the high overall response (+ 400 kg/lactation) resulted in a statistically significant difference (P < 0.05).

6. This trial gave a consistent response with all farms showing a positive effect of treatment. It is probable that by taking alternate cows the coefficient of variation was at a level of about 17% to achieve the recorded statistically significant difference (P < 0.01).

7. In this trial cows were apparently unpaired and there were large differences between control and treated animals in the previous lactation milk yield. In one herd this pre-treatment difference was 1 000 kg, and the average value was 200 kg in favour of the control animals. In such situations one would expect the coefficient of variation to be high and the 5% least significant difference to be far in excess of the reported treatment response of + 173 kg (a value which is lower than the pre-treatment advantage of the controls). Although statistical significance is not stated, it would appear extremely unlikely that a statistically significant treatment effect had resulted.

8. With the close pairing used in this trial one would expect fairly low coefficients of variation, but as only a low response to treatment was obtained the resultant difference would be expected to be non-significant as is stated.

CONCLUSIONS

In the design of this trial the number of animals which could be dealt with was limited, and an approach was made in which the inherent variability involved in the use of milk production data was reduced by restricting the experimental group to one herd, therefore under the same management, environmental and nutritional conditions, and by pairing the animals as far as possible. However, it is clear that the reduction in variability achieved in this way is insufficient to offset the effect of the low numbers of animals then available, and the alternative approach of accepting the high variability and reducing the standard deviation by using much larger numbers of animals is the more successful. This is the basis for the large scale trial currently being conducted by the Agricultural Development and Advisory Service in Britain. Until the results of this trial are available, judgement on the value of anthelmintic treatment of dairy cows in Britain should be suspended, since the evidence to date is conflicting, in contrast to that available elsewhere.

ACKNOWLEDGEMENTS

The authors' thanks are due to Mr. J.N. Merridew for collaboration in organising the trial, and to Mr. J. Wightman for technical assistance. Financial support from Merck, Sharpe and Dohme Ltd., is gratefully acknowledged.

REFERENCES

Bliss, D.H. and Todd, A.C., 1973. Milk production by Wisconsin dairy
    cattle after deworming with Baymix. Vet. Med. and Small Animal
    Clinician 68, 1034-1038.

Bliss, D.H. and Todd, A.C., 1974. Milk production by Wisconsin dairy cattle
    after deworming with thiabendazole. Vet. Med. and Small Animal
    Clinician 69, 638-640.

Bliss, D.H. and Todd, A.C., 1976. Milk production by Vermont dairy cattle
    after deworming. Vet. Med. and Small Animal Clinician 71, 1251-1254.

Cox, D.D. and Todd, A.C., 1962. Survey of gastro-intestinal parasitism in
    Wisconsin dairy cattle. J.A.V.M.A. 141, 706-709.

Fox, M.T., 1979. De-worming of cows - What are the benefits? Vet. Rec.
    105, 315-316.

Harris, B. Jr. and Wilcox, C.J., 1976. Effects of anthelmintics on milk
    production. J. Dairy Sci. 59, 20-21. (Supplement).

McBeath, D.G., Dean, S.P. and Preston, N.K., 1979. The effect of a prepart-
    urient fenbendazole treatment on lactation yield in dairy cows.
    Vet. Rec. 105, 507-509.

McGregor, J.K. and Kingscote, A.A., 1957. A survey of gastro-intestinal
    helminths of cattle in Ontario. Canad. J. Comp. Med. 21, 370-373.

Moore, E.D., Owen, J.R., Dowlen, M.M., Hows, L.D., Richardson, D.O., Smith,
    J.W. and Bennet, S.E., 1974. Comparison of anthelmintic treatments
    for replacement dairy heifers and dairy cows. J. Dairy Sci. 57, 145.
    (Abstracts).

Pluimers, E.J., 1979. Milk production increase following treatment of Dutch
    dairy cattle with thiabendazole. Vet. Quarterly 1, 82-89.

Pouplard, L., 1977. Treatment of gastro-intestinal helminthiasis of the
    dairy cow. 8th Int. Conf. W.A.A.V.P. 150 (Abstracts).

Pouplard, L., 1978. Anthelmintic treatment of dairy cows. Vet. Rec. 103,
    434.

Todd, A.C., Myers, G.H., Bliss, D.H. and Cox, D.D., 1972. Milk production
    in Wisconsin dairy cattle after anthelmintic treatment. Vet. Med.
    and Small Animal Clinician, 67, 1233-1236.

DISCUSSION

Dr. R.M. Jones   *(UK)*

I believe that one of the most important factors in these
comparisons is when the treatments are given. If one is
dealing with autumn calving herds and treatment is given as the
animals are yarded for the winter, then one might expect to get
a beneficial effect, since the wormburden is being removed. That
is assuming that significant infection may not occur in the
yards. This must be compared with animals infected when they
are grazing. Here the effect of treatment can only be transient
in terms of rendering the animal parasite-free because it would
re-infect itself. Have you looked at this?

Dr. R.J. Thomas   *(UK)*

We have analysed our data with respect to season and got
nothing. We analysed for parity, number of lactations, and
again we got nothing. However, basically, we had too few
animals.

THE PREVALENCE OF GASTRO-INTESTINAL NEMATODES
IN DAIRY COWS

[1]D. Barth, [2]D. Bernhard and [3]J. Lamina

[1]Sharp and Dohme GmbH, Katrinenhof,
Walchenseestrasse 8-12, D-8201 Lauterbach,
Federal Republic of Germany.

[2,3]Technische Universität München,
Institut für Tierwissenschaften,
Angewande Zoologie (Entomologie, Fischbiologie, Parasitologie),
D-8050 Friesing - Weihenstephan 12 ,
Federal Republic of Germany.

ABSTRACT

The parasitic nematodes present in the abomasum and small intestine of 198 milk cows sent for slaughter over a period of one year, were counted and differentiated.   In addition, the worm burden of the large intestine of 20 cows and the plasma-pepsinogen levels of 56 cows, were determined.   The results were as follows.

All milking cows were parasitised to a varying degree (up to 225 000 worms), whereas only 13% of them had positive faecal egg counts.   The geometric mean burden of grazing cows was 15 678, whereas that of housed animals was 2 836;   tapeworms (immature Moniezia spp) were present in 12% of the cows.   Of the 14 nematode species found, Ostertagia, Trichostrongylus and Cooperia, were the most common genera;   seasonal variations in adult worm populations confirmed present knowledge of the epidemiology of gastro-intestinal nematodes but an unexpected increase of Ostertagia larvae in the mucosa occurred in winter;   the reasons for slaughter did not significantly influence worm counts;   three and 8 year-old cows had higher worm counts than 5 year-old animals, and there was no statistically significant correlation between worm counts and plasma-pepsinogen levels.

P. Nansen, R.J. Jørgensen, E.J.L. Soulsby (eds), Epidemiology and Control of Nematodiasis in Cattle.
Copyright © 1981 ECSC, EEC, EAEC, Brussels – Luxembourg. All rights reserved.

INTRODUCTION

The worm burden of dairy cows recently has been considered insofar as influences to productivity are concerned. Several investigators have reported increased milk production after treat-ment of cows with anthelmintic drugs (Van Adrichem and Shaw, 1977; Bliss and Todd, 1973, 1974, 1975$_a$, 1975$_b$, 1976, 1977; Kordts, 1971; Pluimers, 1978; Pouplard, 1978; McBeath, 1979; McQueen, 1977; Todd et al., 1972). This effect, perhaps, is contrary to expectations as faecal egg counts of adult cattle normally are low (Barger, 1978; Bliss and Todd, 1975; Boch, 1956; Cox and Todd, 1962; Grisi and Todd, 1978; Jacobsen and David, 1969; Kordts, 1971; Spiess, 1977; Yazwinski and Gibbs, 1975).

There are few published data on the worm burdens of cows and their seasonal distribution. Worm burdens of the abomasum, small intestine and, in some cases, the large intestine of milk-ing cows, are reported here.

MATERIAL AND METHODS

Milking cows (198) killed at the slaughterhouse of Rosen-heim, a typical grassland area in Upper Bavaria, were examined over the period July 1977 to July 1978. Plasma-pepsinogen levels were determined at the same time on 56 of these animals. A 10% aliquot was taken from the contents of the abomasum and exam-ined for worms. The abomasal mucosa was removed and homogenised in a household mixer and a 33% aliquot of this was digested in a hydrochloric acid/pepsin mixture. Larvae in the digested mat-erial were counted under a modified trichinoscope and differ-entiated according to their size. In general, the larvae obtained consisted of larvae smaller than 1 mm (mostly 600 - 800 μm) and larvae between 1 and 2 mm (mostly 1.3 - 1.6 mm). The latter were identified as 4th stage larvae of *Ostertagia ostertagi*, based on the description of Douvres (1956, 1957). The smaller larvae were assumed to be *Trichostrongylus axei* (but this is subject to further study). It is very likely that the majority of larvae were arrested stages since larvae were of a similar size.

For studies of the small intestine, a worm count was done with the first 10 m. For the large intestine the total content was examined (Haffa, 1978). The faeces of each cow was examined for the worm eggs/g ($\bar{e}$pg) by a quantitative flotation method using a NaCl/ZnCl$_2$ solution with a specific gravity of 1.2. Each egg counted represented 10 eggs/g faeces. A blood sample was taken from freshly slaughtered animals and plasma-pepsinogen levels were determined according to the technique of Edwards et al. (1960).

In response to a questionnaire, owners of animals supplied information on their animals regarding, grazing history, the reason for slaughter, the date of last parturition and whether the animals had been treated recently with an anthelmintic.

RESULTS

None of the cows was worm-free, although only 13% of faeces samples were positive in the 10 to 40 epg. Worm counts varied between 40 and 225 500 with a geometric mean of 6 836 worms for all 198 cows (Table 1). Fourteen nematode species were found, but most of the worms belonged to the three genera *Ostertagia*, *Trichostrongylus* and *Cooperia* (Table 2).

The majority of nematodes were found in the abomasum, whereas the small intestine was parasitised in only 55% of the cows. The tapeworms present were immature *Moniezia* spp. of 10 - 40 cm length.

Evaluating the questionnaire showed that cows which had been on pasture had a significantly higher total worm burden ($P < 0.001$) than animals which had been housed during the previous year. The mean worm burden of grazing cows was 15.678 ($\bar{X}$ geom.) whereas of housed animals it was 2 836 ($\bar{X}$ geom.). However, with regard to parasites of the small intestine, there was no significant statistical influence of the grazing history on worm counts. Qualitatively there was no difference between the worm burdens of housed or grazing cows and 3 and 8 - 9 year old cows had significantly (P ≤0.05) more worms than 5 year old animals. Worms, such as *Nematodirus* and *Bunostomum*, which generally occur in young animals, were present in 3 - 9 and 3 - 7 year old cows which suggests there was no influence of age on parasitism by these species. *Cooperia* spp. were present in cows (3 - 15 years) and their number was not subject to seasonal variation.

There was no statistically significant relationship between the various reasons for the slaughter of the cows and the worm counts. However, there was a relationship between the date of parturition and the number of larvae isolated from the abomasal mucosa. Thus, the closer the date of slaughter to parturition, the lower were the counts of larvae from the abomasal mucosa.

A seasonal variation of worm counts was observed in animals which had been on pasture (Figure 1). An analysis of variance showed these variations to be statistically significant (P ≤0.001) - (P ≤0.05). For example, there was an increase of worm counts at the end of the pasture season, with a maximum in November. After housing, worm counts declined but they started to increase again in February, to reach a new peak in May (Figure 1). As *Ostertagia ostertagi* contributed most of all to these seasonal differences, the prevalence of 4th stage larvae and of adults of this species are illustrated in Figure 2.

In permanently housed cows by contrast, no increase in the number of inhibited larvae in the mucosa during winter was found (Figure 3).

Only very few nematodes were found in the large intestine; this organ was worm-free in 12 of the 20 cows examined. Seven cows had *Oesophagostomum radiatum* and one cow 10 *Chabertia ovina*.

The number of samples examined for plasma-pepsinogen levels was small and no statistically significant relationship between

121

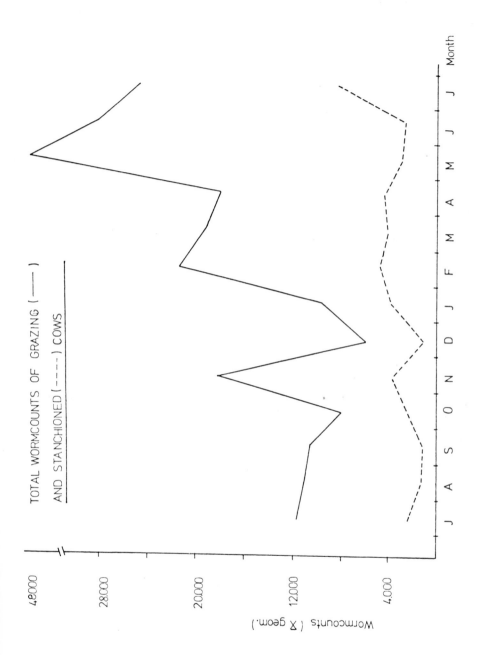

Fig. 1.

122

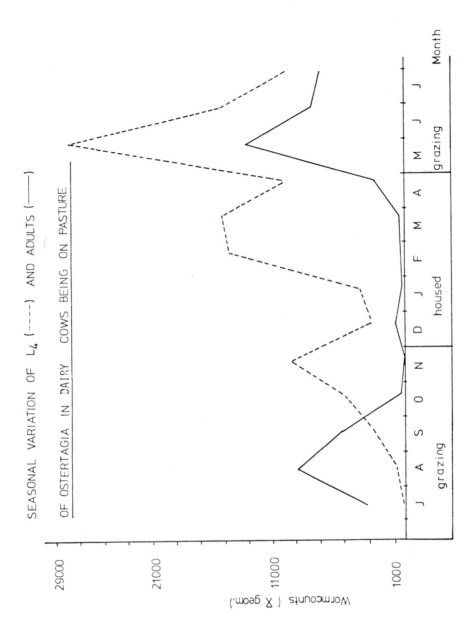

Fig. 2.

123

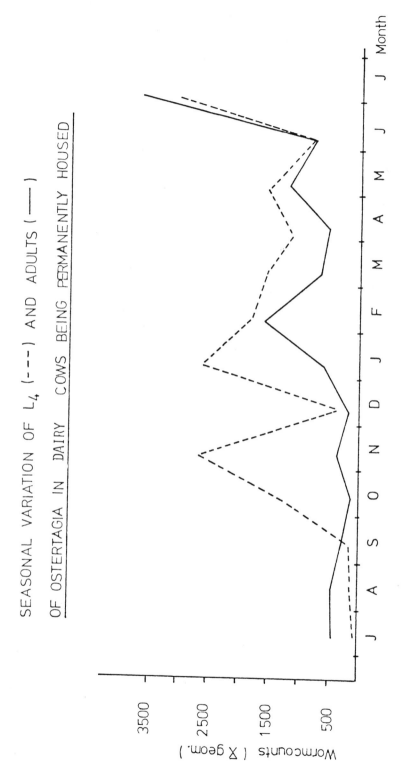

SEASONAL VARIATION OF L₄ (---) AND ADULTS (——) OF OSTERTAGIA IN DAIRY COWS BEING PERMANENTLY HOUSED

Fig. 3.

plasma-pepsinogen level and the number of parasites was apparent (Table 3). Six of the cows investigated had been treated with an anthelmintic during the previous 6 months but their worm burden was not significantly different from the others.

DISCUSSION

The data obtained from faecal examination confirmed low egg counts normally found in cows. However, qualitatively the worm burden in adult cows is comparable to that in younger cattle in Germany (Burger et al., 1966), Austria (Hinaidy et al., 1979) and Switzerland (Eckert et al., 1975). The occurrence of tapeworms was higher than anticipated as investigations from younger cattle showed a low incidence of this parasite (Raffalt, 1955; Neumann and Kirsch, 1968; Hinaidy, 1979)

The observation that 3 and 8 year old cows have a higher worm burden than 5 year old animals, has a parallel in deer. In this species, middle-aged animals have a lower worm burden than young or old deer (Dunn, 1965; Kavasch, 1979; Nilsson, 1971)

In animals which were on pasture during the grazing period the seasonal variations in numbers of adult worms confirms the present knowledge of the epidemiology of gastro-intestinal parasites. However, an unexpected phenomenon was observed in winter in that the number of *Ostertagia* larvae in the mucosa apparently increased while the animals were housed. The origin of these larvae is unknown, but a possible source might be the environment of the cow barn (Wetzel, 1950; Bliss and Todd, 1975). In the case of infection of permanently housed animals, infection probably came mainly from the fresh grass which was brought in daily for the cows during the grazing season.

TABLE 1

WORM BURDEN IN ABOMASUM AND SMALL INTESTINE OF 198 COWS

Parasite	Prevalence (%)	Worm counts	
		Geom. mean ($\bar{x}$)	Range Min/max
Ostertagia spp	100	4 228	10/186 200
Trichostrongylus spp	96	683	7/ 64 740
Cooperia spp	46	116	10/ 25 400
Nematodirus spp	6	42	1/ 2 369
Bunostomum spp	5	7	1/ 720
Haemonchus contortus	0.5	302	302
Moniezia spp	11.6	1	1/ 4

TABLE 2

WORM BURDEN IN ABOMASUM AND SMALL INTESTINE OF 198 DAIRY COWS

Parasite	Occurrence (%)	Worm counts of infested cows	
		Geom. mean ($\bar{x}$)	Range Min/max
Ostertagia ssp (L_4)	96.0	2 322	3/170 500
Trichostrongylus spp (L_4)	81.8	473	3/ 64 740
Ostertagia ostertagi	77.8	1 559	10/ 81 100
Trichostrongylus axei	43.9	1 249	30/ 60 010
Cooperia oncophora	26.8	224	10/ 6 267
Cooperia punctata	23.7	126	10/ 4 412
Cooperia zurnabada	9.1	151	22/ 7 366
Skrjabinagia lyrata	6.6	608	178/ 3 030
Cooperia pectinata	2.5	98	38/ 252
Ostertagia leptospicularis	2.0	608	264/ 2 574
Bunostomum phlebotomum	2.0	14	1/ 47
Nematodirus helvetianus	2.0	28	1/ 2 369
Skrjabinagia kolchida	1.0	528	426/ 657
Spiculopteragia böhmi	0.5	27	27
Trichostrongylus capricola	0.5	23	23
Haemonchus contortus	0.5	302	302

Continued

126

TABLE 2 (Cont)

| Parasite | Occurrence (%) | Worm counts of infested cows | |
		Geom. mean ($\bar{X}$)	Range Min/max
Ostertagia spp ad.*	15.2	221	57/ 1 183
Cooperia spp ad*	12.1	16	10/ 250
Bunostomum spp ad*	2.5	4	1/ 720
Nematodirus spp ad*	3.5	44	1/ 1 258
Moniezia spp imm*	11.6	1	1/ 4

* Species diagnosis was not possible

TABLE 3

WORM COUNTS AND PLASMA-PEPSINOGEN-VALUES OF 56 COWS

Worm counts	No. of animals	Mean plasma-pepsinogen mU of tyrosine ($\bar{X} \pm S$)
0 - 10 000	30	950 ± 398
10 000 - 50 000	16	1 185 ± 280
50 000 - 100 000	6	956 ± 178
>100 000	4	1 880 ± 495

REFERENCES

Van Adrichem, P.W.M. and Shaw, J.C. 1977. Effects of gastro-intestinal
  nematodiasis on the productivity of monozygous twin cattle growth
  performance. I. Milk production, II. J. Anim. Sci., 46, (3), 423

Barger, I.A. 1978. Drenches don't boost milk yields. Rural Res., 99, 25. June.

McBeath, D.G., Dean, S.P. and Preston, N.K. 1979. The effect of preparturient
  Fenbendazole treatment on lactation yield in dairy cows. Vet. Rec.
  105, 507-509

Bliss, D.H. and Todd, A.C. 1973. Milk production by Wisconsin dairy cattle
  after deworming with Baymix. Vet. Med. Small Anim. Clin., 63, 1034-
  1037

Bliss, D.H. and Todd, A.C. 1974. Milk production by Wisconsin dairy cattle
  after deworming with TBZ. Vet. Med. Small Anim. Clin., 69, 638-640

Bliss, D.H. and Todd, A.C. 1975$_a$. The nature of parasitism in dairy cattle.
  World Assoc. for the Advancement of Vet. Parisitology in Thessaloniki,
  Greece, July 14-16, Abstract pp 28-29

Bliss, D.H. and Todd, A.C. 1975$_b$. Milk production losses associated with
  internal parasitisms in dairy cows. PhD thesis, University of Wisconsin,
  Madison

Bliss, D.H. and Todd, A.C. 1976. Milk production by Vermont dairy cattle
  after deworming. Vet. Med. Small Anim. Clin., 71, 1251-1254

Bliss, D.H. and Todd, A.C. 1977. Milk losses in dairy cows after exposure
  to infective trichostrongylid larvae. Vet. Med. Small Anim. Clin.,
  72, 1612-1617

Boch, J. 1956. Zur Frage der Resistenz und Immunität der Wiederkäuer gegen-
  über parasitischen Würmern. Zbl. Vet. Med. 3, 402-418

Bürger, H.J., Eckert, J., Wetzel, H. and Michael, S.A. 1966. Zur Epizootologie des Trichostrongyliden-Befalls des Rindes in Nordwestdeutschland.
  Dtsch. Tierärztl. Wschr. 20, 503-513

Cox, D.D. and Todd, A.C. 1962. Survey of gastro-intestinal parasitism in
  Wisconsin diary cattle. J. A,. Vet. med. Assoc., 141, 706-709

Douvres, F.W. 1956. Morphogenesis of the parasitic stages of *Ostertagia*
  Ostertagi, a nematode parasite in cattle. J. Parisit. 42, 626-635

Douvres, F.W. 1957. Keys to the identification and differentiation of the
  immature parasitic stages of gastro-intestinal nematodes of cattle.
  Am. J. Vet. Res. 18, 81

Dunn, A.M. 1965. The gastro-intestinal helmiths of wild ruminants in Britain. Parasitology, 55, 739-745

Eckert, J. and Eisenegger, H. 1975. Zur Epizootologie und Prophylaxe der Dictyocaulose und der Trichostrongylidosen des Rindes. Schw. Arch. Tierheilkunde, 117, 5, 255

Edwards, K., Jepson, R.P. and Wood, K.F. 1960. Value of plasma-pepsinogen estimation. British Med. Journal, 1, 30-32

Grisi, L. and Todd, A.C. 1978. Prevalence of gastro-intestinal parasitism among milking cows in Wisconsin. Am. J. Vet. Res. 39, 51-54

Haffa, M. 1978. Bedeutung und Vorkommen von Magen-Darm-Helminthen. Diplomarbeit, Weihenstephan, Angewandte Zoologie

Hinaidy, H.K., Prosl, H. and Supperer, R. 1979. Ein weiterer Beitrag zur Gasto-intestinal-Helminthenfauna des Rindes in Österreich. Vienna, Tierärztl. Mschr., 66, 77-83

Kavasch, W.D. 1970. Endoparasitenbefall des Rehwildes im Nördlinger Ries und Behandlungsversuche mit subtherapeutischen Gaben von Phenothiazin, Neguvon und Thiabendazol. Vet. Med. Diss. Munich.

Kordts, E. 1971. Beobactungen über die Leistung von Kühen bei der Parasitenbekämpfung mit "Bilevon R" und "Citarin". Die Milchpraxis, 3.

Neumann, H.J., Kirsch, H. and Kablke, A. 1968. Kritische Beurteilung koprologischer Untersuchungen. Tierärztl. Umschau, 9, 924

Nilsson, O. 1971. The inter-relationship of endo-parasites in wild cervids (*Capreolus capreolus* L.and *Alces alces* L.) and domestic ruminants in Sweden. Acta Vet. Scand., 12, 36-38

Pluimers, J. 1978. Milchleistungssteigerung bei Milchkühen nach Behandlung mit Tiabendazol. Prakt. Tierarzt., 10, (59)

Pouplard, L. 1978. Anthelmintic treatment of dairy cows. Vet. Rec., 103, 434

McQueen, I.P.M., Cottier, K., Hewitt, S.R. and Wright, D.F. 1977. Effects of anthelmintics on dairy cow yields. N.Z. J. Experim. Agric., 5, 115-119

Raffalt, J. 1955. Die parasitären Krankheiten unserer Haustiere im Landkreis Neu-Ulm/Donau. Vet. Diss. Munich

Spiess, H. 1977. Personal communication

Todd, A.C., Meyers, G.H., Bliss, D.H. and Cox, D.D. 1972. Milk production in Wisconsin dairy cattle after treatment. Vet. Med. Small Anim. Clin. 67, 1233-1236

Wetzel, H. 1967. Epizootologische Untersuchungen über den Magen-Darm-
    Strongylidenbefall bei Kälbern. Vet. Med. Diss., Hannover
Yazwinski, I.A. and Gibbs, H.C. 1975. Survey of helminth infections in Maine
    dairy cattle. Am. J. Vet. Res., 36, 1677-1682

DISCUSSION

F.H.M. Borgsteede *(Netherlands)*

I was interested in your mention of large numbers of larvae *Trichostrongylus axei* in the abomasum. A few years ago we had a workshop in Lelystad about the arrest of development for *Trichostrongylus axei*. Many workers did not find any arrest of development at all with regard to *Trichostrongylus axei*. We have never seen any *Trichostrongylus axei* arrested. We have seen a lot of small larvae in the abomasum in the range you describe - less than 1 mm (0.6, 0.7 or 0.8) - and we have examined the structure of these larvae. We think that they are the larvae of free-living nematodes taken in with the food. The structure is not that of arrested larvae of our parasitic nematodes.

D. Barth *(FRG)*

That is interesting. But on the other hand the morphology is very uniform in these tiny larvae. We have been thinking quite a lot as to what these larvae are. As we found the other *Trichostrongylus*, we felt it was more likely that these are *Trichostrongylus* larvae, uniform in structure and size, and they are too small for *Ostertagia* larvae.

J. Jansen *(Netherlands)*

I would like to make a comment on this problem. I think that Dr. Borgsteede is right. *Trichostrongylus* is mainly inhibited in the third stage, so you may overlook the inhibited larvae and see something different as L4.

WORMBURDENS IN ADULT DAIRY CATTLE

F.H.M. Borgsteede and W.P.J. van der Burg

Central Veterinary Institute, Department of Parasitology,
Edelhertweg 13, 8219 PH Lelystad, The Netherlands.

ABSTRACT

Two studies on the wormburden of dairy cattle were carried out. In the first the egg output of cows was estimated within 48 hours after parturition. On basis of larval cultures the mean LPG (larvae per gram faeces) was 8. Larval differentiation showed that Ostertagia spp.*-larvae were the most prevalent (87.9%),* Trichostrongylus spp.*-larvae 47.7%,* Bunostomum spp.*-larvae 13.1%,* Oesophagostomum spp.*-larvae 9.4%,* Cooperia oncophora*-larvae 8.7%,* C. punctata*-larvae 30.5% and* Haemonchus contortus *7.7%.*

In the second study the abomasal wormburden of dairy cows slaughtered at an abattoir at Leeuwarden was examined. Over the period February 12, 1979 until October 1, 1979, 130 abomasa were collected. The presence of the different species was: O. ostertagi *99.2%,* O. leptospicularis *3.1%,* O. circumcincta *0.8%,* Skrjabinagia lyrata *27.7%,* S. kolchida *0.8%,* T. axei *74.6%,* C. oncophora *1.5%,* N. helvetianus *0.8% and* Capillaria bovis *2.3%. The log n transformed mean total number of adult worms was 3 197 and of the early fourth larval stages, 464. There were no obvious differences between age groups with regard to wormburden, state of arrest or stage of development of the worms. The highest percentage of early fourth larval stages were found in February (72%), decreasing in March (62%) April (38%) and May (33%). During summer the percentage was about 20% and in October it rose to 58%.*

INTRODUCTION

The publication by Todd *et al.* (1972), which reported higher milk yields by Wisconsin dairy cattle, after anthelmintic treatment has lead to a number of comparable studies. Some of these showed results similar to those of Todd *et al.* (1972), but others failed to do so. Possible mechanisms of the increase in bulk quantity and quality following anthelmintic treatment has been discussed (Anon, 1978), but there remain a number of inconsistencies. One of these is the wormburden of cows. Only a limited number of studies has been done on this (Bliss and Todd, 1975; Bernard *et al.*, 1978; Guttierres *et al.*, 1979) and it is doubtful whether these results can be applied generally to other countries, regions or management systems.

The present studies were carried out to determine, the faecal egg output and the wormburden of cows in the Netherlands.

MATERIAL AND METHODS

First study: Egg output of cows

In 1978/1979 four farms in the northern part of the country (Province Groningen) and three farms in the south (Province of Noord-Brabant) were selected for study. Rectal faecal samples of 298 cows were taken within 48 hours after parturition. Because egg output was expected to be low a fixed amount of 50 g faeces per cow was cultured, larvae were collected, counted and the genus and species determined, as described by Borgsteede and Hendriks (1973, 1974).

Second study: Wormburdens of cows

Starting on 12 February 1979 until 1 October 1979 and at weekly intervals, four abomasa were collected at random from lactating cows at an abattoir in Leeuwarden (Province Friesland). The abomasa were washed out and the contents diluted and homogenised with a mixing device. A one hundredth aliquot of the contents were sampled and examined. The abomasal mucosa was

scraped off and digested for 4 - 5 hours with a pepsin-HCl
solution at 37° - 40°C. One tenth of the digest was examined.
Worms were collected, counted and determined on the species
level.

RESULTS

Egg output of cows

The distribution of the number of larvae per g of
faeces is presented in Table 1. The untransformed mean on the
Groningen farms was 7.4, in Noord-Brabant 8.7; the total mean
was 7.9.

TABLE 1

DISTRIBUTION OF LPG*-VALUES IN COWS

LPG class	4 Farms Groningen	3 Farms Noord-Brabant	Total
neg	14 (7.4%)	3 (2.8%)	17 (5.7%)
< 1	42 (22.1%)	14 (13.0%)	56 (18.8%)
1	49 (25.8%)	21 (19.4%)	70 (23.5%)
2-5	44 (23.1%)	35 (32.4%)	79 (26.5%)
6-10	18 (9.5%)	15 (13.9%)	33 (11.1%)
11-20	12 (6.3%)	10 (9.3%)	22 (7.4%)
> 20	11 (5.8%)	10 (9.2%)	21 (7.0%)
	190	108	298

*
 LPG - Larvae per g of faeces

The results of the larval differentiation are shown in
Table 2, which indicates the percentage of cattle infected
with different species.

Wormburdens of cows

Table 3 lists the worm species found in 130 abomasa over
the period of study. Table 4 presents the mean wormburden of
the abomasa and the distribution with regard to the age of
animals. Table 5 presents the distribution of the arcsine

TABLE 2

PRESENCE OF COWS FROM WHICH LARVAE OF VARIOUS SPECIES WERE ISOLATED

	Larval type						
	Ostertagia spp.	*Trichostrongylus* spp.	*Bunostomum* spp.	*Oesophagostomum* spp.	*Cooperia oncophora*	*Cooperia punctata*	*Haemonchus contortus*
Groningen 4 farms 190 cows	161 (84.7%)	90 (74.4%)	21 (11.1%)	10 (5.3%)	9 (4.7%)	41 (21.6%)	0 —
Noord Brabant 3 farms 108 cows	101 (93.5%)	52 (48.1%)	18 (16.7%)	18 (16.7%)	17 (15.7%)	50 (46.3%)	23 (21.3%)
Total 7 farms 298 cows	262 (87.9%)	142 (47.7%)	39 (13.1%)	28 (9.4%)	26 (8.7%)	91 (30.5%)	23 (7.7%)

transformed percentages of early fourth stage larvae over the period of study.

TABLE 3

PRESENCE OF WORM SPECIES IN 130 ABOMASA (12.2.79 - 1.10.79)

Species	n	
Ostertagia ostertagi	129	(99.2%)
O. leptospicularis	4	(3.1%)
O. circumcincta	1	(0.8%)
Skrjabinagia lyrata	36	(27.7%)
S. kolchida	1	(0.8%)
Trichostrongylus axei	97	(74.6%)
Cooperia oncophora	2	(1.5%)
Nematodirus helvetianus	1	(0.8%)
Capillaria bovis	3	(2.3%)

Figures in parentheses indicate percentage of abomasa containing the species indicated.

TABLE 4

MEAN WORMBURDEN in 130 ABOMASA (12.2.79 - 1.10.79)

Age class		n	Mean total wormburden	Ibidem ln transf.	Mean number EL-4	Ibidem ln transf.
	<3	25	8 059	3 569	4 820	871
≥3	<4	28	7 654	2 893	3 275	503
≥4	<5	20	4 252	1 901	1 400	334
≥5	<6	14	7 954	3 533	1 677	276
≥6	<7	12	5 235	3 984	1 923	728
≥7	<8	9	9 501	4 817	3 463	224
≥8		22	6 176	3 533	1 400	395
Total		130	6 895	3 197	2 682	464

TABLE 5

DISTRIBUTION OF THE ARCSINE TRANSFORMED PERCENTAGES OF EARLY FOURTH STAGE
LARVAE OVER THE YEAR

Month	n	Mean percentage + SE	Range (min-max)
February	12	72 ± 2.9	37 - 85
March	16	62 ± 4.6	34 - 87
April	15	38 ± 4.8	0 - 75
May	19	33 ± 3.8	0 - 62
June	13	21 ± 4.8	0 - 48
July	20	23 ± 5.1	0 - 100
August	16	19 ± 3.0	0 - 40
September	16	18 ± 2.4	6 - 39
October	3	58 ± 7.1	22 - 65
	130		

DISCUSSION

On the basis of LPG-values in this study, egg counts were
generally very low and with a few exceptions were not detectable
by the methods in use for routine diagnosis in the regional
laboratories of the Animal Health Services in the Netherlands.
However, only 5.7% of the 298 cows in this study were negative.
In the positive cows *Ostertagia* spp.-larvae were most frequently
encountered with *Trichostrongylus* spp. being the second most
frequent. The abomasal parasite, *Haemonchus contortus* was only
seen on farms in the province Noord-Brabant in the south of
the Netherlands. The fact that on the four farms in Groningen
there was no contact between cows and sheep, which was in
contrast to the situation in Noord-Brabant, is probably of more
importance in determining the presence of *H. contortus* in cattle
than the geographical difference. Of the intestinal nematodes
Cooperia puntata-larvae were more prevalent in both provinces than
C. oncophora-larvae, but when *C. oncophora*-larvae were present the
LPG was also usually above average. The same was the case for
H. contortus. Borgsteede (1978) has reported that females of both

species can produce more eggs per unit of time than, for example, *Ostertagia* spp. or *Trichostrongylus* spp. However, the relationship between egg output and worm numbers in older animals probably is more complex than in younger stock.

Based on the results of the first study it was decided to investigate abomasa in the second study only. Although some authors have indicated that generally no more than 500 adult worms of *Ostertagia* spp. are to be found in the abomasum of adult cattle (Anon, 1978), in the present study, with random chosen material, the transformed mean wormburden was 3 197. There was no relationship between age and wormburden and the highest mean burden was found in cows aged between 7 and 8 years. In such older animals, wormburdens will depend on factors such as the management system (zero grazing system versus grazing of cows in the second half of the grazing season on calf paddocks) and immune capacity. Consequently interpretation of the data must be done with care.

The findings in the study with abomasa confirmed those of the faecal examinations, in that *Ostertagia ostertagi* was the most common (99.2%) and *T. axei* was the next, being found in 74.6% of the abomasa. Other species were of minor importance. The absence of *H. contortus* was somewhat remarkable since, of the farms from which the cows came, some must have had sheep on the same pastures. In the Wisconsin studies *H. placei* (identical with *H. contortus* according to Gibbons, 1979), was one of the more important species (Cox and Todd, 1962; Guttierres *et al.*, 1979). Hence the following speculations can be made. Number of *H. contortus* were so low that chances of finding a worm in a 1/100 aliquot were negligible, and secondly, cows having been infected in calfhood, had developed immunity such that *H. contortus* was not able to establish in older cows.

A seasonal pattern of EL-4 stages in the abomasa is evident in Table 5, although the period October - January is lacking. Thus the pattern in older cows is similar to that seen in young stock: higher percentages of EL-4 occurring in autumn and winter, decreasing in spring and being low in summer. The EL-4 in the present study belonged mainly to *Ostertagia* spp. Occasionally very small larvae (< 700 μm) without any structure and with a shape different from that of exsheated infective larvae were found and these were thought to be larvae of free-living nematodes.

ACKNOWLEDGEMENTS

The author wishes to acknowledge the technical assistance of R. Mes, H. de Vries and H. Bouwhuis. Also the co-operation of the veterinary practitioners in Winsum and Valkenswaard is acknowledged, together with the help of the staff of the Animal Health Service and of the abattoir in Leeuwarden.

REFERENCES

Anonymous, 1978. Anthelmintic treatment of dairy cows for *Ostertagia* infection. Veterinary Record <u>103</u>, 103.

Bernard, D., Barth, D. and Lamina, J., 1978. Magendarmnematoden bei Milchkühen. Berliner und Münchener Tierärztlichen Wochenschrift <u>91</u>, 45-46.

Bliss, D.H. and Todd, A.C., 1975. The nature of parasitism in dairy cattle. Paper presented at the Conference of the World Association for the Advancement of Veterinary Parasitology, July 14-16, 1975, Thessalonika, Greece (Abstract 28-29).

Borgsteede, F.H.M., 1978. Observations on the post parturient rise of nematode egg-output in cattle. Veterinary Parasitology <u>4</u>, 385-391.

Borgsteede, F.H.M. and Hendriks, J., 1973. Een kwantitatieve methode voor het kweken en verzamelen van infectieuze larven van maagdarm-wormen. Tijdschrift voor Diergeneeskunde, <u>98</u>, 280-286.

Borgsteede, F.H.M. and Hendriks, J., 1974. Identification of infective larvae of gastrointestinal nematodes in cattle. Tijdschrift voor Diergeneeskunde, <u>99</u>, 103-113.

Cox, D.D. and Todd, A.C., 1962. Survey of gastrointestinal parasitism in Wisconsin dairy cattle. Journal of the American Veterinary Medical Association, <u>141</u>, 706-709.

Gibbons, L.M., 1979. Revision of the genus *Haemonchus* Cobb, 1898 *(Nematoda: Trichostrongylidae)*. Systematic Parasitology, <u>1</u>, 3-24.

Guttierres, V., Todd, A.C. and Crowley, Jr., J.W., 1979. Natural populations of helminths in Wisconsin dairy cows. Veterinary Medicine/Small Animal Clinician, <u>74</u>, 369-374.

Todd, A.C., Meyers, G.H., Bliss, D.H. and Cox, D.D., 1972. Milk production in Wisconsin dairy cattle after anthelmintic treatment. Veterinary Medicine/Small Animal Clinician, <u>67</u>, 1233-1236.

140

DISCUSSION

J. Eckert *(Switzerland)*

Did you see any correlation between the wormburden and the alterations of the abomasum mucosa?

F.H.M. Borgsteede *(The Netherlands)*

No, in older animals all abomasa look the same. It is possible to see areas which *Ostertagia* have penetrated, occasionally an oedematous type mucosa occurs, but usually the abomasa are hardly damaged.

D. Barth *(FRG)*

We have found that based on lesions, nodules and larval counts, there was a very clear correlation between parasite numbers and the number of nodules seen at slaughter. It is unwise to wait too long before examination, since after *rigor mortis* the changes in the mucosa become less clear. But when you look at it just after slaughter, the changes correlate very well with the number of larvae present.

F.H.M. Borgsteede

That is a possibility to be kept in mind. The abattoir of Leeuwarden is about 90 km from Lelystad, where we work, so to get to the abattoir it takes about an hour and collecting the abomasa takes another half an hour; on the way back you have your lunch break before starting work.

J. Armour *(UK)*

It depends on whether the abomasum is oedematous or not. If it is oedematous you have to wait a little while until the oedema subsides before you see the nodules become visible.

J. Euzeby *(France)*

Why did you neglect the counting of *Bunostomum*? Do you think they are not important?

F.H.M. Borgsteede

    No. We only looked at the abomasa and not at the small intestine.

J. Euzeby

    Why?

F.H.M. Borgsteede

    On the basis of the faecal examinations, in the first study, we saw only, say 16% of the cases of the cows were positive for *Bunostomum*. Because of the tremendous mass of work involved in this kind of study, to examine the small intestine of an adult cow would be a major undertaking, we decided to examine only the abomasum.

ORGANISATION OF A LARGE COLLABORATIVE TRIAL ON THE EFFECT
OF ANTHELMINTIC TREATMENT ON THE MILK YIELD OF DAIRY COWS

J.F. Michel[1] and J.R. Mulholland[2]
[1]ADAS, Gentral Veterinary Laboratory, Weybridge, Surrey, UK.
[2]ADAS, MAFF, Great Westminster House, Horseferry Road,
London, SW1P 2AE, UK.

Increasingly insistent claims have been made in recent
years that the milk yield of dairy cows is improved if nematodes
of the alimentary tract are removed by anthelmintic treatment.
Most of the work on which these claims were based was undertaken
in the USA. Smaller experiments have been conducted in Holland,
Belgium, Australia and New Zealand. Most of these smaller
trials have produced results either contradictory or not entirely
convincing. Whether in the UK anthelmintic treatment of dairy
cows is likely to increase their yield is an entirely open
question and three small trials reported recently did little to
resolve the matter.

Nonetheless, first one and later a second commercial firm
in Britain advocated the routine anthelmintic treatment of
dairy cows and the practice was adopted by farmers at a rate
that suggested that before long half the national herd might
be dosed.

Meanwhile, veterinary suregons and advisers of all kinds
were faced with an active demand for an authoritative and
impartial opinion on the subject and were embarrassed by their
inability to provide one. It appeared highly desirable to
obtain conclusive evidence as to whether or not gastro-intestinal
nematode infections were reducing milk yields of dairy cows in
Britain and whether routine anthelmintic treatment prevented
this loss.

The economic benefits to be derived from an adequate
experiment promised to be considerable whatever the result.
If it were shown that dosing was without effect on yield, the

cost of dosing up to half the national herd, some £2.4M
annually, might be saved. Alternatively, if claims made elsewhere were confirmed, an annual benefit of up to £100M annually
might be involved. The guaranteed capitalised benefit of a
conclusive result should therefore lie between £15M and £600M.

It is not, of course, feasible to determine whether
treatment produces any measurable increase because an experiment to achieve this would require an almost infinite number of
cows. But what the practical man wants to know is whether
dosing his cows will increase his profit. Twenty-eight kg of
milk is worth twice the cost of a dose of anthelmintic for a
cow and may be regarded as the smallest increase per head that
would justify dosing the dairy herd. The detection of this
difference between mean lactation yields demands 5 700 cows per
group, provided that the coefficient of variation can be kept
down to 10%. Not all animals entering a trial will complete
the lactation. If wastage can be kept at 25%, the smallest
adequate experiment would require 15 200 cows. This implies
firstly that commercial herds must be used and secondly that
such an experiment is beyond the resources of any single group
of workers.

Collaboration between a number of bodies offered the only
possible means of conducting an adequate trial and a consortium
was therefore formed. This consisted of Agriculture Service,
Veterinary Investigation Service and the Central Veterinary
Laboratory of the Agricultural Development and Advisory Service,
the Veterinary Schools of the Universities of Glasgow, Liverpool
and Cambridge, the School of Agriculture of the University of
Newcastle-on-Tyne, the Department of Applied Zoology of University
College of North Wales, a number of Agricultural Colleges and
a large private veterinary practice. Rothamsted Experimental
Station and the Milk Marketing Boards are also involved.

A very large experiment cannot readily be repeated. It
was decided, therefore, to enlarge slightly the trial above the
minimum size to incorporate features that might provide evidence

of whether an effect on yield, if one could be demonstrated, was due to the removal of worms or to some incidental property of the anthelmintic used. One possible approach was to use several preferably unrelated drugs on the basis that the only property they were likely to have in common would be their effect on worms, and that if all increased milk yield equally this could therefore be attributed to their anthelmintic properties. A second approach was to look for correlations between an effect of treatment on yield and on one or more measures of worm infection in the cow or in her environment.

Inevitably the design of the trial involved compromises between what was desirable and what was feasible. Three anthelmintics, thiabendazole, fenbendazole and levamisole are used, one group being treated with each. There are two control groups, one untreated, the other receiving a placebo. The ratio of three to two between dosed and control animals is the result of a compromise. If the only comparison to be made were between dosed and undosed animals equal numbers would be used. If a comparison between the effects of three anthelmintics were the most important, one quarter of the animals would serve as untreated controls. Thus, there are five groups in the trial, each of 4 000 animals. Allowing for wastage of up to 27% this should ensure that a total of 8 800 dosed cattle and 5 800 undosed control cattle should complete the lactation.

Three different measurements of worm infection were considered. Sufficient resources were not available to undertake pasture larval counts or to estimate levels of pepsinogen in the blood. Faecal egg counts have serious shortcomings but there is evidence that during the periparturient period they give an indication of worm activity. Accordingly it was decided to examine two faeces samples from each cow, one taken on the day she calves and the second two days later. A technique capable of detecting one egg per gram is used.

It was considered preferable that the herdsmen should not know that a placebo was included in the trial nor should they be able to identify which anthelmintic was which. Special formulations of the drugs were therefore used all of which, together with the placebo, were made to look alike.

The cattle are dosed on the day they calve, partly because this is claimed to result in the greatest increase in yield and partly for a simple practical reason. Two of the anthelmintics used are subject to a withdrawal period extending in the case of one of them to 72 hours. The colostrum cannot be sold for human consumption but if treatment were given in mid-lactation compensation would have to be paid for milk rendered unsaleable. This would cost £100 000.

All the cattle used are of the Friesian breed. Further to reduce variation, certain animals are excluded from the trial, namely, heifers calving when less than 21 months old, cows calving for the 7th or subsequent time, cows that have been dry 100 days or more, cattle not producing a live calf or bearing twins.

Since it is not known in advance which cattle will be eligible to enter the trial, they cannot be assigned to their treatment groups until they calve. A procedure was therefore devised to enable the herdsman to allocate animals to their groups at random after blocking by lactation number and calving date. This procedure depends on the use of specialised stationery and corresponding ready-randomised packs of anthelmintics and effectively transfers the possibility of error from the farm to the Central Veterinary Laboratory where the packs were made up. The herdsman is provided with three colour-coded books of forms relating, respectively, to heifers, second and third calvers and to fourth, fifth and sixth calvers. Each form has numbered spaces for ten animals. Boxes of anthelmintics, similarly colour-coded contain correspondingly numbered bottles of anthelmintic. Undosed animals are indicated

in the box by a numbered spacer. Each box contains materials
for five animals, all five treatments being represented but in
random order.

As each cow calves, the herdsman, having satisfied himself that she is not to be excluded, enters her identity number
and the date in the next numbered line on the appropriate form.
He drenches her from the bottle bearing the same number on a
label of the same colour, he takes a faeces sample and puts
it in a correspondingly labelled container packed adjacent to
the drench bottle and two days later takes a second faeces
sample.

Officially recorded herds of more than 100 head were
selected. A high standard of management and keenness to take
part in the trial were the attributes particularly sought
especially if these were likely to be maintained. Even though
owners and herdsmen were well motivated and the procedure to
be followed very simple, it is considered necessary to visit
every farm weekly while animals are calving. The purpose of
these visits is to give support and encouragement, to ensure
that cows are correctly dosed, samples taken and records kept,
also to collect faeces samples, completed forms and empty
containers.

The trial was planned at a time when resources were scarce
and getting scarcer and a number of steps were taken to cut
costs, especially the cost of regular visiting. Thus, larger
herds and fewer of them were chosen, a total of 120 with an
average of 168 cows in each. Preference was given to farms
conveniently situated and visitors were recruited who lived
near or regularly passed these farms. In fact most visits are
made on the way to work and involve no extra travel and the
expenditure of only a few minutes per week. This was made
possible by using many visitors so that each visits only one
or two farms. Indeed, nearly 100 people are engaged in this
activity.

In the same way, diagnostic laboratories, equipped to
handle a fluctuating throughput of work are able to handle a
small additional burden provided this can be dealt with at off-
peak periods. The faecal egg counts are therefore being done
in no fewer than 25 laboratories.

While the use of very many collaborators contributes
greatly to economy, the regulation and standardisation of their
activities represents an exercise in organisation, communication and logistics. The entire operation is under the control
of a project manager who acts through nine regional co-ordinators
These co-ordinations superintend the selection of herds, recruit
farm visitors and arrange where the faeces samples from each
herd are to be examined and how they are to be transported.
They ensure that data comes forward punctually from farms and
laboratories and they scrutinise these data before sending
them on for processing. The average co-ordinator deals with
14 herds, 11 visitors, 3 laboratories and 1 collaborating
organisation outside the public service (for these voluntarily
submit to the same organisation). The Central Veterinary
Laboratory deals with all technical questions, with the
procurement processing and distribution of all materials and
with the standardisation of procedures and laboratory methods.
The Milk Marketing Board provides data of milk yield and
composition in the form of summaries on magnetic tape. Analysis
of the data is undertaken, with the collaboration of the
Statistics Department at Rothamsted, by the Central Veterinary
Laboratory using the Ministry's computer at Guildford.

Lactations starting between 1st January and 31st December
1980 are considered; therefore results of the trial will not be
available until early in 1982.

Many problems in veterinary helminthology require, for
their solution, resources greater than are available to any one
group of workers. This trial may be seen as a study in how to
conduct large collaborative enterprises. A number of points
are already becoming plain. The experimental design appears

not to be too complicated and the procedures to be followed on the farm evidently work. Herdsmen claim that the trial makes very small demands on them and they are making very few mistakes. Up to the time of writing less than 3% of second samples have been missed. It is also evident that an organisation based on the Agricultural Advisory Service structure is effective and that the ratio of three to one between the effort contributed by Ministry of Agriculture personnel and other collaborators is about right. Lastly, the arrangement whereby a technical consultant who has no place in the formal organisation, is in close contact with every stage and level of the operation, is shown to be valuable.

150

GENERAL DISCUSSION

J. O'Shea *(Ireland)*

Could I ask Dr. Thomas to comment on the influence of diet on the ability of worms to depress milk production.

R.J. Thomas *(UK)*

We do not have any idea. There is so little work on the effect of parasitism on metabolism in cattle.

G. Urquhart *(UK)*

How much will Dr. Michel's study cost?

J.F. Michel *(UK)*

It depends on what theories of costing you wish to employ. The amount of money incurred is minimal. The actual cost of materials is less than £12 000 and we are able to give money back to the source from which it came, and we have a fairly substantial sum to give to the cows - who are a deserving class of taxpayers. I should have mentioned something about the cost benefit calculations involved. We are thinking in terms of a capital sum of £15 000 000. By the normal criteria of investment appraisal you can, therefore, justify an investment on this experiment of just under £15 000 000. Supposing we were to show that we have a difference of 5%, then we would be pointing to a loss which again, as a capital sum, would be somewhere around the £350 000 000 mark.

G. Urquhart

It seems to me that it has all got a bit out of hand. The original idea of dosing cows at calving, improving milk yield, is information of a somewhat dubious source. Why would a trial like Dennis Jabobs' (funded by ICI, presumably) or one by Dieter Düwel not solve the problem?

J.F. Michel

The point is that we have had a number of these trials and they have not produced an answer. There has always been an element of doubt about previous results and what we have attempted to do, in this case, is eliminate that doubt - to have an unequivocal answer. Whether we will get it or not, I do not know, but it is an attempt to do so

Let me come back to the cost benefit argument which I think is unanswerable. You might say that all cost benefit analysis is spurious and I would tend to agree with you, but if you accept its validity, then it is unanswerable.

H. de Keyser *(Belgium)*

We have done a trial in Belgium in the following way. We contacted a milk cattle breeding organisation who have 10 000 dairy cows in their Federation. We asked their computer to find us pairs of cows, born in the same month, who were calving for the third, fourth or fifth time, with an insemination date in the same week so that calving was in the same week. We have found 320 pairs of cows and we have treated them in a double blind study with levamisole, or with a placebo. Finally, we had 168 pairs of cows on 62 farms. We now have the results of the first six months of lactation between the treated group and control groups. We have used two methods to compare the results and these have been mentioned by our English colleague, Dr. Jacobs. With these two methods of calculating, there was no difference at all between the two regression curves of the control group and the treated group. This study was an attempt to use a sufficient number of cows and also to eliminate genetic and other variations. Also, these cows had a very low cell count in the milk and hence the role of mastitis in the study was excluded. Additionally, when there was some illness in one cow of a pair, that pair was excluded from the study.

J. Armour *(UK)*

The problem is to explain how 1 000, or even 3 000 worms, mainly *Ostertagia*, can cause this depression in milk yield. What is the pathogenic mechanism? We know that the fourth larval stage is almost non-pathogenic and induces very few changes. Hence, one is considering a few adult worms in a large abomasum. There may be some lesion related to the immune response, but I do not know. The wormburdens mentioned today could hardly produce a disease problem in a susceptible animal.

F.H.M. Borgsteede *(The Netherlands)*

We found that the cows which had the highest production, and which were judged by the farmers to be very excellent cows, had the highest wormburden!

J. Armour

Yes, but what is the pathogenic effect of these burdens? Why should the milk yield be depressed? Unless you have a damaged mucosa and sufficient of the mucosa is damaged, how otherwise can this effect be produced?

G. Urquhart

You are surmising that there is a pathogenic effect. There may be no effect at all. Perhaps you are trying to answer a question that really is not there. If you take the whole spectrum of cows in any country, some will be calving in September, having been out at grass and ingesting massive numbers of larvae, some will be calving in March, having been indoors for six months. Some cows may benefit from anthelmintic treatment if they have a large wormburden. You are making a case on the basis that all cows have 2 000 - 3 000 *Ostertagia* and you are trying to imagine a mechanism for this. I do not think this is the way to approach it.

J. Armour

Sorry, but I think it is. There is the evidence that Dr.
Jacobs showed today in his paper, and also that of David McBeth.
McBeth showed that the ones with the greatest challenge were
the ones that derived the greatest benefit from treatment.

R.J. Thomas

Non-significantly so!

J. Armour

It depends on how you analyse it. If you do it non-para-
metrically, it is significant. Some people would argue that is
the right way to do statistics, others would say the other way.

N. Downey *(Ireland)*

Mr. Chairman, isn't there some danger in using huge numbers
of animals to produce a statistically significant result? It
is the mechanisms involved and the epidemiology involved which
is so important.

J. Armour

Yes, the mechanism is the important thing. Is it the
effect of larval challenge on an immune host which is causing
this? The suggestion is that it is those animals which have
the heaviest challenge which benefit most from treatment.

R.J. Thomas

Yes, I think you would expect that. I am not sure that it
is a valid proposition that there are levels of infection that
are non-pathogenic. The degree of pathogenicity will vary with
the size of the burden but I am not sure at what level you say
that wormburden is non-pathogenic, particularly in relation to
milk production. As O'Shea says, this is very much related to
nutrition and metabolism.

154

J. Armour

However, you know how *Ostertagia* effects an animal; you
know the pathogenic process associated with infection.

R.J. Thomas

But you do not know the effect on metabolism!

J. Armour

What type of metabolism?

R.J. Thomas

Digestible energy. This is really what one needs to know.
One does not need to know the lesion is in the abomasum. The
effect on energy availability, protein availability, to the
animal - that is what we do not know.

J. Armour

That has been done in sheep, has it not?

R.J. Thomas

To some extent, yes.

J.F. Michel

Are you not dealing with partly intangible effects here?

G. Urquhart

I think that Nigel Downey has a very important point. By
using such large number of animals you may, in fact, hide significance. Some herds may, for some reason, be susceptible to
helminthiasis, adult cattle, or they may be calved at a specific
time or under conditions of husbandry which predispose to
larval challenge. Such herds will benefit from treatment.

J.F. Michel

Yes, but are you not assuming that we are going to analyse our data in a very unselective and unenlightened way? We can analyse the data which we will take in a variety of ways: by the age of the animal, by the faecal egg count, by geographical location etc. I would even say that we are fairly confident that statistical work will be well done and is under the guidance, and with the collaboration, of the Physics Department at Rothamstead.

G. Urquhart

I do not know how you picked up the point about larval challenge with your system. On what do you base this?

J.F. Michel

You can only detect a difference, within a herd or within a group, which is related to the number of animals that you are using. If you have not got enough animals you cannot detect the difference. With the number of animals we use we can pick up 28 kg of milk as between all-dosed and all-undosed. If one used smaller groups there would obviously have to be a bigger difference before we could detect it. I would suspect that if we get a result it would be in spring calving heifers. The number of spring calving heifers would be fairly small, so it would have to be a fairly marked result before we, or anyone, could pick it up. However, we would probably be dealing with more spring calving heifers than in previous studies.

R.M. Jones (UK)

What worried me about the use of anthelmintics in dairy cows is that, for reasons other than epidemiological, we need to give the dose just before calving. The dose has got to be given at this time because, with the exception of thibenzole, there is a required withdrawal period. One cannot expect a farmer to discard milk over a number of days and the only time that an anthelmintic can be given is at calving when milk is

discarded because of the colostrum. If one could relate the
time of treatment to the epidemiological situation, to the time
of the challenge of the animals, one might get a completely
different result from treatment before calving. The only data
which has been produced which has shown a statistical difference
(the work of Todd and Bliss) did not, in fact, give the treatment before calving but a number of days after calving when the
animals were reaching peak lactation. They used thibenzole in
their study and, therefore, were able to give the treatment at
a different time. Yet all the studies being discussed here are
concerned with treating just before calving which may not be
the right time, epidemiologically, to give it.

J.F. Michel

The best time would be just after calving. But for practical reasons we cannot give it at any other time because we
would have to compensate farmers for the loss of milk. In our
case it would cost £100 000. However, I would like to make
two points. One is that the concensus seems to be that the most
effective time for treatment is just after calving. Secondly,
the lactation curve is very much influenced by the few days
after calving.

R.J. Thomas

To dose just at calving worries many people. If treatment
was done monthly, or two-monthly, one might expect a result.
Dr. Michel has a point, that the whole lactation curve is
influenced by this early period; that might be the explanation.
The justification for the large-scale trial is partly the conflict between economics, commercial practice and science. One
has to show that the results are statistically significant,
otherwise they do not mean anything. The variation in milk
production of individual cows is large and, therefore, the
size of difference in milk yield required to obtain statistical
significance is relatively large. But the size of difference
that would make it worth the farmer treating is much lower.

The problem is between the difference that would be economically significant and the difference that is statistically significant. Unless you use large numbers you cannot get statistical significance sufficiently sensitive to be applicable at this economically significant difference. That is the reason why one needs to use large numbers of animals.

J. Armour

One thing to do is to study experimental infections in the adult animal. I wonder if Dr. Kloosterman would like to comment on this.

A. Kloosterman *(The Netherlands)*

I am afraid there are only limited data available. Forty-eight heifers were grouped according to bodyweight and age. We did not know anything about their production potential. We had three groups; one group was a control group; the second group was treated with thiabendazole and the third group was infected with ½M larvae (a mixture of *Cooperia* and *Ostertagia*). We did not know anything about production potential of these animals. The infected group milk production started higher than the other groups and the whole lactation curve was flatter than the lactation curve of the anthelmintical treated group and the control animals. The control animals and the anthelmintic treated animals ran fairly parallel; there was no significant difference between groups.

J. Armour

What was the level of infection again?

A. Kloosterman

Half a million larvae. About 20% of them *Ostertagia*.

E.J.L. Soulsby *(UK)*

How many worms would ½M larvae produce?

A. Kloosterman

I have no idea. We did faecal egg counts but there was
no difference between the infected animals and the control
animals. Of course there was a difference between the anthelmintic treated animals and the others.

J. Armour

Had these animals been previously exposed to infection?

A. Kloosterman

No, except perhaps naturally.

J. Eckert *(Switzerland)*

Did you carry out any other examinations to exclude other
factors which may have influenced this result? A statistical
difference does not mean that this is really due to the wormburden. There may be some other factors, for instance differences in food intake; other factors which may also influence
milk production. I think this is a big problem in all these
experiments. There is also the condition of the cow.

A. Kloosterman

We have not looked at the intake of food in these animals.

R.M. Connan *(UK)*

A major effect of *Ostertagia* is on appetite.

J. Armour

Yes! But it requires quite a lot or worms to have an
effect in appetite.

R.M. Connan

There is a general consensus that an effect on appetite is
the major effect of *Ostertagia* infection.

J. Armour

It takes a large dose of larvae to produce an effect on appetite. What do 2 000 worms do?

D.E. Jacobs *(UK)*

It is only in the critical part of lactation that there is an energy gap, where the animal acquires so much nutrient to produce the milk that it cannot, in fact, eat any more; therefore, it is losing bodyweight. We postulated that anything that might effect the appetite of the animal, at this critical point, would have an effect on milk production. Since we know that *Ostertagia* does have this effect - in calves anyway - we have a trial going at this time to measure the food intake of parasitised cows and calves undergoing anthelmintic treatment. It will be another few weeks before we get any results.

J. Armour

What sort of level of infection are you working with?

D.E. Jacobs

These are natural infections. We have not yet found an experimental farm that will allow us to infect their cows.

H.-J. Bürger *(FRG)*

Dr. Kloosterman, at what time did you infect your heifers?

A. Kloosterman

At parturition.

H.-J. Bürger

Directly on the day of parturition? Has anybody done any calculations of the rate of infection of the cows on the pasture? Does anyone have any data?

D. Düwel *(FRG)*

David McBeth has done such counts: larval counts and faecal examinations.

D.E. Jacobs

I presented a chart this morning where we calculated the daily larval intake of cows, throughout the year.

H.-J. Bürger

Have you tried to calculate the correlation coefficiencies between these numbers of larvae and the milk yields?

D.E Jacobs

No.

H.-J. Bürger

Do you intend to do this?

D.E. Jacobs

We do, yes. We have got an enormous volume of data to work through and it may take a few months to sort out.

J. Armour

We have an Ayrshire herd, and there is a problem where milk production is not what it should be. When we examined the pastures, the pasture larval count was between 3 000 and 4 000 larvae/kg of dried herbage on the cow pastures. To me that is beginning to get to a level where we could expect something to happen. But it is a very intensive unit and it is very difficult to get the farmer to rearrange his grazing pattern and, in the cow pastures, they are very heavily stocked. Most of the other pastures we have looked at have been 100 to 200 larvae/kg of herbage.

Dr. J.-P. Raynaud *(France)*

It is difficult to understand how you translate the challenge to the cow. Do you take the actual number of larvae on the pasture and multiply by X number of days, or do you try to follow the animals on the various paddocks they have to cover over a certain time?

D.E. Jacobs

Yes, it is, because it is impossible to get a farmer to comply with an experimental programme. There are all sorts of problems like that. We have been following the cows as they go round the paddocks, sampling the paddocks that the cows are on and trying to work out the daily larval intake at certain times in the year. However, farmers may change their cattle from one field to another and it is almost impossible to get a comprehensive figure over a period of time.

P. Nansen *(Denmark)*

In adult resistant animals you have low egg counts, low pepsinogen levels, minor lesions, but still you have a constant flow of parasites into the animal. I would be interested to know which proportion will complete development in the mucosa and which proportion will be inhibited. Also, how are these larvae affected in the abomasum? Are they rejected when they come into contact with the mucosa?

J. Armour

I think the situation is very similar to that in sheep. In immune ewes there are very few worms present. Due to the leak lesion which develops, and the loss of protein which occurs throughout the GI tract, there is a loss of production which is measurable in wool production.

D. Barth *(FRG)*

I would like to ask a question of Dr. Michel. I understand that you treat the animals at parturition, or a week later, and then you follow them for the whole lactation period. During such a large scale trial I am sure you must have had arguments why you should not follow a 100 day period only.

J.F. Michel

No. Because the official milk recording scheme makes it easy to do either.

D. Barth

Can you get an interim result as well so you can evaluate 100 days and, in addition, the 300 days?

J.F. Michel

To some extent we can. Unfortunately it is common practice now, when recording herds, not to weigh milk every day at every meal but to weigh and sample milk only once a month. That really does complicate the issue, because that month is determined, not in relation to calving, but in relation to a set monthly interval. But, to some extent, we do get the interim figures and it may be possible to adjust them.

D. Barth

This raises the question, why did you not have an extra group with a repeated treatment?

J.F. Michel

This is largely a question of the cost in compensating people for loss of milk.

J. Armour

And numbers!

J.F. Michel

Numbers would not be impossible but inconvenient. The essence of the trial is that it must be simple to operate.

G. Urquhart

In his paper, Dr. Michel has mentioned that the practice of dosing milking cows is already widespread in Britain. I wondered if this is generally true of Britain and other countries.

J. Armour

It is certainly true in our area of Scotland.

G. Urquhart

Is this quite a recent development?

J. Armour

It has been a reflection of advertising by pharmaceutical companies over the last two to three years. When we look for farms for trials, we find that numerous people say that they are using anthelmintic treatment already.

G. Urquhart

And this is all due to advertising?

J. Armour

Absolutely!

R.M. Connan *(UK)*

Absolutely!

R.J. Thomas

Oh yes. There is a lot of dosing being done at the moment. This is due to advertising and what is being shown. This is the whole point of <u>not</u> doing Dr. Michel's trial.

J. Armour

A negative answer would, in a way, be a good thing for the national economy.

J.F. Michel

I can say, with some accuracy, how many cows were dosed against gastro-intestinal nematodes in 1978. It was about a third of a million. That was really before the advertising campaign started. I would expect it to be substantially more now.

J. Armour

After Dr. A.C. Todd visited New Zealand, the sales of anthelmintics to dairy cows rocketed. It was fantastic.

G. Urquhart

As regards the analogy with sheep, how far has it been studied, say from abattoir studies, that pregnant cattle lose their immunity, possibly in late pregnancy, and may acquire numbers of inhibited or non-inhibited larvae due to reinfection? There is not much evidence of a spring rise in egg count is there, in calving?

J.F. Michel

Yes, there is!

J. Armour

Yes, but it is very low compared to sheep.

J.F. Michel

Yes, there is, but it is a peri-parturient rise.

G. Urquhart

How significant is it?

J. Armour

It was first reported in Corsica.

G. Urquhart

Scores of pregnant cows must go to abattoirs every day. It should be easy to establish wormburdens.

J. Armour

In our present studies, burdens are almost nil. I am sure there must be marked differences between one part of Britain and another, or one part of Europe and another.

E.J.L. Soulsby

I am quite surprised to see the figures quoted by Dr. Barth and Dr. Borgsteede for worms in the abomasa. My experience was that it was difficult to find any worms in the abomasa of adult cattle. Were the cows that you examined, Dr. Barth, from high yielding large herds, or were they from small farms? These numbers seemed extraordinarily high to me, but perhaps I am just out of date with what to expect in terms of dairy cattle and their wormburdens.

D. Barth

The animals did not come from herds with a high milk yield. They were ordinary farms, 5 - 30 cows per farm, and there was nothing special about them apart from being in a grazing area. This means that they were either grazing outside or the grass was brought in. The average milk yield was about 3 800 litres, very much below the average farm.

H.J. Over *(The Netherlands)*

Is there any evidence in your material that all the farms where, according to Professor Soulsby, you had this rather high number of *Ostertagia* had a different type of treatment for the younger cattle?

D. Barth

I do not know the exact grazing history.

H.J. Over

In terms of applications of the anthelmintic, there are different types of farms where it is done every year, perhaps two or three times a year in young calves.

J.W. Hansen *(Denmark)*

Is it possible to pair the animals in such a way that you have, in one group, animals who have never experienced a parasite, and milking cows who have a natural infection and have gained some immunity, and then compare the milk production in those two groups. It could provide an answer as to the influence of the parasites.

D. Barth

This has been done by Paul van Adrichem, in Holland and Belgium, when he used his identical twins - there were 80 twins - and one group was treated regularly, every fortnight, and the other twins were held as a control. There were very obvious differences between the first lactation yields.

J.W. Hansen

That is not really my meaning. In milking cows, it does not have to be the first lactation period; there must be some difference in cows experiencing infection and cows that have not experienced infection.

J. Armour

You are asking the difference between cows which experience an infection for the first time and cows which have previously been exposed and then experience a similar infection?

J. Eckert

I would like to ask a question with regard to the timing of treatment. Farmers are advised to treat the animals at parturition but how do you prevent them from treating the animals later? What is your practical experience in this respect

This seems to me to be a very important point. Even if there was a general recommendation for treating the cows at parturition, I am convinced that some farmers may treat them later. What is the recommendation of this group with regard to the residues in the milk?

J. Armour

I would have thought that this is fairly well covered by the legislation in various countries. To my knowledge, and certainly in Britain, there is no 'on the spot' testing for anthelmintic residues, such as is done for antibiotics.

E.J.L. Soulsby

But it might well be.

J. Armour

It may come. I think Professor Soulsby is right; it is one possible development in the future.

D. Barth

As far as thiabendazole is concerened there is no withdrawal period so you can use it whenever you want. In addition, however, there is no influence on milk. This was confirmed by the new law.

J.F. Michel

In Britain one must regard that as a temporary situation.

R.M. Jones

I think it is probably inevitable that we will go the way of the FDA and sometime introduce monitoring of residues in milk and beef in spot tests which would have to be performed by the authorities rather than by the industry.

J. Armour

We get about 400 cows per annum for post mortem in the abattoir at the veterinary school in Glasgow. In one or two of these, animals have got heavy wormburdens - 150 000, 200 000 or 300 000. Inevitably, these animals are suffering from other conditions, such as lymphosarcoma which has an effect on the immune system. So there seems to be an inter-relationship between susceptibility to helminth infection and immune status.

E.J.L. Soulsby

Did Dr. Thomas say that for an economic significance one would need less of a difference in milk yield than for a production significance?

R.J. Thomas

Yes.

E.J.L. Soulsby

With regard to some of these data presented this morning, from the economic point of view would they be significant?

R.J. Thomas

Yes. I think Dr. Michel worked out the level that one would need to get an economic return. This is relatively low.

J.F. Michel

We have said that there is a benefit for the farmer if he shows an increase due to dosing of 28 kg. Half of this is the cost of the drug, the other half is the cost of administering it. The data which we have seen obviously indicate increases in yield considerably greater. The problem is that there is no statistical significance attached to them.

R.J. Jørgensen *(Denmark)*

I have been concerned about the large number of animals
necessary for such a trial. Have you calculated how many cows
a farmer must have in order to benefit from treatment?

J.F. Michel

We are suggesting that an intelligent farmer would ask
for a substantial difference before he thought it worth dosing.
That may be, but we are concerned with the National Herd. If
we are honest public servants we have got to think of the
National Herd as being one herd of 2.8M cows, not counting
Scotland. I am not certain of the number of cows in Scotland.
In England and Wales it is 2.8M.

J. Armour

The mean herd size in Scotland, of course, is double of
that in England and Wales! Eighty compared with 48.

T. O'Nuallain *(Ireland)*

Did I understand Dr. Michel to say that the herds that he
was using in the scheme were all big herds?

J.F. Michel

Yes, the average size is 168. We were looking for herds
with more than 100 cows. We have, in fact, got two of 98 and one
of 540.

T. O'Nuallain

How would this influence the benefit to the farmer of a
small herd? What proportion of the cows in the UK are in the
small herds?

J.F. Michel

I think the benefit, or lack of benefit, is going to be the
same. The situation is that we do not know if the treatment is

to be of benefit or not. Yet we have been discussing, in great
detail, how great the benefit is to be and what it is due to.
Let it first be shown whether there is a benefit.

J.-P. Raynaud

Could you explain the sort of techniques you recommend?

J.F. Michel

We are trying to standardise techniques. We are using
a flotation technique for faecal examination with a sensitivity
of one egg/g of faeces.

J.-P. Raynaud

You start with 5 g or 10 g?

J.F. Michel

We start with 4.5 g.

J.-P. Raynaud

That's British!

J.F. Michel

There are historical reasons for this associated with
the size of McMaster chambers.

H.-J. Bürger

Dr. Barth what is the explanation for the different
percentages of 4th stage larvae in the abomasa? You had
relatively low percentages of inhibited larvae in the abomasa
around December or so, and then you had decreasing percentages.
What is your explanation for that?

D. Barth

    We had an increase up to the middle of October and then,
suddenly, when they were housed there was a decrease. I think
it is a question of housing. New infection stops when animals
are getting silage and hay. But soon there is an overcrowding
effect; there is a tendency for farmers to house too many
animals and then we may have the infection transmitted indoors.

H.J. Over

    We are talking about autopsy results. We do not know
much about the selection the farmer has made and it would be
unwise to draw conclusions on the epidemiology based on such
data. For example, in older animals the incidence is somewhat
higher compared to the middle age group. It may be that a
higher proportion of older animals are sent for slaughter than
in the summer months.

F.H.M. Borgsteede

    I think that the infection pattern of cows is the same
as it is in calves. They are turned out in spring and take up
small numbers of larvae. The great mass of larvae is picked
up by cows after the mid-summer increase around the months of
September and October (at least in our country) and that is the
explanation why in wintertime you have high numbers of arrested
larvae and only small numbers of adult worms. During the
wintertime, the number of adult worms decreases faster than
the numbers of the arrested larvae. Therefore, through the
winter the percentage of larvae increases but the absolute
number decreases.

J. Armour

    I would like to ask Dr. Raynaud to comment on the problem
of worms in adult cows. In your paper you described the
clinical problem in adult cattle in France. How do you account
for the vary large wormburdens in some of these cows,
particularly just after calving?

J.-P. Raynaud

This has been found in Charolais cattle in an area of
France where the animals are raised almost wholly out of doors.
These animals are submitted to a very high challenge because of
permanent pasture and high stocking rate etc. Diarrhoea
following the calving is common. Post mortems and worm counts
on these animals show high numbers of parasites. In Normandy,
very high numbers of worms are found at the time of calving in
slaughtered animals.

J. Euzeby *(France)*

So far we have talked only about infection in dairy cows.
I should like to talk about beef cattle. In several parts of
France, and chiefly around Lyon, we have a very big problem
with cattle that have just finished second and third grazing
seasons. I refer to those which have sub-clinical infections.
There is a very big difference between the meat production of
these animals, even with sub-clinical infection, and those
which are not infected by larval oesophogastomiasis. Even in
the big areas where there is larval oesophagostomiasis it is
often quite focal. Sub-clinical larval oesophagostomiasis may
make a major difference in meat production.

J. Armour

Would anyone like to comment on the problem of larval
oesophagostomiasis in cattle? And the possible inter-relation-
ships?

G. Urquhart

This larval oesophagostomiasis in adult cattle: is this
an immune reaction, or is it a primary exposure?

J. Euzeby

No, it is not a primary exposure. These cattle have
already experienced two to three grazing seasons in the same
place and it is probably an immune reaction process.

H.-J. Bürger

As far as I know there is a disturbance to the metabolic metabolism of some minerals, in the animal, due to fluorosis, but I do not know if there is any connection with the immunological system of anything else.

SESSION 3

EPIDEMIOLOGY I

Chairman: J. Eckert

SIGNIFICANCE OF NEMATODIASIS IN CATTLE GRAZING ON ALPINE PASTURES[1]

J. Eckert, R. Perl and F. Inderbitzin

Institute for Parasitology, University of Zürich,
Veterinary Laboratory, Kanton Graubünden, Chur/Switzerland.

ABSTRACT

Epidemiological studies carried out in 1979 near Chur and Arosa (Kanton Graubünden/Switzerland) showed the following: Third stage larvae of cattle trichostrongylids (Ostertagia, Cooperia, Nematodirus) *can overwinter on high alpine pastures (2 000 - 2 400 m altitude) at least until mid June. Egg counts, serum pepsinogen levels and worm burdens of 6 tracer calves indicated that trichostrongylid infections were subclinical in calves and cattle grazing at a low stocking rate (0.5 animals/ha) on high alpine pastures. At the end of the grazing period on high alpine pastures (mid September) 31% and 57% of two groups excreted* Dictyocaulus *larvae.*

[1] Supported by Bundesamt für Veterinärwesen, Berne (Project No. 012.79.3)

INTRODUCTION

Information on the significance of nematodiasis in cattle grazing on alpine pastures in Europe is scarce. Therefore, an epidemiological study was conducted in 1979 in a mountainous area of Chur and Arosa, Kanton Graubünden, in the south-eastern part of Switzerland.

EXPERIMENTAL DESIGN AND METHODS

Animals and grazing management

Examinations were carried out in two groups of animals:

Group A1 comprised 136 winter-borne Swiss Brown female calves which had been raised indoors on 7 farms. At the beginning of the trial in April 1979 the animals were 3 - 6 months old. Of this group, 50 calves were selected at random for the study.

Group A2 comprised 25 calves, 4 - 6 months old, and 90 female cattle of the second grazing season, 13 - 18 months of age. Each 20 calves and cattle were included in the trial.

The grazing management was a rotational system which is based on the succession of plant development on alpine pastures at different altitudes.

As indicated in Figure 1, calves of groups A1 were first grazed, as small subgroups, on 'home pastures' close to the farms in May or later in June for 15 - 46 days. At the beginning of July all animals proceeded to a common 'high alpine pasture' at 1 800 - 2 500 m altitude where they remained for 75 days. Due to heavy snowfall in September the animals had to be housed for some days. Later, they were grazed on 'intermediate alpine pastures' or 'home pastures' for 31 - 48 days until the housing period in mid November. The animals of group A2 were grazed according to a similar scheme in Figure 2.

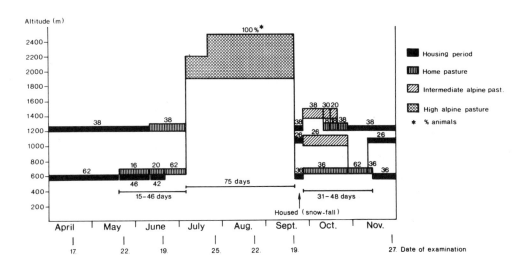

Fig. 1.   Grazing management of calves (Group Al: Aroseralp) 1979

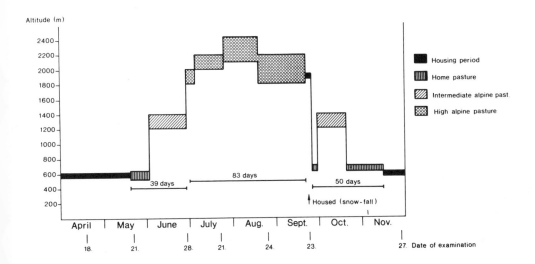

Fig. 2.   Grazing management of calves (Group A2: Alp Wolfboden)

The 'high alpine pastures' are extensive, mountainous
natural pastures which have been used for cattle grazing for
35 - 75 years. The stocking rate is low, about 0.5 animals/ha.
The ground is mostly dry with some moist places near a lake
and ponds and creeks which also serve as drinking places for
the animals.

Methods

The following methods were employed in the study. The
Baermann technique was used for the recovery of nematode larvae
which had overwintered in cattle faecal pats on pasture. Counts
of gastro-intestinal nematode eggs and coccidia oocysts were
made by the modified McMaster technique using 4 g faecal samples.
Dictyocaulus larvae were counted by the Baermann technique in
faecal samples of 30 g per animal. Serum pepsinogen values
were determined by the method of Hirschowitz (1955) and post
mortem examinations of tracer calves were undertaken according
to Eisenegger and Eckert (1975).

Meteorological data (Figure 3) were obtained from the
weather-station at Arosa (1 864 m) which is situated in a
distance of about 2 km from the high alpine pastures which were
grazed by groups A1 and A2.

RESULTS

The following results were obtained:

Overwintering of larvae

Table 1 presents the viable third stage larvae of *Ostertagia*,
Cooperia (C. oncophora-type) and *Nematodirus* that could be isolated
in mid June 1979 from cattle faecal pads that had overwintered
at 1 950 - 2 350 m altitude on high alpine pastures. Such
pastures had not been used by domestic ruminants for 8.5 months,
i.e. since end of September 1978.

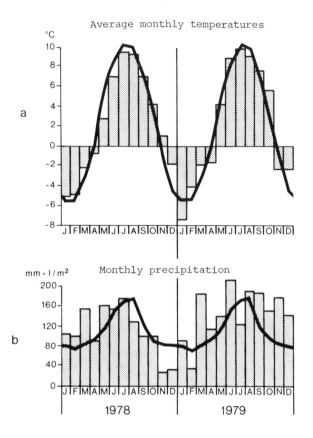

━ = average of 40 (a) or 75 (b) years

Fig. 3. Meteorological data of Arosa (1 864 m)

Egg counts

Figure 4 presents the gastro-intestinal nematode egg counts in calves. These were very low until June. An increase was observed in July, 3 or 4 weeks after the beginning of grazing on high alpine pastures, but the average counts did not exceed 100 per g. The maximum individual count was 500 per g. Up until the end of the high alpine grazing period in September there was only a slight increase of egg excretion. At the beginning of the housing period in November, egg output was unchanged in group A1 and had decreased in group A2.

TABLE 1

OVERWINTER SURVIVAL OF TRICHOSTRONGYLID LARVAE IN FAECAL PADS ON HIGH
ALPINE PASTURES NEAR AROSA. Sampling dates: June 13 and 14, 1979

Alpine pasture	Altitude (m) of sampling place*	Number of samples	Living third stage larvae		
			Ostertagia	*Cooperia*	*Nemato-dirus***
A1: Aroseralp	1 950	5	–	+	–
	2 000	5	+	–	+
used until end	2 100	5	+	+	+
of September 1978 by calves	2 150	10	+	+	+
of 1st grazing	2 200	5	–	–	–
season	2 250	5	–	+	–
	2 350	5	–	+	–
A2: Wolfboden	1 950	10	–	–	–
used until end	2 050	10	–	–	+
of September 1978 by calves	2 200	10	–	–	–
of 1st and cattle	2 350	5	–	+	–
of 2nd grazing season	2 400	5	–	–	–

*
  Each sample of about 200 g cattle faeces represents one faecal pad in a
  different location.

**
  Recovered by Baermann technique.
  +: at least one sample positive,   –: no larvae recovered.

   A similar pattern of egg excretion was observed in
cattle, but egg counts and the percentage of egg excreting
animals were lower.

Serum pepsinogen levels

   Average pepsinogen levels in calves are presented in
Figure 5. They remained under 1 unit of tyrosin per 1 during
the housing and grazing period. The maximum individual value
was 2.4 units obtained in September. In cattle average levels
did not exceed 1.25 units.

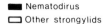

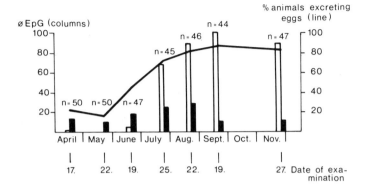

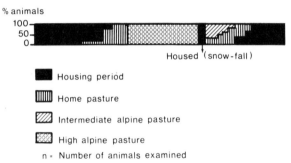

Fig. 4. Excretion of Trichostrongylid eggs in calves of Group Al
(Aroseralp) 1979

Excretion of lungworm larvae

In calves excretion of lungworm larvae was first observed
end of July during grazing on high alpine pastures (Figure 6).
At the end of this period, 31% and 57% of the animals in the
two groups were excreting *Dictyocaulus* larvae. Only 1 of 18
cattle were found to excrete lungworm larvae in July.

Other parasites

High percentages of calves (up to 100%) were excreting
coccidia oocysts during the grazing season. In May, 5 of 8
calves of one farm had oocyst counts of 70 000 - 310 000 per g
of faeces. Later, the average faecal oocyst counts in all

184

calves were around 500 - 1 000 per g.   Cattle had lower counts.

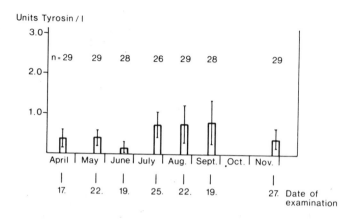

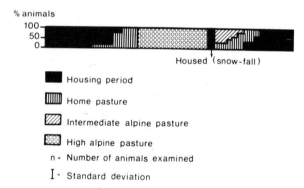

Fig. 5.   Average serum pepsinogen levels in calves of Group Al (Aroseralp)
1979.

Clinical signs

Thorough clinical examinations could not be done.
However, sporadically, soft faeces and coughing was observed
in a few calves in August and September.   Only one of 136
calves of group Al exhibited distinct clinical signs of
trichostrongylidosis and dictyocaulosis.

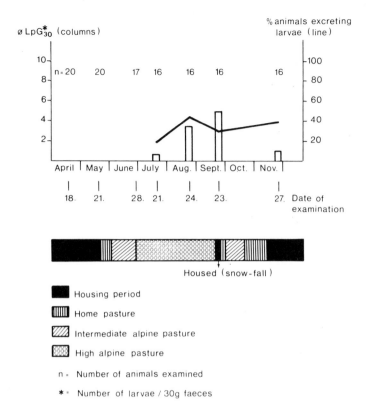

Fig. 6. Excretion of lungworm larvae in calves of Group A2 (Alp Wolfboden) 1979.

Tracer calves

Groups each of two calves raised helminth-free, 5 - 6½ months old, were grazed together with the calves of group A1 on a high alpine pasture for 25 days in July, August or September, respectively. The first group was put on pasture on the first day of the high alpine grazing period, i.e. after 8½ months of winter-rest. Before slaughter the animals were kept indoors for 25 days under conditions designed to prevent infection.

The results (Table 2) indicate that the first and the following groups acquired subclinical infections of abomasal and small intestinal trichostrongylids and some lungworms.

TABLE 2

WORM BURDENS OF TRACER CALVES GRAZED ON HIGH APLINE PASTURE Al

Grazing period (1979)	Calf no.	No. of trichostrongylids					Lungworms	
		Abomasum[1] ad.*	imm.*	Small intestine[2] ad.	imm.	Total	ad.	imm.[3]
July 6 –	95	4 800	760	1 280	100	6 940	0	2
July 31	97	2 860	1 460	600	0	4 920	0	0
July 31 –	96	3 060	60	660	320	4 100	0	3
Aug. 25	98	1 620	0	700	20	2 340	0	2
Aug. 25 –	99	1 820	120	7 360	40	9 340	85	7
Sept. 19	100	3 620	760	3 720	860	8 960	67	12

[1] *Ostertagia ostertagi* 87.8%, *Ostertagia leptospicularis* 0.3%, *Skrjabinagia lyrata* 11.7%, *Trichostrongylus axei* 0.2%.

Percentages represent averages of all 6 animals.
Immature stages: Mostly developing 4th stages of *Ostertagia* spp., a few inhibited.

[2] *Cooperia oncophora* 42.8%, *Cooperia zurnabada* 9.4%, *Nematodirus helvetianus* 47.8%.

Percentages represent averages of all 6 animals
Immature stages: Developing 4th stages.

[3] Inhibited 5th stages.

* ad.: adults, imm.: immatures.

DISCUSSION

These results indicate that third stage larvae of
Ostertagia, Cooperia and *Nematodirus* can overwinter on high alpine
pastures of 2 000 – 2 400 m altitude until mid June, i.e. for
at least 8½ months. The epidemiological role of these larvae
has not yet been determined but it can be speculated that the
larvae may contribute to the infection risk on high alpine
pastures. Boch and Spiess (1979) were not able to demonstrate
survival overwinter by end of June i.e. after about 10 months

of winter rest of trichostrongylid larvae on cattle pastures
at 780 - 1 772 m altitude in Bavaria. Nevertheless, in
Switzerland, appreciable numbers of trichostrongylid larvae
can overwinter on midland pastures at 700 - 1 200 m altitude
for 7 - 7½ months (Eisenegger and Eckert, 1975).

The egg counts of calves under alpine grazing conditions
follow the same pattern as occurs in midland (Eisenegger and
Eckert, 1975) and lowland areas (Michel, 1976) in Europe.

Egg counts, serum pepsinogen levels and worm burdens of
tracer calves indicated that the trichostrongylid infections
in calves and cattle grazing at a low stocking rate on alpine
pastures constituted subclinical infections.

The data indicate that transmission of trichostrongylids
and lungworms occur on high alpine pastures during July until
end of September. It appears that lungworms may be disseminated
from the common high alpine pastures to midland or lowland
farms previously free of *Dictyocaulus* by calves.

REFERENCES

Boch, J. and Spiess, A., 1979. Chemoprophylaxe und Weidewechsel als
    wirksame Massnahmen zur Verhinderung klinischer Helminthosen bei
    Jungrindern auf Gemeinschaftsweiden (Allgäuer Alpen). Berl. Münch.
    Tierärztl. Wschr. 92, 293-296.
Eisenegger, H. and Eckert, J., 1975. Zur Epizootologie und Prophylaxe
    der Dictyocaulose und der Trichostrongylidosen des Rindes. Schweiz.
    Arch. Tierheilk. 117, 225-286.
Hirschowitz, B.I., 1955. Pepsinogen in the blood. J. Lab. Clin. Med.
    46, 568-579.
Michel, J.F., 1976. The epidemiology and control of some nematode infections
    in grazing animals. Adv. Parasit. 14, 355-397.

DISCUSSION

J. Armour *(UK)*

Where do you think the lungworm infection came from in the calves?

J. Eckert *(Switzerland)*

Our experience from this study and others shows that some animals with a lungworm infection come to graze on the common alpine pasture. There were animals from two farms which were infected at the beginning of the grazing season. At the end of the grazing season on the high alpine pasture a rather high percentage were excreting lungworm larvae. However, you must consider that this was only one faecal examination, and we found that about 30 - 57% were excreting lungworm larvae; there were probably more but we did only one faecal examination and we may have missed a rather high proportion.

J. Armour

So you think that the initial excretion of lungworm larvae came from infection which had been taken in on the pastures of the lower grazing area?

J. Eckert

Yes. I must add that, in Switzerland, we have no indication as yet that overwintering of lungworm larvae is of epidemiological importance. These animals may acquire the lungworm infection on pastures of lower altitudes and these pastures may be contaminated by older animals.

J. Euzeby *(France)*

Are there any wild animals in these places?

J. Eckert

Yes, there are wild animals: roe deer and also some other wild ruminants. But we were very careful in selecting only the faecal pats of cattle which could be identified for the overwintering studies. Also the species determination, in the tracer animals, indicated that we found typical cattle parasites; mostly *Ostertagia ostertagi, Cooperia oncophora*. We found no species which were typical of wild animals.

J. Euzeby

At the moment I am carrying out a survey in the French Alps about the parasite elements of wild animals. Some of them are common to both wild animals and sheep. Perhaps they can act as a reservoir.

J. Eckert

We do not exclude the idea that roe deer, for example, would be able to contaminate cattle pastures with lungworm larvae. They may be responsible for a first contamination of the pasture; this cannot be excluded. However, with regard to the overwintering trichostrongylid larvae, we are quite sure that we isolated the larvae of cattle parasites.

J. Euzeby

As far as lungworms are concerned I was able to find *Dictyocaulus eckerti* - I don't think it is yours!

J. Eckert

I don't think it is a valid species.

J. Euzeby

I found it in wild animals - but this one has not been transmitted to sheep, so far.

E.J.L. Soulsby *(UK)*

How does the structure of the high alpine pasture differ from a low alpine one, in terms of soil, mat and plants, etc?

J. Eckert

There are big differences. The high alpine pasture are practically natural pastures - not fertilised except in some small areas. Under these conditions the plants grow differently. As it is a natural pasture, and not improved, the stocking rate is lower.

E.J.L. Soulsby

From one of your slides it appeared that there might be a very dense microclimate of the mat just on the soil surface. Would that be so?

J. Eckert

It was about the end of August when the picture was taken and the plants were already very short. As the temperature gets rather low during the night the grass growth is rather limited at this time. However, in July, for example, there may be a high humidity in the microclimate of the mat.

H.J. Over *(The Netherlands)*

Is there any reason why, in the alpine region, the stocking density could not be increased by introducing fertiliser?

J. Eckert

There are some alpine pastures which are called 'improved' pastures, and there the stocking rate is higher. In this area there was a pasture with a higher stocking rate. There we were of the impression that the nematode infections were of subclinical to clinical intensity. I think the stocking rate can be increased, but parasitism may also be increased under these conditions.

R.J. Thomas *(UK)*

Do you think these infections in the calves are significant in checking the growth rate. Early exposure might be important in subsequent immunity rather than in causing disease problems at the time.

J. Eckert

In comparison with animals grazing on lowland pastures, we would designate these infections as sub-clinical, according to the low pepsinogen levels and also according to the low worm burdens. In lowland pastured animals we obtained pepsinogen levels of about 4 or 5 tyrozine units per litre, and much higher worm burdens. I do not believe that the sub-clinical infections, in these studies were significant to the performance of the animals.

RECENT RESULTS ON EPIDEMIOLOGY OF NEMATODE INFECTIONS IN BEEF AND DAIRY CATTLE IN FRANCE

[1]J.-P. Raynaud, [2]C. Mage, [3]J.P. Le Stang and [4]R.M. Jones

[1]Agricultural R & D Station, Pfizer International,
37400 Amboise, France.
[2]I.T.E.B., 87100 Limoges, France.
[3]E.D.E. Maison de l'Elevage, 23700 Bernay, France.
[4]Pfizer Central Research, Sandwich, Kent, UK.

ABSTRACT

Beef herds: a type of breeding and production typical of this enterprise in France was investigated. Eleven calves (first year on pasture; suckling, then weaned) and 42 heifers were sacrificed between April and November. Moreoever, egg counts and performances were checked on 157 calves and 392 heifers in a field trial concerned with strategic treatments. Calves were infected late in the season, mainly by Ostertagia. Treatment was given at the time of housing.

Early in the season the heifers showed a self-cure and after July the number of parasites increased significantly (mainly Ostertagia, then Trichostrongylus axei and Cooperia). Two treatments were given in July – August and September – October.

Dairy herds: an experiment was conducted in a typical intensive breeding system (Normandy, Western France). Twenty calves were raised on two permanent pastures and additional calves were used as tracers.

Ostertagia and Cooperia were the main parasites responsible for pasture contamination and calf infections. An 'early July rise' of larval counts, high enough to induce clinical symptoms, was well controlled by treatments. To appreciate the pasture contamination, herbage samplings or tracer calves could be used. They are of equivalent value, but the latter gives information on retarded larvae picked up late in the season. The value of this information for understanding the parasitism of continuously grazing animals has still to be examined.

P. Nansen, R.J. Jørgensen, E.J.L. Soulsby (eds), Epidemiology and Control of Nematodiasis in Cattle.
Copyright © 1981 ECSC, EEC, EAEC, Brussels – Luxembourg. All rights reserved.

INTRODUCTION

Two studies on nematodiasis in cattle were performed recently. One involved beef cattle in central France (Limousin) where helminth infections were investigated in single suckled calves as well as in heifers. The second study was performed in dairy herds in western France (Normandy) where the larval contamination of pastures was studied by means of tracer calves and pasture sampling. In addition, the effect of parasitism on performance and clinical conditions was investigated.

BEEF CATTLE (CENTRAL FRANCE)

Management

The calves were born during the period December - March, while the cows were housed. In April, cows and calves were turned out to graze on permanent pasture which was divided into paddocks. The same rotational system was used for cows and calves as well as for heifers. Each paddock was grazed for 7 - 14 days and then left ungrazed for approximately 3 weeks. The stocking rates were 0.8 - 1.2 livestock units/ha, which equals 1 cow plus her calf/ha. For the heifers the stocking rate was 4 animals/ha.

In October - November the calves were weaned and separated into various production groups.

Female calves, selected for breeding, were housed until April. Intensive feeding was applied for those intended for fattening, whereas older heifers and steers were outwintered on pasture.

Calves: few worms were found in calves sacrificed in mid-August (Table 1), and only in animals sacrificed at weaning in autumn could the level of parasitism be considered 'average' (Raynaud et al., 1974). Similarly, faecal egg counts were low. Eggs may be detected in June. In July only 7% of the calves had counts of more than 150 epg.

TABLE 1

WORM COUNTS AND FAECAL EGG COUNTS OF SUCKLING BEEF CALVES FROM PERMANENTLY GRAZING HERDS

	August 20th	October 1st
Number of animals	5	6
Age (months)	6 - 7	7 - 8
Average weight (kg)	195	250
WORM COUNTS		
Haemonchus total	8 (0 - 40)	0
Ostertagia Ad. + L_5	2028 (870 - 3040)	1770 (260 - 6140)
L_4	1986 (1080 - 3130)	8592 (1510 - 14532)
% L_4/total *Ostertagia*	49% (35% - 70%)	83% (61% - 98%)
Trichostrongylus axei total	0	0
Cooperia total	888 (150 - 2320)	2748 (602 - 6940)
Nematodirus total	594 (320 - 2120)	1077 (48 - 6302)
Oesophagostomum total	0	0
Trichuris total	8 (2 - 25)	1 (0 - 3)
TOTAL WORM COUNTS	5512 (3282 - 9035)	14188 (7400 - 17690)
FAECAL EGG COUNTS (epg)	189 (75 - 315)	262 (15 - 735)
Dictyocaulus total worms	15 (0 - 50)	89 (0 - 370)

It appears from Table 1 and Figure 1 that worm counts were low and that the majority of worms were found as arrested larvae in October.

Worm counts and egp for the period mid-August to the following November are shown in Figure 2.

Anthelmintic treatment of calves was done with Tetramisole injected at 15 mg/kg. The results presented in Table 2 show that treatment given in July, August or September resulted in slight but non-significant increases in live weight and daily weight gains.

Based on this, we would only advise treatment at housing in order to improve health and feed conversion in calves during the winter.

<u>Heifers</u>: during the second grazing season the most important phases of parasitism in the young heifers were:

1.   A 'self-cure' phenomenon, i.e. a loss of worms between April and July. In early July there was a minimum of worms and lesions and a minimum percentage of L_4/total *Ostertagia* of 1 - 21%.

During the first half of the grazing season, the parasitism was the same as that of calves at housing: mainly *Ostertagia*, then *Cooperia*, but *Dictyocaulus* was eliminated.

2.   A new intake of parasites from September on: 34 974 worms per calf in September, 40 735 in November (Table 3).

At the same time the epg of faeces were so low that it was of no value to assess the parasitism of the heifers.

Ostertagia remained an important and significant parasite, but *Trichostrongylus axei* was ranked No. 2, and *Cooperia* No. 3.

Abomasal nodules

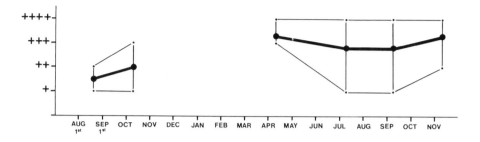

$$\frac{\text{Ostertagia L}_4}{\text{Total Otertagia}} \quad 100\ \%$$

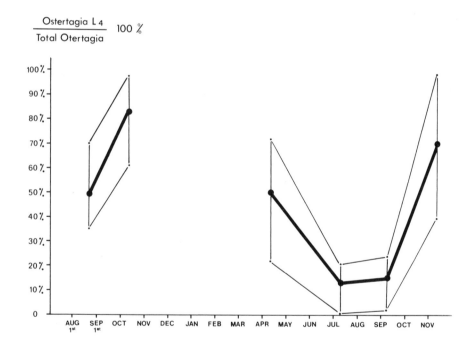

Fig. 1: Abomasal lesions and % L_4 on total *Ostertagia* in Limousin calves and heifers.

198

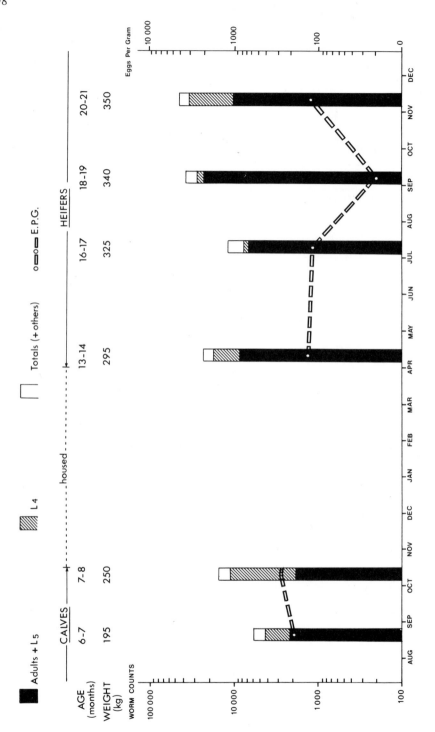

Fig. 2: Worm counts and epg in Limousin calves and heifers.

TABLE 2

LIVE WEIGHT (LW) AND DAILY WEIGHT GAIN (DWG) OF SUCKLING CALVES TREATED IN
JULY, AUGUST OR SEPTEMBER WITH TETRAMISOLE INJECTIONS

| | October | |
	LW (kg)	DWG since treatment
Treatment in July		
3 farms in Creuse		
27 control calves	238	961 g
27 treated calves	241	1000 g
difference	+ 3 kg	+ 4%
Treatment in August		
1 farm in Haute-Vienne		
32 control calves	219	871 g
31 treated calves	224	952 g
difference	+ 5 kg	+ 9%
Treatment in September		
1 farm in Haute-Vienne		
20 control calves	246	1054 g
20 treated calves	250	1127 g
difference	+ 2 kg	+ 7%

Again, *Dictyocaulus* could be considered as being absent from the
heifers.

Major findings on 20 - 21 month old heifers, sacrificed
on November 10 (Figure 1), were extensive nodular lesions,
the large percentage of L_4 in the *Ostertagia* population (average
70%, range 40 - 99%), and the fact that two animals out of 12
(16%) had typical *Oedematous Ostertagiosis* as described by Raynaud
and Bouchet (1976). As originally described, the *Ostertagia*
counts for those animals with extensive lesions were low:
17 000 or 18 000 developing stages only (adults + L_5).

An anthelmintic trial was conducted on 392 heifers on 17
farms in the same area, the animals being randomised by groups

TABLE 3

WORMS COUNTS AND FAECAL EGG COUNTS OF YOUNG BEEF CATTLE IN THEIR SECOND GRAZING SEASON (PERMANENTLY GRAZING HERDS)

	April 10th	July 8th
Number of animals	6	12
Age (months)	13 - 14	16 - 17
Average weight (kg)	295	325
WORM COUNTS		
Haemonchus total	17 (0 - 100)	21 (0 - 100)
Ostertagia Ad. + L$_5$	8349 (1010 - 12900)	6480 (840 - 20400)
L$_4$	8375 (410 - 32600)	936 (10 - 5400)
% L$_4$/total	50% (22% - 72%)	13% (1% - 21%)
Trichostrongylus axei total	1677 (60 - 4300)	1303 (0 - 4800)
Cooperia total	4195 (0 - 10600)	2243 (0 - 13700)
Nematodirus total	0	38 (0 - 460)
Oesophagostomum total	15 (0 - 50)	18 (0 - 40)
Trichuris total	0	0
TOTAL WORM COUNTS	22627 (1520 - 57700)	11040 (1380 - 30112)
FAECAL EGG COUNTS (epg)	127 (0 - 350)	116 (0 - 400)
Dictyocaulus total	0	0

(Continued)

TABLE 3 (Cont/d)

WORM COUNTS AND FAECAL EGG COUNTS OF YOUNG BEEF CATTLE IN THEIR SECOND GRAZING SEASON (PERMANENTLY GRAZING HERDS)

	September 7th	November 10th
Number of animals	12	12
Age (months)	18 – 19	20 – 21
Average weight (kg)	340	350
WORM COUNTS		
Haemonchus total	0	0
Ostertagia Ad. + L_5	21962 (2080 – 325250)	9889 (50 – 25800)
L_4	3970 (110 – 8300)	22581 (580 – 116000)
% L_4/total	15% (2% – 24%)	70% (40% – 99%)
Trichostrongylus axei total	8393 (100 – 44700)	5163 (0 – 19800)
Cooperia total	445 (0 – 2300)	3051 (0 – 24800)
Nematodirus total	192 (0 – 2300)	50 (0 – 600)
Oesophagostomum total	15 (0 – 50)	1 (0 – 10)
Trichuris total	0	0
TOTAL WORM COUNTS	34974 (3780 – 92540)	40735 (1130 – 153030)
FAECAL EGG COUNTS (epg)	21 (0 – 50)	125 (0 – 800)
Dictyocaulus total	0	0.2 (0 – 2)

of 2: non-treated and treated. The treatment groups received
Tetramisole on 2 - 13 July and Thibenzole on 7 - 14 September.
Egg counts were of no value to appreciate the possible effect
of the treatment as very few animals had epg higher than 150.
However, on 24 non-treated animals (12% of the total), clinical
cases of gastro-intestinal parasitism were found between
August and September, and these animals were treated individually

No disease was seen on the systematically treated animals,
and the average gain was about 9 kg/heifer, compared with the
control (Table 4).

This difference was non-significant, but the major interest
of the treatment is that it was done at the right time to avoid
any pathology.

Another important problem detected in heifers was the very
severe *Ostertagiosis* lesions found on some animals about mid-
November. The September treatment should be followed by a
strict pasture management scheme to avoid contamination or,
if necessary, premature housing to avoid such a severe handicap
on 2-year-old heifers.

Conclusion for the Limousin area

Suckling calves are worm-infected later in the season
than comparable weaned animals of the same age which are put
on the same pasture; it is only in September - October that
the level of worms/calf is 'average'.

Heifers show a 'self-cure' and in July they have the
minimum amount of parasites. But the number increases significantly, and pathology could be expected from August onwards,
and then during wintering.

Strategic anthelmintic treatments are advised at housing
for calves, and in July - August and September - October for
heifers.

TABLE 4

BEEF HERD (LIMOUSIN) HEIFERS TREATED IN JULY (2 - 13) AND SEPTEMBER (7 - 14); AVERAGE PERFORMANCES, LIVE WEIGHT IN kg (LW) IN 17 FARMS : 196 X 2 = 392 HEIFERS. HAUTE-VIENNE 1975 - 1978

| | 7 JULY | 12 SEPTEMBER | | 8 NOVEMBER | | DWG |
	LW	LW	Gain since July	LW	Gain since July	July - Nov
Controls	328.7	339.8	11.1 kg	363.9	35.2 kg	307 g
Individual treatments?	O	+ on 24 animals (12%) in August - September for digestive strongyles		O		
Treated (July + September)	327.7	343.1	15.4 kg	371.8	44.1 kg	367 g**
Individual treatments?	O	O		O		
Difference vs controls			+ 4.3 kg		+ 8.9 kg**	

** Difference highly significant at the P = 0.05 level

DAIRY HERDS (NORMANDY) - MATERIALS AND METHODS

Experimental calves and management

A permanent pasture of 2.2 ha, previously grazed by cattle for a number of years, was divided into two paddocks called 'W' and 'Y', respectively.

Castrated 'Normand' calves were reared worm-free indoors. The initial weight was 136 - 182 kg. Two groups of 10 'test calves', equivalent in average weight and range weight, were turned out on 8 May in the two paddocks (1.1 ha for 10 calves). An additional 14 calves were reared worm-free indoors and used as tracers at monthly intervals. When put on pasture, the tracer calves were comparable in weight to the continuously grazing calves.

The calves were set stocked on the experimental paddocks W and Y. According to local practices they were fed a concentrated mixture of cereals. With this system the quantity offered was high when available pasture was scarce and *vice versa* (from 1.5 to 2.5 kg/head/day).

Tracers

One worm-free tracer calf was introduced into each paddock at turnout, removed two weeks later, and housed for 3 weeks before slaughter for worm counts. Another tracer calf was introduced into each paddock every 4 weeks thereafter. The last pair of tracers was put out on 24 October.

Herbage larval contamination

Herbage samples for larval counts were taken from each paddock every 4 weeks. The sampling and processing followed those of Taylor (1939). Before processing the samples were subjected to two soakings on two successive days.

Supervision and sampling of calves

The calves were individually weighed and faecal samples were taken every 2 weeks. They were closely observed for clinical signs of parasites. Clinical cases of parasitic gastro-enteritis and relapses were treated with pyrantel tartrate (25 mg/kg). The period of observation was terminated on 8 November when the animals were housed.

Calculated intake of larvae by the tracer calves

We estimated the daily feed intake of tracer calves when put on pasture. It was expressed in dry matter for both the concentrate and the herbage. The ranges for herbage were about 2 - 4 kg/d, and this generally increased from start to finish. We then calculated the 'theoretical total larvae intake' for the 2 weeks they were on pasture, for the two major species and for the total. This was compared with the actual worm burdens in tracer calves.

RESULTS

Larval counts on herbage

Ostertagia and *Cooperia* were found in all samples (Tables 5 and 6). Other species were found irregularly. *Trichostrongylus* was found 9 times out of 14 at a rate of up to 10.8%, *Bunostomum* twice out of 14 times at up to 4.0%, and *Oesophagostomum* once at 3.7%.

In April, before turnout, both pastures carred small numbers of larvae: 354 or 763 *Ostertagia* and 173 or 451 *Cooperia* per kg dry herbage. They disappeared in June, but started to rise again in early July (4 July).

Pasture 'W' (Table 5): after the early July rise, *Cooperia* became slightly predominant, except for a peak on August 29 when *Cooperia* appeared to have doubled (compared with the previous result and the following one) and *Ostertagia* appeared to have been multiplied by 5.

TABLE 5

LARVAL COUNTS ON HERBAGE AND WORM COUNTS OF TRACERS. DATA FROM PASTURE 'W' IN A DAIRY HERD IN NORMANDY

Time	L3/kg dry herbage		Dry herb. ingested for 14 days	Calculated intake of L3 /tracer calf		Worm counts of tracers					
						Ostertagia			Cooperia		
	Ost.	Coop.		Ost.	Coop.	Ad.+L5	L4	$\frac{L4 \times 100}{Total}$	Ad.+L5	L4	$\frac{L4 \times 100}{Total}$
April 28 – May 23	364	173	30.8	11211	5328	4080	0	0	320	0	0
June 6 – June 20	37	11	36.4	1347	400	190	0	0	60	0	0
July 4 – July 18	321	154	44.8	14381	6899	12375	0	0	1875	0	0
Aug. 1 – Aug. 16	1194	1563	55.5	66267	86746	58500	260	0.4%	14300	40	0.3%
Aug. 29 – Sep. 12	10417	3943	53.2	554184	209768	66200	550	0.8%	13900	9000	39.3%
Sep. 26 – Oct. 10	2015	1906	50.4	101556	96062	21600	48500	69.2%	26300	28300	51.8%
Oct. 24 – Nov. 7	5405	8186	35.0	189175	286510	47800	246500	83.8%	10900	14500	57.1%

TABLE 6

LARVAL COUNTS ON HERBAGE AND WORM COUNTS OF TRACERS. DATA FROM PASTURE 'Y' IN A DAIRY HERD IN NORMANDY

Time	L3/kg dry herbage		Dry herb. ingested for 14 days	Calculated intake of L3 /tracer calf		Worm counts of tracers					
	Ost.	_Coop._		_Ost._	_Coop._	_Ostertagia_			_Cooperia_		
						Ad.+L5	L4	$\frac{L_4}{Total} \times 100$	Ad.+L5	L4	$\frac{L_4}{Total} \times 100$
April 28 – May 23	763	451	26.6	20296	11997	3150	0	0	1030	0	0
June 6 – June 20	24	24	40.6	974	974	1095	0	0	680	0	0
July 4 – July 18	108	88	44.8	4838	3942	5460	0	0	1600	0	0
Aug. 1 – Aug. 16	1908	2432	52.5	100170	127680	18000	220	1.2%	55100	600	1.1%
Aug. 29 – Sep. 12	6208	1967	56.0	347648	110152	10200	130	1.3%	30400	5000	14.1%
Sep. 26 – Oct. 10	2803	3628	53.2	149120	193010	5000	41000	89.1%	7000	39200	84.8%
Oct. 24 – Nov. 7	9591	14678	57.4	550523	842517	32300	178000	84.6%	27000	93800	77.5%

The range of these post July values could be considered as 'average'.

Pasture 'Y' (Table 6): This was very similar to W, but the August 29 peak was slightly less important with normal values for *Cooperia* and a level multiplied by 3 for *Ostertagia*.

Worm burdens in tracer calves

The calves put on pasture in May, June and July carried very few worms and the information obtained on the parasitism existing on pasture is of little interest. The fact that no arrested larvae were found should be noted.

Plot 'W' (Table 5): in August the worm burden had reached a significant level and it was dominated by counts of about 60 000 - 70 000 adults and L_5 of *Ostertagia*. The August and early September tracers were in poor condition and diarrhoeic. In early September a small percentage of *Ostertagia* were in the form of arrested larvae (less than 1% of the total population) whereas 30% of *Cooperia* arrested L_4 were found.

The tracers put on pasture for 2 weeks on September 26 or October 24 suffered a very heavy parasitism. When sacrificed, they were in poor condition and diarrhoeic. The carcases were cachectic and the percentage of arrested larvae was high: at the end of September 69% of the *Ostertagia* and 52% of the *Cooperia* specimens were arrested. At the end of October, 84% of the *Ostertagia* , i.e. 246 000, were found to be arrested.

At the end of the season *Cooperia* L_3 were more abundant than *Ostertagia* in the pasture, whereas the corresponding tracers harboured 10 times more *Ostertagia* than *Cooperia*.

Plot 'Y' (Table 6): the comments are similar to those for pasture W, but *Cooperia* was relatively more important in the tracers here, and the percentage of retarded *Cooperia* larvae was higher in late season.

Comparison between L_3/kg herbage and worm burden of tracers

From Tables 5 and 6 it may be concluded that:

- the two values used for estimating L_3 on herbage are similar and follow the same pattern
- there is a parallelism between herbage L_3 counts and worm counts in tracers, and the patterns are very close.

Performance (Figures 3 and 4)

For both groups which had an average bodyweight of 155.5 kg when turned out on May 8, the growth curve was comparable to that obtained on the same experimental farm for the preceding 10 years (Jolivet et al., 1973, 1974; Le Stang et al, 1976). A linear growth was seen until August 15, then loss of weight and obvious signs of parasitic gastro-enteritis appeared. Individual treatments were necessary from August 30 until September 18. All the animals were treated and the large majority were re-treated between September 11 and October 24. These treatments allowed the animals to maintain their performance until wintering in early November, as some compensatory growth was seen at the end of the grazing season. An early rise in egg counts was found on July 4 when about 100% of the animals excreted eggs at an average count of 260 - 288 epg, with the highest counts being 600 - 800 epg.

CONCLUSION

Gastro-intestinal parasitism in continuously grazing calves was well reflected by herbage larval counts and by worm counts of tracer calves.

Ostertagia and *Cooperia* were found to be the main parasites responsible for pasture contamination and calf infections.

The animals excreted eggs which were responsible for an early July rise of larvae counts, high enough to induce clinical symptoms.

210

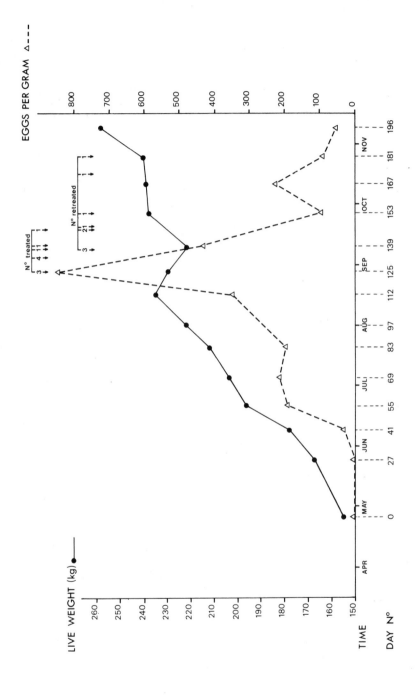

Fig 3.   Mean live weight and egg counts of 10 continuously grazing calves (Pasture W) given supplementary feeding. The indicated individual anthelmintic treatments were given to suppress clinical parasitism.

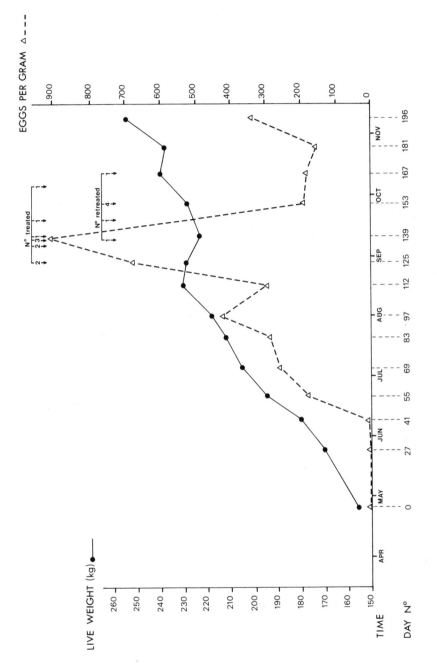

Fig 4. Mean live weight and egg counts of 10 continuously grazing calves (Pasture Y) given supplementary feeding
The indicated individual treatments were given to suppress clinical parasitism.

As the animals were individually treated, their performance was satisfactory at the end of the grazing season. However,
at that time, the animals ingested enormous amounts of parasites,
the majority of which remained as retarded larvae.

The contamination of the pasture can be well followed,
either with herbage sampling or by using tracer calves. There
is a parallelism between the two parameters, but tracers give
unique information on the possible amount of retarded larvae.
But this information does not correlate with the actual parasitism of test animals over the same period.

The fact that, without any other treatment, the animals
had a satisfactory growth and no clinical disease during
wintering, and had not suffered dramatically from the actual
heavy parasitism present when withdrawn from the pasture, will
be examined later. As with heifers in beef herds, this could
be explained by immunity and a 'self-cure' phenomenon.

REFERENCES

Jolivet, G., Le Stang, J.P. and Delcure, J., 1973. Etude de l'incidence des
strongyloses digestives sur la croissance des jeunes bovins au pâturage.
Expérimentations en élevages. Rec. Med. Vét., 124, 11. 1351-1375.

Jolivet, G., Le Stang, J.P. and Delcure, J., 1974. Etudes le l'incidence des
strongyloses digestives sur la croissance des jeunes bovins au pâturage.
Expérimentations en station. Rec. Med. Vét., 125, 3, 319-349.

Le Stang, J.P., Jolivet, G. and Delcure, H., 1976. Prophylaxie des strongyloses des jeunes bovins au pâturage. Brochure 48 pages publiée par
l'I.T.E.B., Paris.

Mage, C., 1979. Etude du parasitisme en troupeau de vaches allaitantes.
Brochure I.T.E.B., 144 pages, No. 79071.

Raynaud, J.-P., Laudren, C. and Jolivet, G., 1974. Interpretation épidémi-
ologique des Nematodoses gastro-intestinales bovines évoluant au
pâturage sur animaux 'traceurs'. Ann. Rech. Vétér., 5, (2) 115-145.

Raynaud, J.-P. and Bouchet, A., 1976. Bovine ostertagiosis, a review.
Analysis of types and syndromes found in France by post mortem examinations and total worm counts. Ann. Rech. Vétér., 7, (3), 253-280.

DISCUSSION

N. Downey *(Ireland)*

Did I understand you to say that you got symptoms in the second year in the Limousin breed in the heifers, but not in the second year in Normandy?

J-P. Raynaud *(France)*

May we discuss the parasitism risk in the Limousin and the Charolais breeds? Charolais is more intensive in the system of breeding, so they may have more problems. The only problems with the calves occur very late in the season, but the majority of the larvae occur in heifers, on 2nd year infected animals, early in the season or late in the season. In the Normandy system it is mainly the second part of the first year which is very critical; August to September. What is the importance of the *Ostertagia* inhibited larvae, because on the tracers we have found very high amounts? Probably the tracers overestimate this aspect on the available L3 which become inhibited. It is not exactly related to the problems found on the principal animals.

R.M. Connan *(UK)*

Is the difference between these two systems not the difference between single suckling calves, which do not get a very heavy infection in their first season and come out to graze in their second still with some susceptibility, and calves grazing together as a family group? In the Normandy situation however, calves receive a fairly heavy challenge in their first grazing season and come out to their second with a very significant resistance?

J-P. Raynaud

I would like to refer to the results presented by Professor Eckert. What is the significance of the tracer calf? If you put a tracer calf in the middle of ten calves in one hectare, you can see there is a correlation. We are happy with the correlation You could put the same tracer calves on ten hectares or on twenty

hectares of the pitch, because the amount of infection on the
pasture is so diluted. Suckling calves are milk fed for the
main part of the year and so this delays the intake of the larvae
and the acquisition of immunity. But what is the significance
of tracer animals in those extensive systems, I do not know. I
have no experience of them.

RECENT DANISH STUDIES ON THE EPIDEMIOLOGY OF BOVINE PARASITIC BRONCHITIS*

R.J. Jørgensen

Institute of Veterinary Microbiology and Hygiene,
Royal Veterinary and Agricultural University, Bülowsvej 13,
DK-1870 Copenhagen V, Denmark.

ABSTRACT

Epidemiological studies on verminous bronchitis were carried out by weekly observations and sampling of groups of calves and the plots grazed by them. Twenty-one calves were given a light initial infection of Dictyocaulus viviparus *in May and turned out to graze on the same day in three groups of seven calves each on plots of different sizes. Moderate patent infections developed in all calves and gave rise to pathogenic pasture larval contaminations after 5 to 6 weeks. Although the magnitude and the horizontal distribution of the pasture contamination varied between the plots, severe outbreaks were observed in all three groups, resulting from prepatent superinfections. The discrepancy between the pasture results and the clinical observations was explained by favourable climatic conditions and large individual variations.*

A second experiment was conducted by turning out eight susceptible calves on 1st August on an adjacent plot which had not been grazed and from where a hay crop had been taken. Four of these calves excreted lung-worm larvae four weeks later. This was explained by field-to-field transmission shortly after turning out. A resulting moderate pasture larval contamination was recorded during weeks 5 and 6. It gave rise to an outbreak during weeks 8 to 10. There was a tendency that the calves which did not excrete larvae during the first 6 or 7 weeks, became more affected than the calves which were responsible for the pasture larval contamination. The pasture contamination which was high in autumn, was followed into the next grazing season. The number of infective larvae per kilo of herbage dropped markedly before and after a period with frost and snow and reached an extremely low level in May, whereas the larval contamination of a pasture

* These studies were supported by the Danish Agricultural and Veterinary Research Council.

sample stored during the winter on a hay loft dropped markedly when the herbage dried out in mid-winter.

The infection in the first experiment which culminated in mid-summer, became undetectable in the pasture samples taken in late autumn, and no larvae were detected in the faeces of eleven calves available during the stabling period. One specimen of D. viviparus was recovered from the lungs of one out of 5 calves slaughtered in May. The remaining six calves turned out into their second grazing season on the same paddock grazed by them the previous year, but no larvae were detected in their faeces or in the pasture. Similarly, no signs of infection were observed in the lungs of two tracer calves or in the faeces of 4 calves which were turned out simultaneously on the same paddock during the second year of observation.

INTRODUCTION

Bovines are infected with lungworms by grazing pastures contaminated with *D. viviparus* larvae originating from dung pats of infected animals. Jørgensen (1980a) found that the horizontal distribution of larvae in the pasture depends on climate and on the fact that a short lived larval contamination may reach high levels in the herbage near faecal pats. The finding of such an uneven distribution of larvae may indicate that the pasture infectivity is influenced not only by climate and the numbers of larvae passed in faeces, but also by the concentration of faecal pats.

The first experiment reported in the present paper focussed on the possible effect of different stocking rates on the herbage contamination and infectivity. Observations on the infection in this experiment were extended into the next grazing season in order to study over-wintering.

During the first grazing season (1978) observations were also carried out on a neighbouring plot grazed by susceptible calves from 1st August to see whether they would acquire the infection.

Two more experiments, one on the role of *Pilobolus* fungi, the other on the importance of early versus late turning out, combined with tactical use of anthelmintic treatments, were carried out in 1979. They will be reported briefly here and will be published elsewhere in greater detail.

MATERIALS AND METHODS

Site

An experimental field which had not been grazed for the last five years was used. It carried a moderate trichostrongyle larval contamination originating from liquid manure which had been spread each spring. The last application was in March

1978. Otherwise the field had been used for hay production. The following numbers of Trichostrongyle L_3 were found per kg of fresh/dried herbage collected at random in spring: 3rd March: 810/3, 388, 19th April: 212/912, 19th May: O/O.

Experiment 1 was carried out in the southern end of the field dividing that part into three plots of the following sizes: Plot 1: 0.5 ha, plot 2: 0.75 ha, and plot 3: 1 ha.

Experiment 2 was carried out on the northern part of the field. A hay crop was taken on 24th June, and it was divided into plot A (0.5 ha) and plot B (1.5 ha). None of the plots had been grazed earlier the same year. They were separated from the plots of experiment 1 by an electric fence.

Animals, experimental design and management

Experiment 1 included 21 indoor reared female Red Danish dairy breed calves with a mean body weight of 130 kg (range 100 - 185 kg). The calves were divided into 3 groups of 7 calves each. All calves were artificially infected with third stage larvae at a dose rate of 2 - 3 per kg bodyweight on 23rd May. All groups were turned out on the same day to graze separately on the three plots. Thirty per cent of each plot was fenced off on 6th June and re-opened on 11th July to regulate grass availability. From 19th September the fences between the plots were removed and on 14th October the grazing experiment was terminated.

Experiment 2 involved eight indoor reared Friesian female calves with an average bodyweight of 170 kg (range 135 - 200 kg). They had been fed intensively and were all in a correspondingly good state of nutrition. On 1st August the calves were turned out on plot A. It was grazed close after approximately one month and on 19th September the calves were moved to plot B where grass was abundant throughout the experiment. Experiment 2 was terminated on 11th October.

Faecal examinations

Samples were taken per rectum at weekly intervals. Ten grams of faeces from each animal were baermannised according to Nevenič et al. (1962) for 24 hours and the number of *D. viviparus* larvae present in the sediment recorded as larvae per 10 grams of faeces (LP10G).

Pasture examinations

Two herbage samples were picked from each plot at weekly intervals according to Jørgensen (1980b) and washed in a cement mixer. Grass free sediments were obtained and processed further according to Jørgensen (1975). Before processing, each sediment was split into two and processed separately to reduce variation. The number of infective *D. viviparus* larvae per kg of fresh herbage was calculated.

Post mortem

Lungs were perfused by a modification of the technique described by Inderbitzin (1976).

Climate

Recordings of temperature, rainfall and sun hours were obtained from a meteorological station situated 500 m from the experimental field. The climate during the 1978 grazing season is shown in Figure 1. The first five weeks were relatively warm, sunny and dry. Week 6 was particularly wet, cool and cloudy. After a dry, warm and sunny August, the weather changed again around 1st September.

RESULTS

Experiment 1

Grass availability

Differences in grass availability were first noted on 13th June. This and further observations are summarised in Table 1.

220

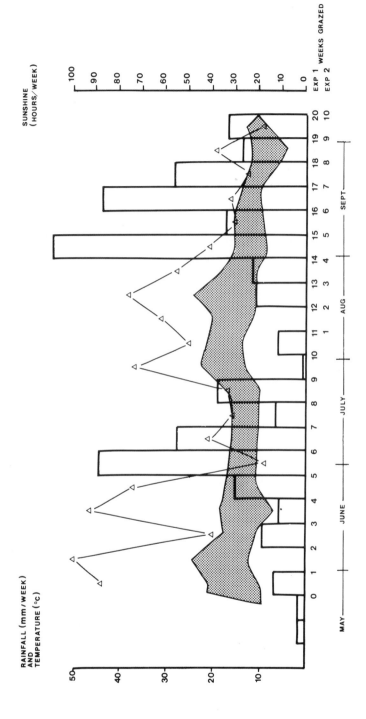

Fig. 1. Climatic recordings during 1978 grazing season. Mean weekly maximum and minimum temperatures (shaded area) recorded 2 m above ground level; hours of sunshine (-o-) and millimeters of precipitation (histogram) per week.

TABLE 1

SUMMARY OF OBSERVATIONS ON GRASS AVAILABILITY IN EXPERIMENT 1

Date	No. of weeks grazed	Observations
13th June	3	Plot 1 grazed closer than plot 3.
20th June	4	Obvious differences in grass availability according to stocking rates.
7th July	7	Plot 1 grazed close. Areas of 50 - 100 cm diameter around faecal pats partly grazed. Slightly more grass on plot 2. Plot 3 grazed close on 1/3 of its area only; herbage around faecal pats ungrazed.
1st August	10	The lush herbage around faecal pats on plot 1 constituted 30 - 50% of the area, but 80 - 90% of the herbage on the plot.

Clinical observations

The clinical observations are summarised in Table 2. On 11th July an outbreak in all 3 groups was observed, and the calves were allowed access to extensions with non-contaminated pasture. However, one calf (calf number 2) had ceased to graze and died three days later. Four calves (numbers 17, 24, 26 and 28) were all in a critical stage and therefore it was decided to treat all animals with an anthelmintic[*]. Despite the treatment 5 calves died or were euthanised during week 8. A marked improvement was observed among the survivors approximately 4 days after treatment. After week 9 the general condition of the calves was good with the exception of one calf (number 15), but coughing was heard, particularly after the calves were exercised. Calf number 15 coughed throughout the summer and its general condition remained poor.

[*] Fenbendazole 10% susp. (Panacur (R), Hoechst), 7.5 mg per kg bodyweight per os.

TABLE 2

SUMMARY OF CLINICAL SIGNS OBSERVED AMONG THE CALVES OF EXPERIMENT 1 DURING THE EARLY PART OF THE GRAZING PERIOD

Date	No. of weeks grazed	Observations
30th May	1	Elevated respiration (up to 120/min.) in some calves. Sunny weather.
6th June	2 3+4+5	The first coughs were heard. The only signs of verminous bronchitis were occasional coughs.
4th July	6	Coughing heard more frequently in most calves. Particularly after exercise. One calf (number 22) observed to hyperventilate.
11th July	7	Most calves appeared dull. Signs of verminous bronchitis in all three groups. Three calves (number 2, 26 and 24) showed low respiratory rate, but their respiration was pumping.

Faecal larval counts

The first larvae were detected in 6 of the calves after the third week. All calves were positive after four weeks. Details of the faecal examinations for larvae are shown in Table 3 and Figure 2. During the fourth and fifth weeks a uniform pattern of the same magnitude was observed between individuals and therefore also between the groups. The further course of the mean larval excretions of the groups up to the outbreak was dominated by large individual variations. Reshedding of larvae was observed in most calves approximately 4 weeks after treatment. It was at an extremely low level except in calf number 15 which excreted larvae in large numbers in late August and early September.

Herbage larval contamination

Lungworm larvae were first detected in herbage samples taken on plot 1 after the fourth week and on plots 2 and 3 after the fifth week. The further course of the herbage contamination with lungworm larvae is shown in Figure 3. On all three fields the contamination increased markedly during

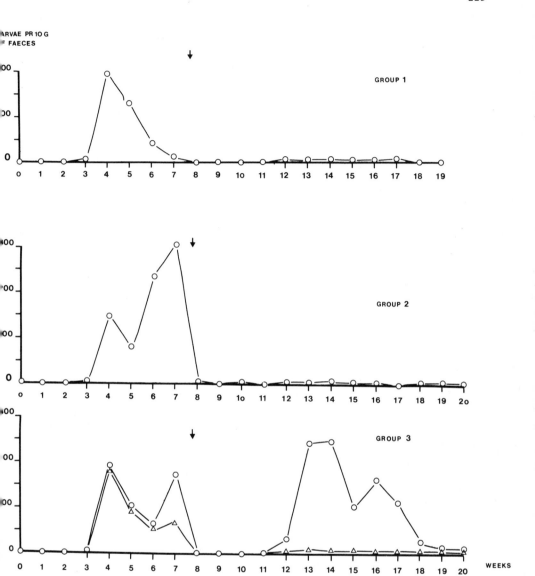

Fig. 2. Mean faecal larval counts of three groups of calves (experiment 1).
All calves were artificially infected on 23rd May, the day of
turning out, with 2 - 3 infective *D. viviparus* larvae per kg of
bodyweight. Triangles show mean counts of group 3 minus calf
No. 15. Arrows indicate anthelmintic treatments (Panacur®).

TABLE 3

FAECAL LARVAL COUNTS PER 10 g OF FAECES (LP 10 G) OF 3 GROUPS OF CALVES (EXPERIMENT 1)

	Weeks grazed after artificial infection and turning out																				
	0	1	2	3	4	5	6	7	8	9	10	11	12	13	14	15	16	17	18	19	20
Group I No. of calves positive	0	0	0	1	7	5	5	4	0	0	0	0	2	3	1	1	1	1	0	0	0
No. of calves examined	7	7	7	7	7	7	7	7	5	5	5	5	5	5	5	5	5	5	5	5	5
Mean LP 10 G	0	0	0	0.6	196	93	24	6	0	0	0	0	0.6	3	0.2	0.2	0.4	0	0	0	0
Group II No. of calves positive	0	0	0	3	7	7	6	7	3	0	1	0	3	3	3	2	3	0	1	1	2
No. of calves examined	7	7	7	7	7	7	7	7	6	6	6	6	6	5	5	5	5	5	5	5	5
Mean LP 10 G	0	0	0	0.6	151	82	273	309	0.8	0	0.2	0	2	3	8	6	2	0	1	0.6	0.4
Group III No. of calves positive	0	0	0	1	7	7	7	4	0	0	0	0	3	3	5	4	5	2	4	2	4
No. of calves examined	7	7	7	7	7	7	7	7	6	5	5	5	5	5	5	5	5	5	5	5	5
Mean LP 10 G	0	0	0	1	193	103	66	170	0	0	0	0	30	245	449	105	163	114	28	9	12
Group III minus calf No. 15 Mean LP 10 G	0	0	0	3	184	97	54	66	0	0	0	0	1	12	2	2	3	0.3	2	0.3	2

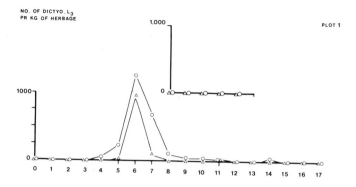

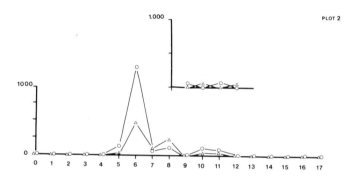

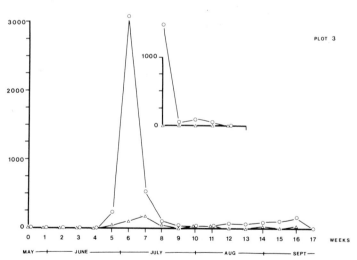

Fig. 3. Herbage contamination with lungworm larvae on plots 1, 2, and 3 of experiment 1. Results of separate sampling of extensions (not grazed 6 June – 11 July) are inserted: o samples taken 5 cm from faecal pats: △ samples taken at least 100 cm away from faecal pats.

week 6, peaked after the 6th week and dropped rapidly during
the next one or two weeks. By comparing the peaks occurring
on 4th July on the three plots it appears that it was of the
same magnitude near faecal pats on plots 1 and 2 whereas
considerably more larvae were recovered from plot 3. The
contamination away from faecal pats appeared, peaked, and
decreased simultaneously with the contamination close to faeces,
but at a lower level. On plot 1 it constituted approximately
80% and on plots 2 and 3 approximately 30% and 3%, respectively,
of the contamination close to faeces. With the exception of
a few larvae recovered close to faeces after week 14, no
larvae were detected on plot 1 after the 12th week and onwards.
During the same period no larvae were recovered from plot 2,
whereas on plot 3 low numbers were recovered from most samples
taken in late summer.

Pooled samples were picked on plot 1 plus plots 2 and 3
in autumn and early winter. Low numbers (3 - 28 per kg herbage)
were recovered. The last sample, taken on 12th December, was
negative.

Infective trichostrongyle larvae were also enumerated in
the samples taken in order to compare fluctuations occurring in
both groups of parasitic larvae. The results are presented in
Figure 4. Although this contamination was high in early spring
(see Materials and Methods) only few larvae were recovered
during the first month of grazing. During the second month a
pattern similar to, but less uniform than the one observed
with lungworm larvae, was observed. Large fluctuations in
numbers appeared in late summer, particularly on plots 1 and 2.
The horizontal distribution of this contamination did not show
a distinct pattern, although most larvae were recovered near
faecal pats on most dates.

Post mortem examinations

The lungs of the five calves which died during week 8 were
all found to be over-inflated with lung emphysema and petecchial

227

NO. OF TRICHO. L_3
PR KG OF HERBAGE

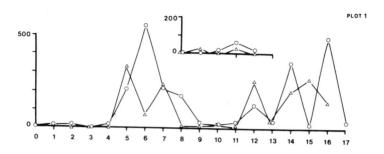

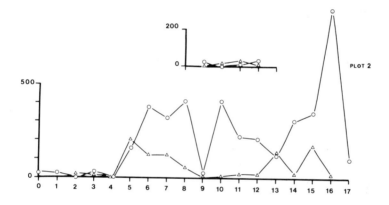

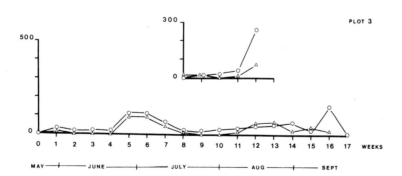

Fig. 4. Herbage contamination with infective trichostrongyle larvae on
plots 1, 2 and 3 of experiment 1. Results of separate sampling
of extensions are inserted. o samples taken 5 cm from faecal
pats. Δ samples taken at least 100 cm away from faecal deposits.

and lobular bleedings. Perfusion revealed very few visible worms in the air passages. The details of the macroscopic and microscopic examinations of material collected by perfusion are included in Table 4. The size distribution of recovered lungworms from two calves with a reasonable number of worms is included in Figure 5.

TABLE 4

WORMS RECOVERED BY PERFUSION OF LUNGS OF CALVES WHICH DIED OR WERE EUTHANISED. 'OTHER SPECIES' INCLUDES IMMATURE NEMATODES, MOST OF THEM WITH A *Cooperia-Ostertagia* TYPE OF MORPHOLOGY.

| Experiment | Calf No. | Date | Lungworms | | Other species |
			> 3 cm	Total	
I	2[*)	14th July	15	1 298	30
I	28[*)	16th July	30	1 949	25
I	17[*)	16th July	0	555	10
I	8[*)	17th July	0	78	15
I	13[*)	20th July	0	305	5
II	42[**)	10th Oct.	350	864	150

[*) Treated with fenbendazole (Panacur ®, Hoechst) on 14th July.
[**) Treated with same on 10th October.

Further observations during stabling and during the second grazing season

Eleven of the calves, including number 15, were available for further observations after the grazing experiment was terminated. Calf number 15 was observed to cough during the winter. Faecal examinations of this calf on 29th November revealed 2 LP 10 G, whereas all other calves were negative. All calves were negative on the following dates during stabling: 31st January, 14th February, 8th and 20th March, 3rd and 19th April, 1st and 8th May. Five calves were slaughtered on 17th May. Perfusion of their lungs revealed one specimen (5 mm) of *D. viviparus*.

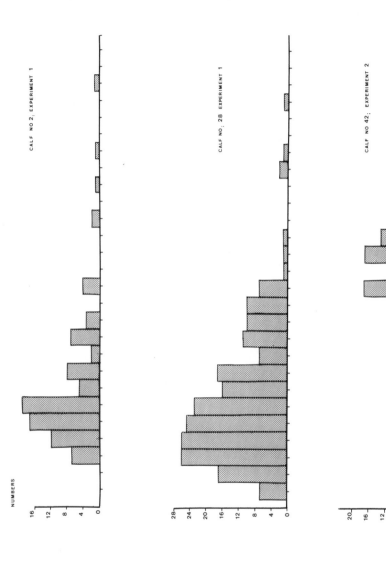

Fig. 5. Size distribution of worms recovered from lungs of calves numbers 2 and 28 of experiment 1, determined during the 8th week of grazing, and of calf number 42 of experiment 2, determined after 10 weeks of grazing

The remaining 6 animals, including number 15, were turned out on 22nd May, 1979, together with six susceptible calves on the field used the previous year (the fences between plots 1, 2 and 3 were removed). Two of the calves were grazed for the first two weeks only. They were stabled for two weeks, then slaughtered and examined for *D. viviparus* by perfusion of their lungs. Both were negative. Weekly sampling of the grazing heifers and calves as well as the pasture grazed by them during May, June, July and August failed to reveal any *D. viviparus* larvae. Number 15 coughed at intervals; otherwise no signs of respiratory disease were observed. (During the same period and therefore under the same climatic conditions, outbreaks of verminous bronchitis occurred on the northern part of the field (Jørgensen, 1980c) initiated by over-wintered larvae originating from experiment 2).

Experiment 2

Clinical signs and *post mortem* examination

The first coughs were heard after eight weeks (26th September). Hyperventilation was first noticed one week later (3rd October). During the next few days some of the calves developed signs of severe verminous bronchitis. On 10th October one of these calves (number 42) ceased to graze, to drink and to pass faeces and it was euthanised on the same day. Its lungworm burden is included in Table 4 and Figure 5. The experiment was terminated when the remaining calves were treated on 11th October.

Faecal and herbage examinations for *D. viviparus* larvae

The results of the individual faecal examinations are shown in Table 5, and the mean larval count is presented in Figure 6, which also shows the pasture larval contamination.

Randomly collected herbage samples were also taken at weekly intervals before the calves were turned out. They were all negative except on 4th July, where a contamination of 20 larvae per kg of herbage were found (compare peak occurrence

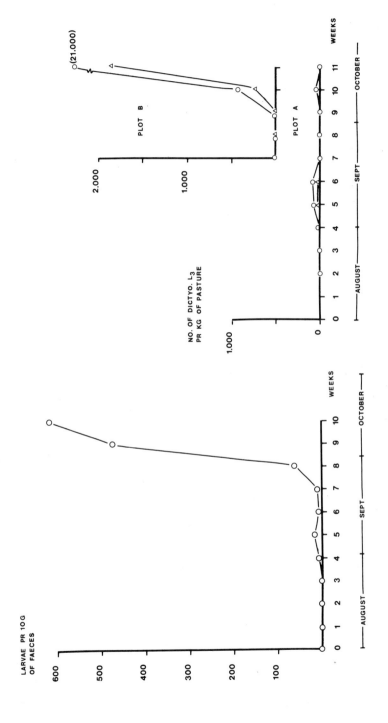

Fig. 6. Mean faecal larval counts (left) and pasture larval contamination (right) of experiment 2. The calves were turned out on 1st August and moved from plot A to plot B on 15th September. Herbage samples were picked near (o) and away (Δ) from faecal pats.

of the pasture contaminations of experiment 1 as shown in
Figure 3).

TABLE 5

INDIVIDUAL FAECAL LARVAL COUNTS PER 10 g OF FAECES OF 8 SUSCEPTIBLE CALVES
TURNED OUT TO GRAZE ON 1st AUGUST (EXPERIMENT 2). THE PLOT HAD NOT BEEN
GRAZED PREVIOUSLY. AN OUTBREAK HAD BEEN RECORDED ON ADJACENT FIELDS
(EXPERIMENT 1)

Calf No.	August		September				October	
	Weeks grazed:							
	0 - 3	4	5	6	7	8	9	10
41	0	0	0	0	14	49	1 203	3 443
42	0	0	0	0	0	116	1 137	11 608
43	0	0	0	0	6	208	1 231	431
44	0	2	3	1	17	130	82	235
45	0	6	1	0	0	21	79	180
46	0	19	30	2	1	17	23	6
47	0	0	0	0	5	10	1	1
48	0	5	101	31	3	29	6	12

After four weeks of grazing larvae were detected in the
faeces of four of the calves as well as in the herbage picked
close to faecal pats. From Table 5 it appears that larvae
were not detected in the remaining calves until they had grazed
for 7 or 8 weeks. An initial pasture contamination was
observed on plot A (Figure 6). It culminated during week 6.
The increased larval excretion during weeks 8, 9 and 10 resulted
in an extremely steep rise in the pasture larval contamination
of the grazed plot (plot B) close to as well as away from
faecal pats.

Herbage larval contamination of plot B during the winter 1978 - 1979

The late occurrence of high numbers of viable *D. viviparus*
larvae on plot B made it possible to quantitate the contamination
during the following winter. Forty randomly selected faecal
pats were each marked with an iron fencing post to facilitate

their recognition. The results of the pasture examinations are shown in Figure 7. The lungworm larval counts dropped rapidly in autumn and in spring, whereas apparently the larvae resisted frost and snow. The pattern observed was similar in samples picked close to as well as away from the pats. The trichostrongyle pasture contamination showed a different pattern. It did not decrease in the autumn, and low but significant numbers were recovered in late April - early May close to faecal pats. Away from faeces a reduction was observed between autumn and spring.

As a supplement to the samples collected on the field during the winter five kg of grass were collected on 17th November near faecal pats and left on an unheated hayloft. In January the herbage appeared dry. The number of viable lungworm larvae found per kg of dried herbage is shown in Table 6. The table shows that the numbers dropped more rapidly than those on the field. The most marked decrease took place when the sample turned into hay.

TABLE 6

LUNGWORM LARVAL CONTAMINATION OF A GRASS SAMPLE STORED UNDER DRY CONDITIONS ON AN UNHEATED HAYLOFT. THE SAMPLE WAS PICKED ON 17TH NOVEMBER AROUND FAECAL PATS OF A HEAVILY CONTAMINATED FIELD (PLOT B OF EXPERIMENT 2).

	4th Dec.	12th Dec.	19th Dec.	9th Jan.	6th Apr.
Dictyo. L_3/kg of dried herbage	1 975	1 350	1 100	68	10

DISCUSSION

Experiment 1   The purpose of infecting the calves artificially was to introduce the infection at a low initial level considered to be comparable to a natural over-wintered pasture larval contamination. The mild clinical symptoms observed during the first 6 weeks were undoubtedly the result of this infection. The rapid aggravation of the clinical condition of most calves during weeks 7 and 8 was unexpected.

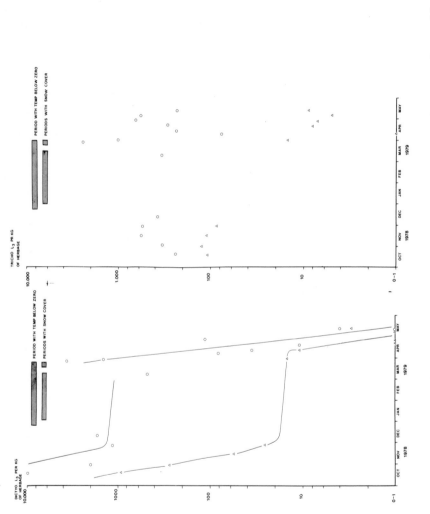

Fig. 7. Viable *D. viviparus* L_3 and trichostrongyle L_3 quantitated on the same herbage samples collected during the period October 1978 – May 1979 from plot B of experiment 2. o samples taken 5 cm from faecal pats. △ samples taken at least 100 cm away from faecal droppings.

The dull appearance together with the very limited larval excretion of some of the diseased calves during the outbreak and the low number of macroscropically visible worms in the calf that died before treatment was given did not preclude that other causes of disease could be involved. However, from the details of the *post mortem* and of the herbage examinations it was obvious that the clinical condition in all three groups was caused by a severe prepatent superinfection.

By comparing Figures 2 and 3 it appears that the larval excretion of the three groups in late June resulted in pasture peaks which occurred with a remarkable regularity on the three plots considering the uncertainty with which pasture larval counts are obtained. This indicates that the climatic conditions were particularly favourable during this period.

The differences in the pasture contamination between the plots at their peak occurrence may be seen in relation to stocking rate and grass availability. On plot 3 where the vegetation was high on most parts of the plot, the new generation of lungworm larvae and the overwintered trichostrongyle larvae showed marked differences in their horizontal distribution. It is likely that uniform moisture conditions were responsible for the uniform distribution of the trichostrongyle larvae. The horizontal distribution of the lungworm larvae was on the other hand poor. If lungworm larvae are predominantly *Pilobolus* translated (Robinson, 1962) then the high contamination near faecal pats of plot 3 may be explained on the basis that a high proportion of larvae-carrying sporangiae were caught after their discharge in the high vegetation near the pats. The differences between the plots in the lungworm larval contamination away from faeces may be explained by a simple dilution effect, since the sizes of the areas sampled are inversely correlated to stocking rate. This contamination away from faeces is of particular interest. It is this part of the pasture which is preferred by cattle and it is therefore grazed predominantly, provided sufficient herbage is available on it.

Differences in clinical conditions or larval excretion similar to the differences in the pasture contaminations could not be demonstrated between the groups of the present experiment however. There are two possible explanations for this. Firstly, the contamination reached pathogenic levels on all three plots due to the very favourable climatic conditions for translation during weeks 5 and 6. Secondly, any such differences were overshadowed by large individual variations seen between the relatively small number of calves within each group. The particular course of infection in calf number 15 is interesting. Apparently protective immunity failed to develop, resulting in poor clinical condition throughout its first grazing season and in raised pasture contamination of plot 3 in late summer due to high levelled reshedding of larvae.

Experiment 2 It has been mentioned in the past that fields which have not been grazed for a prolonged period in summer and from which a hay crop has been taken, can still be infective to grazing stock (Michel and Shand, 1955). This was confirmed recently in the detailed study by Duncan et al. (1979) where two possibilities were mentioned as obvious explanations to the presence of lungworm larvae on such fields in August, i.e. prolonged survival of larvae and windborne field-to-field transmission of larvae by *Pilobolus* sporangiae. In the present study the demonstration of a few larvae in the herbage of plot A on 4th July, i.e. before it was grazed, obviously originated from the neighbouring plots of experiment 1 where the pasture contamination culminated on the same date, since no cattle or deer were present within a distance of several kilo-meters from the experimental area. Similarly, the transmission of the infection to the calves within a few days after turning out shows a very efficient and rapid mode of spread which is not contradictory to the *Pilobolus* theory.

The fact that only some calves acquired patent infections initially is similar to observations made by the author in 1974 (Jørgensen, 1980a) and in 1979 (Jørgensen, 1980c), and shows that the initial infection was at a low level. The calves harbouring patent infections gave rise to a pasture contamination during weeks 5 and 6. It is likely that the uptake of these larvae boosted the larval excretion 3 weeks later which again resulted in extremely high pasture larval counts after a further week. Similarly to the previously mentioned studies there is a tendency that the calves which did not acquire patent infections initially were suffering most during the second cycle of the infection. Therefore the phenomenon may be of general interest in the understanding of large individual variations seen in the onset and severity of verminous bronchitis in grazing stock.

The survival of the lungworm infections beyond the first grazing season

In experiment 1 the infection culminated in early July and became undetectable in faeces and herbage samples at the end of the year. Although one specimen was found in the lungs of one calf slaughtered in May, reshedding of larvae in faeces was not detected. The negative result of the second year's observations showed that the infection did not over-winter in the heifers nor in the pasture. In experiment 2 the pasture contamination culminated on plot B in the autumn. Although it decreased rapidly, it was at a high level at the beginning of the winter. By comparing the pasture results with the hay loft observations it appears that the infective larvae were more susceptible to dry conditions than to the climatic conditions on the field during the period with frost and snow. The sharp drop in the pasture contamination in spring is interesting because it seems as if the larvae die around the time where animals are normally turned out. This is in contrast to trichostrongyle larvae which may survive dry periods (Figure 4, weeks 5 and 6). The epidemiological significance of the rapid disappearance of the lungworm larvae in spring was investigated further in experiment 4 (see Addendum).

238

ADDENDUM

Two other experiments on lungworms were presented by the author during the meeting:

Experiment 3   This experiment which was carried out in 1979 by H. Rønne and C. Helsted in co-operation with the author, showed that in the absence of *Pilobolus* fungi the proportion of lungworm larvae translated from faecal pats was extremely low, and consequently the pasture infectivity towards susceptible tracer calves was greatly reduced (8 : 1) compared to the normal situation where *Pilobolus* fungi were present. The details of this experiment will be published and discussed elsewhere.

Experiment 4   A combined epidemiology and control experiment was carried out on plot B of experiment 2 in 1979. Calves turned out on 8th May all picked up over-wintered larvae. Their larval excretion gave rise to a pasture contamination reaching pathogenic levels during weeks 5 and 6, followed by an outbreak two weeks later. Another group of calves turned out on 22nd May to graze separately on the same field showed a lower level of infection and some calves did not become infected initially. Clinical disease was prevented in sub-groups by anthelmintic (tactical) drenching after the sixth and the eighth week on pasture. This experiment will also be published and discussed elsewhere (Jørgensen, 1980c).

ACKNOWLEDGEMENT

I wish to express my sincere thanks to Mr. Niels Midtgaard and Mrs. Karen Madsen for their technical assistance.

REFERENCES

Duncan, J., Armour, J., Bairden, K., Urquhart, G.M. and Jørgensen, R.J.,
  1979. Studies on the epidemiology of bovine parasitic bronchitis.
  Vet. Rec. 104, 274-278.

Inderbitzin, F., 1976. Experimentell erzeugte Entwicklungshemmung von
  Dictyocaulus viviparus des Rindes. Thesis, University of Zürich,
  Switzerland.

Jørgensen, R.U., 1975. Isolation of infective *Dictyocaulus* larvae from
  herbage. Vet. Parasitol. 1, 61-67.

Jørgensen, R.J., 1980a. Epidemiology of bovine dictyocaulosis in Denmark.
  Vet. Parasitol, 7, 153-167.

Jørgensen, R.J., 1980b. Monitoring pasture infectivity and pasture
  contamination with infective stages of *Dictyocaulus viviparus*.
  Proceedings from CEC-Workshop on 'The epidemiology and control of
  nematodiasis in cattle', Copenhagen 4th to 6th February, 1980
  (in press).

Jørgensen, R.J., 1980c. An experimental study on the epidemiology and
  prevention of naturally acquired verminous bronchitis. Acta Vet.
  Scand.

Michel, J.F. and Shand, A., 1955. A field study of the epidemiology and
  clinical manifestations of parasitic bronchitis in adult cattle.
  Vet. Rec. 67, 249-266.

Nevenič, V., Jovanovič, M., Sokolič, A., Cuperlovič, K. and Movsesijan, M.
  1962. A simple method for finding out *Dictyocaulus filaria* larvae.
  Veterinarski glasnik 16, 203-209.

Robinson, J., 1962. *Pilobolus* spp. and the translation of the infective
  larvae of *Dictyocaulus viviparus* from faeces to pastures. Nature,
  London 193, 353-354.

A NEW ASPECT OF THE EPIDEMIOLOGY OF
PARASITIC BRONCHITIS IN CALVES

J.L. Duncan and G.M. Urquhart

Wellcome Laboratory for Experimental Parasitology,
University of Glasgow, Veterinary School,
Bearsden Road, Bearsden, Glasgow, G6I IQH, UK.

For many years it has been considered that clinical out-breaks of parasitic bronchitis arose from two sources. First, that a proportion of cattle in their second or subsequent year were lightly infected with adult lungworms and contaminated the pasture with larvae immediately preceding the use of the pasture in the same year by susceptible calves.

Secondly, and perhaps more commonly, from infective larvae overwintering on vacated pastures in sufficient numbers to produce the disease in calves turned out to grass for the first time in May; in this case either the numbers of over-wintered larvae were sufficient to produce clinical signs by themselves or, alternatively, they gave rise to sub-clinical patent infections the larvae of which after becoming infective were responsible for the disease.

This second hypothesis although providing an explanation of why parasitic bronchitis commonly occurs after calves have been at pasture for 2 to 4 months, takes no account of the relatively rapid development of immunity to *D. viviparus* infection and has always been regarded by us with some reservations.

The purpose of this paper is to suggest a new explanation of the origin of outbreaks of parasitic bronchitis on grassland vacated during the winter and only grazed by susceptible calves the following May.

The design and the results of the experiments from which these observations were made were published recently (Duncan

P. Nansen, R.J. Jørgensen, E.J.L. Soulsby (eds), Epidemiology and Control of Nematodiasis in Cattle.

et al., 1979). For this reason only an outline of these is given and readers should consult the original publication for details.

Basically the observations were made over two years on a three hectare pasture where there was a history of repeated outbreaks of parasitic bronchitis.

On the 1st May 1976 two tracer calves were grazed for 17 days on the pasture which had been empty since the previous November. At the subsequent necropsies one calf had no lung worms and the other twelve. On the 17th May the pasture was divided equally and two groups of seven calves, one vaccinated with Dictol (Glaxovet, London) and the other unvaccinated, turned out to graze on the separate plots.

Within 42 days i.e. June 28th the unvaccinated calves developed clinically apparent parasitic bronchitis, larvae being recovered from their faeces 7 days later. By August three of the calves had died of the disease. Within the vaccinated group coughing was also observed in some calves although this subsided as did their respiratory rate within a few weeks.

The origins of this outbreak were rather puzzling. Despite the almost complete absence of infection on the pasture during the first half of May as shown by the two tracer calves (herbage examination for larvae was also negative at this time) a clinical outbreak occurred within 42 days on calves grazed immediately afterwards i.e. there was not enough time for any light infection to become patent and recontaminate the pasture.

Subsequently, one of the plots was closed in September and at the beginning of May was grazed by three tracer calves for one month. At necropsy, three weeks later, no evidence of lungworms was observed. Thereafter a hay crop was taken from the plot in July and in mid-August it was grazed by a further

three tracer calves for one month. Between three and four
weeks later, two of these developed clinical signs of parasitic
bronchitis and at necropsy 4 150, 621 and 101 lungworms were
recovered from the lungs of the calves.

There seemed to be two possible explanations for this
outbreak. First, that the grass on the plot had become
contaminated by lungworm larvae transported by windborne
spores of *Pilobolus* spp. (Robinson, 1962). Secondly, that a
proportion of larvae on the pasture from the previous year had
survived but were not available on the pasture when grazed by
the three tracer calves in May and were not removed with the
hay crop. This, in turn, suggests that these larvae may have
overwintered in the soil and had only emerged onto the pasture
in July. There was little chance that they had survived over
this period in dung-pats since these had disintegrated
completely during the winter.

In summary, one of these episodes of clinical disease
occurred in June and the following year in late August. In
both cases there was evidence that the pastures were free or
almost so of lungworm larvae during the weeks immediately
preceding their being grazed by the calves which developed
parasitic bronchitis.

It is suggested that infective *D. viviparus* larvae overwintering in the soil might have emerged onto the pasture in
May and in July respectively during these two years.

We are attempting to test the validity of this theory
by the examination of core samples of soil, at fortnightly
intervals over a period of twelve months, from a pasture of
which an outbreak of parasitic bronchitis had occurred. If
confirmed, this explanation would go a long way towards
explaining the susceptibility of calves to lungworm infection
despite their having been at grass for two or three months and
having an opportunity to acquire immunity.

These observations also suggest that current anthelmintic regimens for the control of bovine ostertagiasis are unlikely also to prevent lungworm infection. In neither of the outbreaks described i.e. one in June and the other on aftermath in August would one have anticipated the strategic use of anthelmintics for parasitic gastroenteritis.

REFERENCES

Duncan, J.L., Armour, J., Bairden, K., Urquhart, G.M. and Jørgensen, R.J., 1969. Studies on the epidemiology of parasitic bronchitis. Veterinary Record, 104, 274-278.

Robinson, J., 1962. *Pilobolus* spp. and the translation of the infective larvae of *Dictyocaulus viviparus* from faeces to pasture. Nature, 193, 353-354.

DISCUSSION

F.H.M. Borgsteede *(The Netherlands)*

Everyone who has a culture of lungworm in his laboratory
has problems with the passages. You need a lot of passages
every year - in our laboratory we need five - to maintain
lungworm infection. In a refrigerator they stay alive in
water for two or three months. How can you explain the survival
of *Dictyocaulus* larvae in the soil for almost a year? In the
laboratory, under ideal circumstances, one cannot achieve lungworm larval survival for longer than half that time.

G. Urquhart *(UK)*

If the larvae do survive in the soil from September until
August then the circumstances in laboratory conditions are
not ideal. Perhaps there are more suitable conditions in the
soil for example in the herbage mat. Larvae are difficult to
keep in a viable condition, particularly in water; however
they do survive on grass perfectly well.

R.J. Thomas *(UK)*

It is puzzling that larvae appear late in the season. I
am quite prepared to believe it is possible that they will
survive in soil, although they do not in the laboratory,
because I have a feeling they are better adapted to survival
in soil than they are in Petri dishes. But it's still puzzling
that they appear so late in the year, especially when the soil
warms up normally much earlier leading to events such as the
nematodirus hatching of nematodiasis eggs. On sheep pastures,
we tend to find that the overwintered larval pasture count goes
down, and it is relatively low. We get a rise around April or
May which looks like activation of dormant larvae from somewhere, however this occurs when, meteorologically, you would
expect it. It is a bit puzzling therefore with the present
experiment that it should occur so late in the year.

G. Urquhart

    I am not suggesting that they appeared just before these calves went out because the tracer calves went out in May. Conceivably, the larvae could have appeared in June, July or August. The point is that they were not removed by the taking of a hay crop. One might have anticipated most of them would have been removed by this.

R.J. Thomas

    This suggests that it was a July activation.

J. Eckert *(Switzerland)*

    We have found, under our conditions in the midlands with tracer calves that there was no infection of tracer calves until the end of June. The first lungworms were picked up in July or the beginning of August. But in this connection I have one question. Did the tracer calves also pick up trichostrongylid infections? Secondly, what about water-borne infections. Dr. Duwel showed, many years ago, that lungworm larvae may be transported by water and acquired by the animal as a water-borne infection.

G. Urquhart

    These calves were kept free of gastro-intestinal parasites in the first experiment, by thiabendazole treatment every fort-night. In the second year the tracer calves were not treated in any way, so they may have picked up very small numbers of *Ostertagia* in the three weeks on pasture. As far as water-borne transmission goes: we certainly have plenty of water at the experimental site, but I do not think it flowed from field to field.

J-P. Raynaud *(France)*

    In your experience, if you had calves vaccinated early in the season, is it possible these animals would not be challenged by pastural infection? If you had put such animals

on the pasture in August/September do you think they would
have retained their immunity?

G. Urquhart

There has only been one experiment done on duration of
immunity. Cows were vaccinated and experimentally challenged,
I believe one month, and four months afterwards. There was a
very high degree of immunity, protection falling from approximately 97% to 92%. Yes, there would be immunity, as far as
can be assessed from the published evidence.

R.M. Jones *(UK)*

There seem to be two alternatives regarding the source
of the lungworm larvae: either they were on the pasture all
the time, or there was an external source. For example, do
wild ruminants play any part at all in bringing in lungworm?

G. Urquhart

I do not know! Certainly not to the extent that would
precipitate an outbreak.

R.J. Jørgensen *(Denmark)*

I have a question on the survival of larvae in the
pasture or on the grass. At one point you said that the
number of larvae seemed to drop very rapidly, but later on
you said that they persist quite well. Could you explain?

G. Urquhart

It was an observation based on your own work. In view
of the way larvae increase on pasture in spring and then disappear from pasture, can one assume that they disappear into
the soil? It is remarkable in the way that they just disappear
and cannot be found by the best-known techniques; larvae
cannot be found during the April/May/June period.

R.J. Jørgensen

I think those things are correct, of course. It is a central point in the epidemiology that, though one discusses the majority of larvae, how they disseminate and, how they disappear, nevertheless, we have also to consider the few larvae which may survive; the proportion of larvae which may go somewhere else - as you say, possibly into the soil and which may be responsible for the initiation of disease.

G. Urquhart

I think this is true. Very small numbers of lungworms will cause clinicial signs. I agree, yes.

H.-J. Bürger (FRG)

Mr. Bunke in our laboratory has shown, in laboratory experiments, that the death rate of *Dictyocaulus* larvae is very high during the first days, including first stage larvae as well as the third stage larvae. This depends upon the temperature at which the larvae are kept. If larvae are kept at relatively high temperatures of 25°C, the majority of larvae will die very rapidly. At a relative humidity of 95% they will be killed in a very short time also. These conditions are similar to those we have in summer, outside, and which may explain, at least in part, why large numbers of larvae disappear from the pasture so rapidly. This was the situation when we sampled a couple of pastures which were heavily contaminated by some sick animals. The larvae disappeared from the pasture very rapidly although we looked at them at close intervals. However, when we maintained the larvae at a 5°C, or even below that, we were able to keep a small proportion of these larvae alive for half a year. This may be the answer to your question.

PARASITOLOGICAL EFFECT OF ALTERNATE GRAZING OF CATTLE AND SHEEP[1]

F. Inderbitzin, J. Eckert and H.R. Hofmann

Institute for Parasitology, University of Zürich,
Association for the Advancement for Forage Crop Production,
Zürich, Switzerland.

ABSTRACT

Preliminary results of a 4 year trial on alternate grazing of cattle and sheep carried out on a pre-alpine pasture in Switzerland indicated that the use of sheep pastures by cattle during the second part of the grazing period (July – September) resulted in reduced faecal egg counts and serum-pepsinogen levels in cattle. This effect was pronounced if the calves were treated with fenbendazole (7.5 mg/kg body weight) before a change of pasture at the beginning of July.

The alternate grazing appeared to be advantageous also for a well balanced plant population on pasture.

[1] Supported by the Government of the Kanton of Zürich

INTRODUCTION

Reports from Great Britain, Norway, Australia and other countries (Barger, 1978) indicate that sequential stocking of a pasture by cattle and sheep may lead to reduced burdens of gastrointestinal nematodes and better weight gains in both animal species. The major reason for the efficacy of this system of alternate grazing appears to be the relative host specificity of sheep and cattle trichostrongylids.

In some areas of Switzerland, and other countries, it is difficult to provide 'safe' pastures in parasitic control programmes. Therefore, a 5 year trial was initiated in Spring 1976 to study the parasitological effect and other aspects of alternate grazing of cattle and sheep. After 4 years, preliminary results are presented here with special reference to cattle.

EXPERIMENTAL DESIGN AND METHODS

Animal groups.

Cattle and sheep for the trial were divided into 4 groups (Table 1). Cattle of group K grazed only on cattle pastures and sheep of group S only on sheep pastures during the whole grazing period. The cattle group KS began to graze on cattle pastures in May, and this group was moved in July to sheep pastures which had been used from May to July by sheep of group SK. Similarly, sheep of group SK grazed on sheep pastures in May and were moved in July to the cattle pastures grazed previously by cattle of group KS.

Each year new groups of cattle, which were 5 - 6 months old in May, were introduced into the experiment at the beginning of the grazing period. The cattle had been raised indoors and were adapted to grazing conditions about 1 month before the experiment on a clean or slightly contaminated pasture.

TABLE 1.

ANIMAL GROUPS AND EXPERIMENTAL DESIGN

| Group | Grazing | | Number of animals |
	Duration (in weeks)	Management	
Cattle K	May-September (19-20)	only cattle pasture	6-8
KS	May-July (9-11) July-September (8-10)	cattle pasture sheep pasture	6-8
Sheep S	May-September (19-20)	only sheep pasture	lambs 8-13 ewes 8-10
SK	May-July (9-11) July-September (8-10)	sheep pasture cattle pasture	lambs 8-15 ewes 8-10

The same ewes were used throughout the experiment, but every year 3 to 4 old animals were replaced by younger ones. Every year the lambs which were born in winter or Spring were included into the experiment.

Pastures and grazing management.

The trial was conducted in a pre-alpine area in the Kanton of Zürich. The pasture, at 900 - 1000 m altitude, was divided by fences into 5 sections, each of four paddocks, to accommodate the 4 experimental groups. Each animal group was allocated to 5 different paddocks, each being grazed sequentially for about 4 to 10 days, so that the group returned to the first paddock on average after about 30 days. The total pasture area comprised 2.7 ha. The stocking rates of the pasture were comparable for the 4 animal groups. Anthelmintic treatment was not applied during the experiments in the first 3 years of the trial. In 1979 all groups were treated in July with one dose of fenbendazole (7.5 mg/kg body weight, 10% suspension Panacur®).

Methods.

The following techniques were used:

Counts of gastrointestinal nematode eggs were made using a modified McMaster technique utilising 4 g faecal samples

Determinations of serum pepsinogen levels followed the method of Hirschowitz (1955) as modified by Jennings (pers. communication).

Post mortem examination of 6 cattle and 10 lambs were conducted at the end of each grazing period (Eisenegger and Eckert, 1975).

Body weights were determined 5 - 7 times during each grazing season and the plant population, dry matter contents of the herbage and the contents of nutritive substances were determined.

RESULTS

The following results were obtained:

Egg counts of cattle.

In the first 2 years of the experiment (1976, 1977) (see Figure 1) average egg counts were comparatively low, and no significant differences were present between cattle grazing only on cattle pastures (K group) and those of the KS group which used sheep pastures in the second half of the grazing season. In 1978 egg counts of the K group appeared to be generally higher than in the KS group, but the differences were only statistically significant at the end of July, in August and mid-September.

In 1979 (see Figure 2) egg counts of cattle were low after anthelmintic treatment in July in both groups. An increase was observed in the K group during August and September being finally higher than in the KS group. In September the differences were statistically significant.

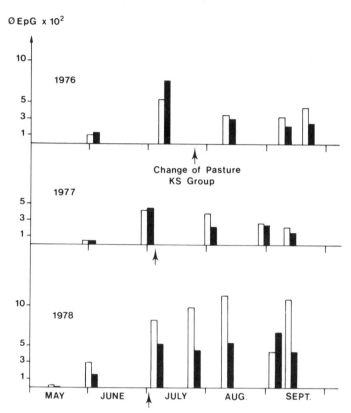

□ Only Cattle Pasture (K) n = 6 - 8

■ May - July : Cattle Pasture
July - Sept. : Sheep Pasture } (KS) n = 6 - 8

ØEpG x 10²

1976

Change of Pasture
KS Group

1977

1978

MAY   JUNE   JULY   AUG.   SEPT.

Fig. 1. Average counts of trichostrongyle eggs in cattle.

Serum-pepsinogen values of cattle.

Examinations of the pepsinogen levels were carried out in 1978 and 1979 only. The values were below 1 unit (= u) tyrosin/ℓ in May and June 1978 (Figure 3). A marked increase occurred in the K group at the beginning of July and was consistent with the increase of egg counts. The values of this group were significantly higher during July and August as compared with the KS group. In the same period a continuous increase in the KS group was observed. At the end of the grazing period in September the values of both groups did not differ markedly.

254

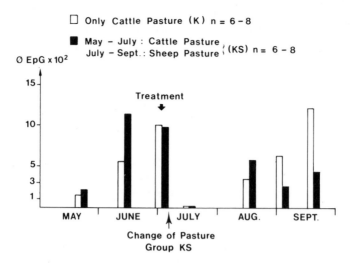

Fig. 2. Average counts of trichostrongyle eggs in cattle 1979.

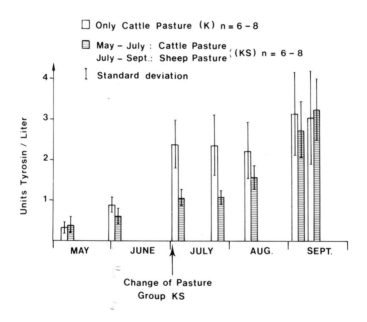

Fig. 3. Average serum-pepsinogen levels of cattle 1978.

At this time average values of about 3 units with maximum individual levels of 4.819 u were observed.

In 1979 (Figure 4) the pepsinogen values were relatively low until July. In August and September high levels were measured in the K group which had been treated in July but remained on the same contaminated pastures. On the other hand there was no increase of the pepsinogen values in the KS group which also had been treated but which had been moved thereafter to sheep pastures. The differences in August and September were significant.

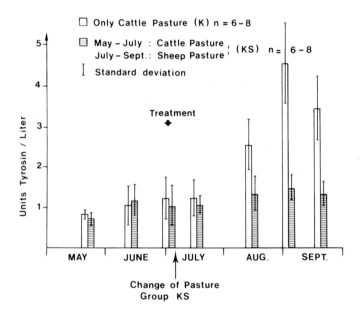

Fig. 4. Average serum-pepsinogen levels of cattle 1979.

Post mortem examination of cattle.

The worm counts only reflect the status at the end of the grazing period as animals were slaughtered at this time. Individual counts varied widely, and no significant differences were observed between the average worm counts of the K and KS groups.

256

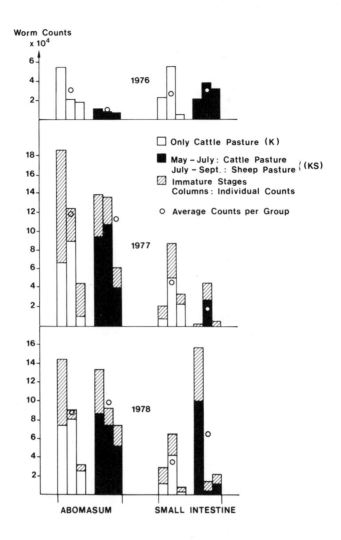

Fig. 5.   Total counts of trichostrongylids of cattle slaughtered:
September, end of grazing season.

Nematode species differentiation is not yet completed,
however, preliminary data indicate that cross transmission of
sheep nematodes to cattle was of a limited nature. The worm
burdens of cattle examined in 1978 consisted mainly of typical
cattle trichostrongylids, such as *Ostertagia ostertagi, Cooperia
oncophora, C. zurnabada* and *Nematodirus helvetianus* ; only small
numbers of *Haemonchus contortus* were found, and no *Trichostrongylus*
species were present.

Body weight gains.

The average daily weight gain of group KS was better in every year of the study compared with the K group. However, the differences were not statistically significant, which was probably due to the small number of animals and to the wide individual variations.

Plant population.

The flora of the paddocks had altered during the first 3 years of the trial, especially in the paddocks grazed only by sheep or only by cattle. In these paddocks plants which are refused by the corresponding animal species increased in number.

This happened, for example, with the graminaceous species *Festuca rubra* which was found twice as often in the paddocks grazed by sheep only, as compared with the paddocks grazed only by cattle. Vice versa, the herb species *Alchemilla vulgaris* was found to have doubled in density on paddocks grazed only by cattle compared with pure sheep paddocks.

CONCLUSIONS

From these preliminary data the following conclusions can be drawn:

The egg output in the K and KS groups was not markedly different in the first two years of the experiment. In 1978 and 1979 the cattle of K group (without pasture change) excreted more eggs in July, August and September, but the differences were not always statistically significant.

Serum-pepsinogen levels indicated that moving of cattle at the beginning of July from their permanent pasture to sheep pastures reduced abomasal damage as compared with cattle remaining on the same pasture. This effect was more pronounced if the animals were treated before changing of pasture.

The system of alternate grazing described here is advantageous for the achievement of a well balanced plant population
on pastures.

REFERENCES

Barger, I.A., 1978. Grazing management and control of parasites in sheep.
    In: The epidemiology and control of gastrointestinal parasites of
    sheep in Australia. Donald, A.D., Southcott, W.H., Dineen, J.K., eds.,
    pp 53-63, CSIRO Division of Animal Health, Melbourne.

Eisenegger, H. and Eckert, J., 1975. Zur Epizootologie und Prophylaxe der
    Dictyocaulose und der Trichostrongylidosen des Rhindes. Schweiz. Arch.
    Tierheilk. 117, 255-286.

Hirschowitz, B.I., 1955. Pepsinogen in the blood. J. Lab. Clin. Med. 46,
    568-579.

DISCUSSION

F.H.M. Borgsteede *(The Netherlands)*

We have done a comparable experiment, though not in a bovine situation. Have you any idea of what happened with the lambs? The weight gain in lambs in our experiments grazed alternately with cattle and was much higher that it was for cows.

F. Inderbitzin *(Switzerland)*

In lambs we only have data for egg output and worm burdens at slaughter. We have no pepsinogen levels. Therefore, it is more difficult to assess the effect in the lambs. The preliminary results indicate a more marked effect in cattle than sheep.

J. Armour *(UK)*

We have been doing similar experiments. We obtained a 90% reduction in worm burdens when there was a transfer of cattle onto sheep pasture, compared to when cattle were maintained continuously on cattle pasture and 17% of worm burdens in cattle were sheep parasites.

F. Inderbitzin

We were interested to find, at least to date, that only cattle worms were recovered in our cows.

J. Armour

In our studies 17% of the *Ostertagia* were *O. circumcincta*. It would be interesting to keep the parasite going in cattle for a 5 - 6 year period to see whether or not there was an adaptation to an alternative host.

J. Eckert *(Switzerland)*

I think we can say here that over 90% of the trichostrongylids in the abomasum were *Ostertagia ostertagi*, definitely, and also some *Ostertagia leptospicularis* and *Skrjabinagia lyrata* were present. It was surprising that there were no sheep parasites.

F. Inderbitzin

We were surprised also not to see marked differences in the worm counts. In July and August the pepsinogen levels were significantly different and I think that, had we slaughtered cattle at this time too, we would have found differences in worm counts.

J. Armour

Yes, our pepsinogen results were very similar.

F.H.M. Borgsteede

I think that if you had slaughtered at this time you would also have found large numbers of trichostrongylids.

H.J. Over *(The Netherlands)*

Have you ever mown those pastures? Or were they permanently grazed? I wondered about the change in vegetation.

F. Inderbitzin

They were never mown. They were only grazed by cattle. Since agronomists were involved in this trial, there was rather an overstocking of the pasture. The whole experimental area was only 2.7 ha. At times we had to feed concentrates because of the overstocking.

H.J. Over

Therefore, when the grazing period ended in September, between September in year number one and May of year number two, the grass was not cut?

F. Inderbitzin

It was not cut.

SESSION 3

EPIDEMIOLOGY II

Chairman: J.F. Michel

FLUCTUATIONS OF HERBAGE INFESTATION ON CALF PASTURES AND WEATHER FROM 1973 TO 1979

H.-J. Bürger

Institute of Parasitology,
Hannover School of Veterinary Medicine,
Bünteweg 17, D 3000 Hannover 71, Federal Republic of Germany.

ABSTRACT

Duplicate herbage samples were taken from pastures at the Mecklenhorst state farm from July 1973 to December 1979 at two week intervals during the grazing season and at longer intervals during the rest of the year. Larvae of gastro-intestinal nematodes were counted. Each pasture was grazed three or four times per year for approximately one to two weeks by cattle, mainly calves during their first grazing season, but occasionally by older stock. Weather records of the nearby official weather station at Hannover-Langenhagen were compared with the fluctuations of larval counts.

The number of larvae per kilogram of dry herbage was generally high in February or March, this decreased considerably during March and April and was negligible from the beginning of May to at least the beginning of July. Larval counts rose again to substantial levels between late July and early October. An additional increase to produce high levels occurred on many pastures during October or November.

The first increase during (late) summer coincided with or was preceded by a period of cool and rainy weather with at least 20 mm of precipitation evenly spread over a period of approximately one week.

P. Nansen, R.J. Jørgensen, E.J.L. Soulsby (eds), Epidemiology and Control of Nematodiasis in Cattle.

INTRODUCTION

It is well established that in many parts of the world with a temperate climate, herbage contamination with infective larvae of gastro-intestinal nematodes follows a seasonal pattern. This has been demonstrated in the northern part of the Federal Republic of Germany (Bürger, 1976) and these investigations have now been extended to include an additional three years so that data for seven years will be presented here.

MATERIAL AND METHODS

The technique used for the survey was that described by Sievers Prekehr (1973). Duplication herbage samples were taken from pastures at intervals (2 weeks during the grazing season and 4 to 8 weeks during the winter depending on weather conditions e.g. snow and ice). The pastures were at the Mecklenhorst state farm near Hannover and were grazed by groups of calves which were moved to a new paddock at 1 to 2 week intervals and were returned to a previously grazed paddock 3 or 4 times a year. Occasionally, individual pastures were grazed by older cattle in early spring or in autumn. The pastures which were selected for the presentation of data are those on which the increase of herbage contamination in the summer was early and pronounced.

Weather data were obtained from the official weather bureau at the Langenhagen airport which is close to the farm. The farm also maintains records of precipitation and air temperature.

RESULTS

There was a basic pattern of high larval counts in March, then decreasing numbers of larvae during spring and negligible numbers from the end of May until July or even later. Herbage contamination increased again after the middle of July, however, this rise occurred at different times of the season in different years (Figure 1). For example, larval counts were high at the

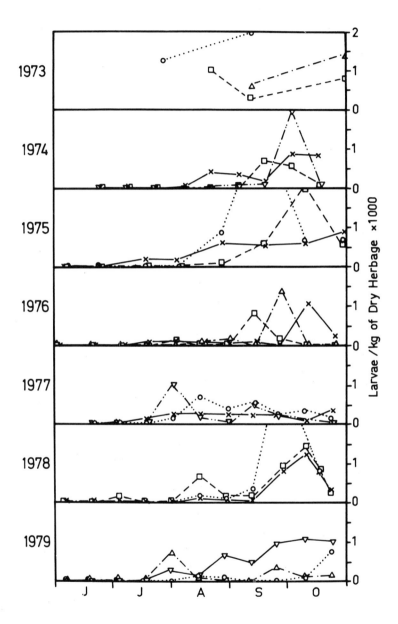

Fig. 1. Increase of herbage infestation on individual calf pastures
(O, △, □, ▽, X) in different years.

end of July in 1973, whereas high numbers of larvae occurred
only at the beginning of October in 1974 (with the exception of
moderate counts on a single pasture). In 1975, a moderate
number of larvae were present at the end of August and these
increased further during September and persisted through the
autumn. In contrast, negligible numbers of larvae were
detected until the autumn in 1976 and some pastures remained
almost free of larvae until October or November. An early rise
occurred at the end of July in 1977 and also in 1979 but this
occurred in August in 1978.

The rise in herbage contamination occurred similarly on
all pastures in most years, though 1976 was an exception to
this. This was true not only for the pastures on our experimental farm but also for other pastures which were at least
15 km from the experimental farm (Bürger, 1976). Further
investigations have shown that pasture contamination is similar
over much larger areas at similar times (Bürger, unpublished).
A comparison of the weather records and the herbage contamination
disclosed that the first increase of herbage contamination was
usually preceeded by, or coincided with, an extended period of
rain which resulted in 20 mm or above in approximately a week.
However, rainfall was not reflected in increased larval counts
if it occurred in June or the first half of July, however,
precipitation from the end of July which extended over two
successive days was followed regularly by rising herbage
contamination (Figures 2 - 8). Thus in 1979, heavy rains fell
during late July and a moderate increase of herbage infestation
was observed at that time (Figure 2). In 1978, there was a
wet, increasingly cooler period in early August and this was
followed by a small, temporary rise of larval counts and a long
wet period in September was followed by very high counts
(Figure 3). In 1977 substantial rains fell in late July and
larval counts of pasture rose immediately thereafter (Figure 4).
In 1976 the year was extremely dry until November. Rainfall
consisted of isolated heavy thunderstorms and herbage
contamination remained low generally on the majority of pastures
until November, although isolated peaks on selected pastures

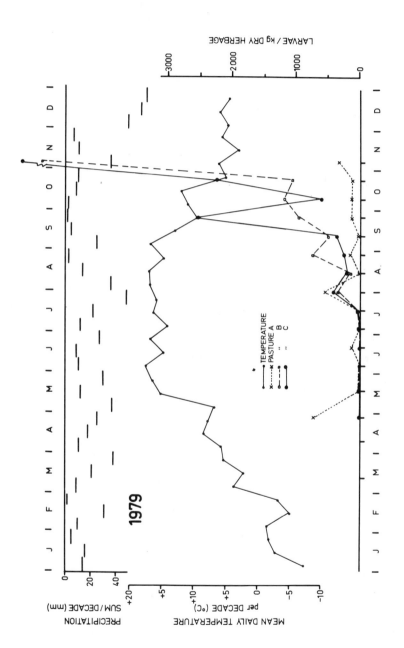

Fig. 2. Herbage infestation with infective larvae of gastro-intestinal nematodes on calf pastures and weather data.

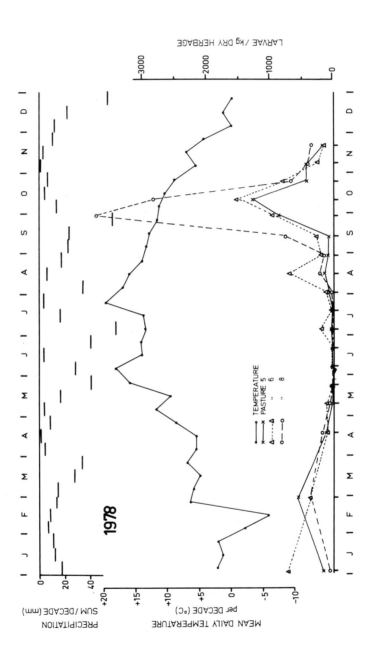

Fig. 3.   Herbage infestation with infective larvae of gastro-intestinal nematodes on calf pastures and weather data.

269

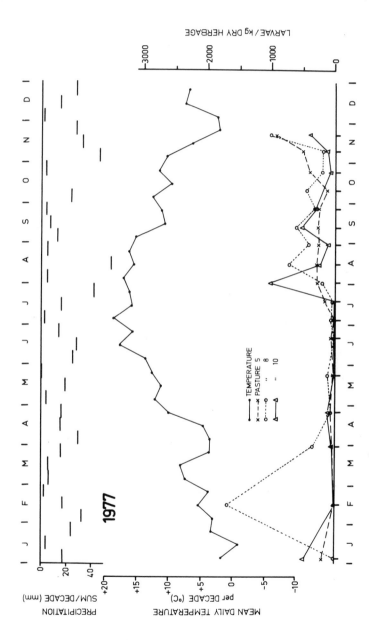

Fig. 4. Herbage infestation with infective larvae of gastro-intestinal nematodes on calf pastures and weather data.

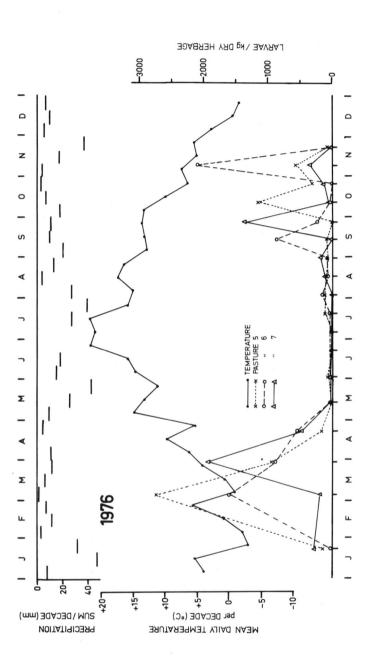

Fig. 5. Herbage infestation with infective larvae of gastro-intestinal nematodes on calf pastures and weather data.

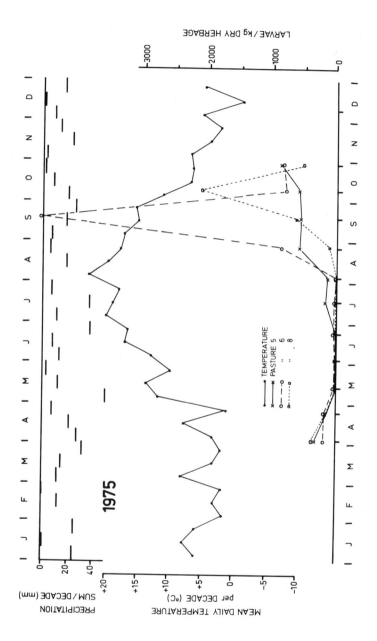

Fig. 6. Herbage infestation with infective larvae of gastro-intestinal nematodes on calf pastures and weather data.

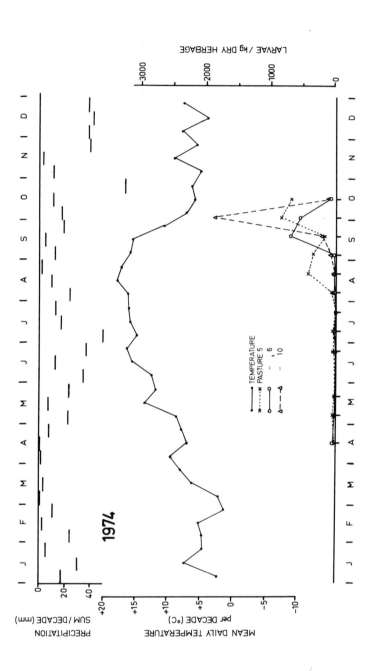

Fig. 7. Herbage infestation with infective larvae of gastro-intestinal nematodes on calf pastures and weather data

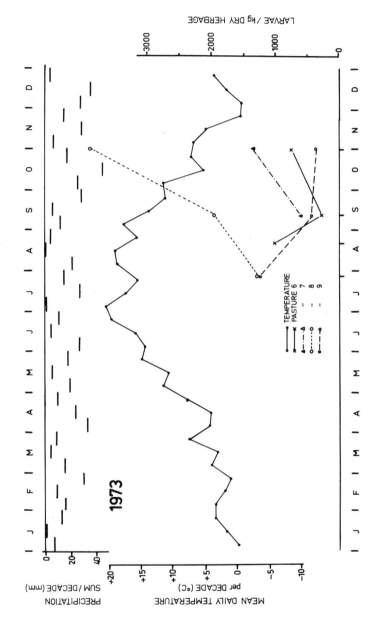
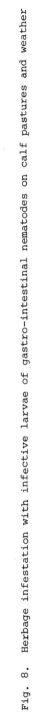

Fig. 8. Herbage infestation with infective larvae of gastro-intestinal nematodes on calf pastures and weather data.

occurred, but these had disappeared by the next sampling time
(Figure 5). In 1975 there was hardly any rain from the middle
of July unitl August. An increasing herbage contamination was
detected only at the end of August following sustained rainfall
around 10 August (Figure 6). In 1974 heavy rainfall during two
days in August resulted in total precipitation of 24 mm, but
otherwise the summer was dry until September. One pasture had
moderate larval counts in August while with the other pastures
the larval counts rose in September after a period of extended
rainfall (Figure 7). In 1973 high larval pasture counts in
late July followed two weeks of rainfall and increasingly cooler
weather from the middle of that month onwards (Figure 8).

These findings indicate that herbage contamination rose to
moderate levels generally after the middle of July but it
depended on the occurrence of rainfall spread over a period of
two successive days.

Other trends include a decrease in larval pasture counts
on most pastures after an early peak in late July or August in
1977 and 1979; this conicided with relatively dry periods from
August through October. However, herbage contamination increased
further, from moderate levels of 500 to 1 000 larvae/kg of dry
herbage in late summer, to considerably higher levels from late
September to November in other years e.g. 1973, 1975 and 1978.
Sustained rainfall occurred during September or October in
these years.

DISCUSSION

The following implications arise from the present studies.

The concept of dosing and providing animals to fresh
pasture for the control of parasitic gastro-enteritis depends
on the provision of clean pasture, usually aftermath. However,
grass may not have grown sufficiently following hay production
and in the absence of satisfactory aftermath farmers ask for

alternatives. The present study indicates that moving livestock in late July accompanied by dosing will be possible under
the conditions in the Hannover area, and this may be postponed
in some years.

On farms where two cuts for silage have been taken in
spring and early summer, a third crop will not be available
earlier than August, thus providing clean pasture only later
during the season.

The present data indicate that a further rise in the
level of herbage contamination may occur in late September or
October. This was particularly evident on some permanent
pastures, and it might be safer to remove the calves from these
pastures in late September or early October, particularly if
extended rains occur at that time.

Anthelmintic treatment is given at times in late
September when some animals have started scouring. This
practice, empirical as it is, may obviate a second rise in
herbage contamination even though it neglects the reduction in
weight gains that may occur after the midsummer rise and which
is often not noticed by the farmer.

The most important finding of this survey is that the
increase of herbage contamination in the middle of the summer
does not occur at a fixed date and the time of increasing
herbage contamination depends on the amount and duration of
rainfall after the middle of July. We have been able during
the last three years to inform the farmers about the time when
their calves fall at risk from trichostrongyle infections. We
would be in a better position to advise when we can concentrate
our efforts on grass sampling etc. following the critical
rainfall.

REFERENCES

Bürger, H.-J., 1976. Grasuntersuchungen auf ansteckungsbereite Tricho-
    strongylidenlarven in Niedersachsen. Symposium über Leberegel-,
    Magendarmwurm- und Lungenwurmbekämpfung bei Rindern. Husum, 28.-30.9.
Siever Prekehr, G.H., 1973. Methode zur Gewinnung von III. Strongyliden-
    larven aus dem Weidegras. Vet. med. Dissert., Hannover, 59 p.

THE ROLE OF THE SOIL AS A POTENTIAL RESERVOIR FOR
INFECTIVE LARVAE OF *Ostertagia ostertagi*

J. Armour, K. Bairden, I.M. Al Saqury and J.L. Duncan
Department of Veterinary Parasitology,
University of Glasgow, UK.

INTRODUCTION

During investigations into the epidemiology and control of
bovine parasitic bronchitis and ostertagiasis we have observed
outbreaks of these diseases when young cattle were introduced
onto silage or hay aftermath grazing in later summer. In
one outbreak, helminth-free calves were grazed on a hay aftermath in August and developed clinical signs of parasitic
bronchitis within 3 weeks of grazing (Duncan et al., 1979). In
another, calves grazed on a pasture with low number of
Ostertagia ostertagi infected larvae (L3) were treated with the
anthelmintic, levamisole (ICI Alderley Edge, Macclesfield,
England) and transferred to a silage aftermath in late July.
A marked increase in *O. ostertagi* L3 numbers on the aftermath
occurred within 7 days of the calves being introduced and
clinical ostertagiasis occurred 4 weeks later (Bairden et al.,
1979). In both these outbreaks the aftermath pastures had not
been grazed by livestock since the previous autumn and the
interval between entry to the aftermath and clinical or other
evidence of infection precluded the possibility of the calves
themselves being responsible for cycling of the infection.
The source of infection in these outbreaks was obscure but one
possibility considered by us and previously suggested by
Nelson (1977) in relation to *Dictyocaulus viviparus* larvae, was
the existence of a reservoir of infective larvae in the soil
which had persisted from previous grazing seasons.

To ascertain whether trichostrongyle larvae existed and
persisted in the soil we examined samples of soil taken at
regular intervals from permanent cattle pastures over the 12
month period August 1978 through July 1979. As infective

P. Nansen, R.J. Jørgensen, E.J.L. Soulsby (eds), Epidemiology and Control of Nematodiasis in Cattle.

larvae of *O. ostertagi* were regularly present in these soil
cores we attempted to quantitate more accurately the numbers
present by examining a greater number of samples during the
period October 1979 to January 1980.

MATERIAL AND METHODS

In the first series of observations (Experiment 1) 10 soil
samples were removed at monthly intervals from a plot of 0.3
hectares between August 1978 and July 1979. Individual soil
samples had an area of 28 sq. cm. and a depth of 10 cm. of soil
plus about 0.5 cm. of root/mat and surface herbage (core
samples). Each sample we divided into four layers namely:
1) herbage; 2) root-mat; 3) upper 5 cm. of soil and 4) lower
5 cm. of soil. The divisions from each sample were aggregated
and examined by the technique of Bairden et al. (1980, these
proceedings). The numbers of infective larvae of *O. ostertagi*
present were expressed as L3 per 10 soil cores.

In the second series (Experiment 2), 125 core samples
were removed at each sampling from another permanent cattle
pasture of 0.8 hectares. The decision to remove 125 samples
was based on the variation in larval numbers between samples
and from this data the number required to provide statistically
meaningful results of a quantitative nature was derived.
Sampling was carried out in October and November 1979 and in
January 1980. The samples were treated in the same manner as
in Experiment 1 and aggregate samples of each layer processed
as before. The numbers of *O. ostertagi* L_3 in this instance were
expressed as L3 per hectare.

RESULTS

The total numbers of *O. ostertagi* L_3 recovered from
different layers of the 10 soil cores removed at monthly
intervals in Experiment 1 are shown in Figure 1. Larvae were
present at each sampling and there was some indication that the
numbers increased in all layers during June.

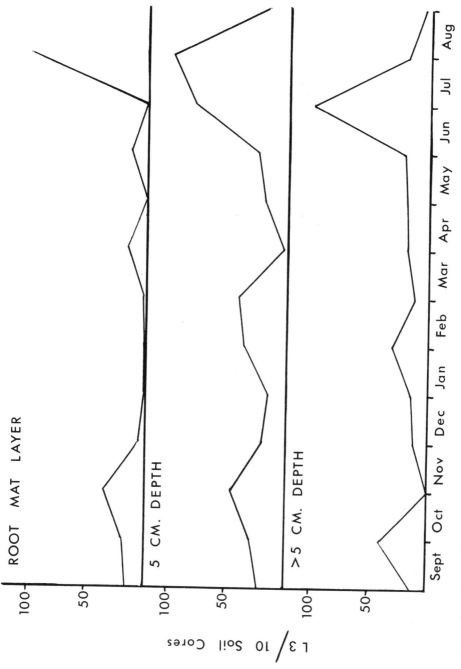

Fig. 1. *O. ostertagi* L_3 recovered from soil cores during 1978 – 1979.

Larvae were also consistently present in the different fractions of the core samples taken in Experiment 2 and are shown in Figure 2. Extremely high numbers (37×10^6) were present in the root mat and soil layers in October and although a marked reduction occurred in the numbers present on the herbage in November and January several million L_3 (25×10^6 and 17×10^6 respectively) were still present in the soil layers.

DISCUSSION

The most significant finding from these two experiments is that *O. ostertagi* L_3 were consistently present in the soil cores examined. In the three samplings from which quantitative data was obtained the numbers of L_3 present were considerable and if only a proportion migrated to the soil surface and onto the herbage these would be sufficient to precipitate ostertagiasis as suggested by our original observation on an outbreak of ostertagiasis on aftermath grazing (Bairden et al., 1979). It is also probable that the larval numbers recorded are an underestimate since losses undoubtedly occur during processing.

It is of course impossible to judge if these L_3 do ever return to the soil surface although the trend of the graph shown in Figure 1 suggests that they do so; also, Fincher and Stewart (1979) working in the U.S.A. have recently demonstrated that if bovine faeces containing *O. ostertagi* eggs are buried to a depth of 12.5 cm. under pasture or beneath 15 cm. of soil in the laboratory, then L_3 develop and migrate vertically through the soil. It is therefore possible that the increase in L_3 numbers in June shown in Figure 1 may have originated from deeper in the soil and we may require to sample deeper than 10 cm. to recover the entire larval pool in the soil.

Whether vertical migration of larvae occurs independently under natural conditions or requires the aid of transport hosts such as earthworms, as observed by Grønwold (1979) is not definitely known as yet but this is an area we are currently investigating.

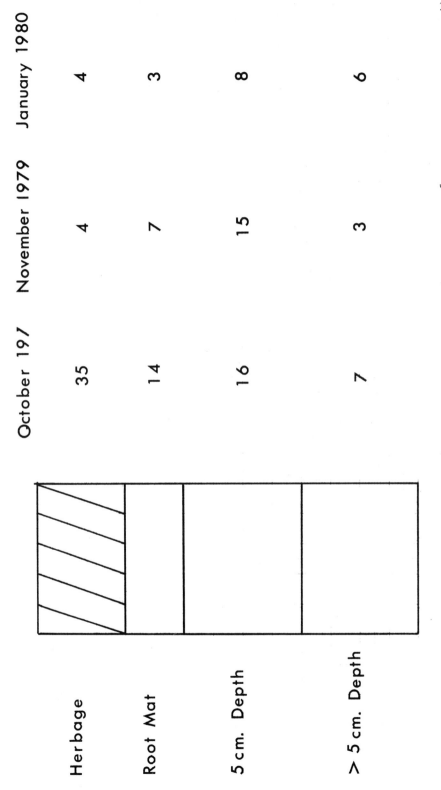

	October 197	November 1979	January 1980
Herbage	35	4	4
Root Mat	14	7	3
5 cm. Depth	16	15	8
> 5 cm. Depth	7	3	6

Fig. 2. Estimated numbers of *O. ostertagi* L_3/hectare of soil, root mat and herbage x 10^6.

Finally, it would be interesting to know if our observation on larvae in soil reflect a local situation occurring only under certain climatic conditions and specified soil types or whether it is a more general phenomenon. If the latter were true and vertical migration occurs then some reconsideration may have to be given to currently advocated control measures.

REFERENCES

Bairden, K., Parkins, J.J. and Armour, J., 1979. Bovine ostertagiasis; A changing epidemiological pattern. Veterinary Record, 105, 33-35.

Duncan, J.L., Armour, J., Bairden, K., Urquhart, G.M. and Jørgensen, R.J., 1979. Studies on the epidemiology of bovine parasitic bronchitis. Veterinary Record, 104, 274-278.

Fincher, G.T. and Stewart, T.B., 1979. Vertical migration by nematode larvae of cattle parasites through soil. Proceedings of the Helminthological Society of Washington, 46(1), 43-46.

Grønvold, J., 1979. On the possible role of earthworms in the transmission of *Ostertagia ostertagi* third stage larvae from faeces to soil. Journal of Parasitology, 65, 831-832.

Jørgensen, R.J., 1975. Isolation of infective *Dictyocaulus* larvae from herbage. Veterinary Parasitology, 1, 61-67.

Nelson, M., 1977. Where do lungworms go in wintertime. Veterinary Record, 101, 248.

Oakley, G.A., 1979. Delayed development of *Dictyocaulus viviparus* infection. Veterinary Record, 104, 460.

DISCUSSION

J.F. Michel *(UK)*

This is an extremely important subject. The crucial
question is whether or not one will be able regularly, to show
an increase in herbage infestation from soil derived larvae or,
in fact, whether one will be able to demonstrate it at all.

J. Euzeby *(France)*

What about the role of beetles as pasture cleaners or
scavengers?

J. Armour *(UK)*

As pasture cleaners or scavengers or for moving the larvae
about? There are two possibilities here. I believe what you
were suggesting was the breaking up of the faecal pats by dung
beetles. Or are you talking about the movement of larvae?

J. Euzeby

No, I am talking about the role of beetles as pasture
cleaners; this has been investigated and some workers maintain
that beetles can clean the pastures of larvae.

J. Armour

Well, it is the faeces that they remove, isn't it? I
think they may play a role in the movement of larvae possibly
earthworms may do the same.

J.-P. Raynaud *(France)*

Have you any results of herbage sampling which can be
related to your data?

J. Armour

Yes. The fall in number of larvae is very similar to
that detectable on the herbage. In the first slide I showed
you there was a marked drop in November/December. Dr. Michel's

284

work suggests that the greater numbers occur in February/
March and the decline is a little later - but that might be
due to a regional temperature difference.

P. Nansen (Denmark)

If we look on potential transport mechanisms in the cow
pats we may consider a number of possibilities, e.g. dung
beetles, flies and earthworms. When one looks on the activity
of these organisms there seems to be somewhat like a succession
of occurrence in the dung. Fresh dung pats are attacked
primarily by various beetles and flies. After some weeks
earthworms arrive and gradually the insect activity declines.
The arrival and activity of the earthworms are more or less
coincident with the development and occurrence of third stage
nematode larvae. In many fields the earthworm activity increases
in late summer and autumn. This led one of our students to
look in closer detail on the role of earthworms in the transmission of larvae from faeces.

Infective larvae could be recovered in the intestine of
earthworms and in earthworm faeces. In a separate experiment
comparing larvae transmission from dung pats containing and
not containing earthworms, respectively, a striking difference
was demonstrated in both horizontal and vertical transmission
of larvae onto herbage and into soil. It would be interesting
to know the overall role of earthworms in the transmission of
the infection in the grazing season as well as the transmission
from season to season.

R.J. Thomas (UK)

Previous studies in Scotland, on the rate of removal of
faeces by earthworms, indicate the turnover is quite marked.
I did some small-scale experiments with Nematodirus eggs in
faeces and their removal by earthworms. There was a fairly
high rate of removal of faeces pellets by earthworms and the
distribution of Nematodirus eggs, was most evident in the top

2 cm. of soil. I would image, that at times of the year when
Trichostrongyle eggs are developing very rapidly they may be
removed by earthworms and be distributed in the soil. The
situation with larvae may be more complicated. However, I
would agree with Peter Nansen that earthworms may be very
important in the transmission of larvae.

J. Armour

This is a theory of my colleague Dr. Frank Jennings!

J.F. Michel

I am wondering what proportion of the faeces of an earthworm ends up on the surface or below the surface of the soil?

R.J. Thomas

It depends on the species of earthworm. Some are surface
casters and others are not. Generally, earthworms do not go
deeply into the soil and hence casts occur on the surface and
in the upper layers of the soil. Casts deposited on the surface,
are composed of very fine material, which will be absorbed into
the top soil rapidly.

P. Nansen

The experiments were analysed by the Jørgensen technique
and there was no reduction in viability of larvae during their
passage through earthworms.

E.J.L. Soulsby *(UK)*

Two points come to mind. Work done many years ago by
T.W.M. Cameron, in Canada indicated the survival of horse
strongyle larvae in the soil over the summer. Gemmell in
New Zealand has demonstrated rapid contamination of pasture
with tapeworm eggs (up to about 100 m^2 in ten days) from a
single source of infected dog faeces. He believes this is due
to rapid transport of eggs by invertebrates. If that is the
case with tapeworm eggs with larvae that are motile, one might

have rapid transfer of infective material in the soil and across the soil. One might even have transport of eggs into the soil. Have you any thoughts about the eggs being carried down into the soil and developing there?

J. Armour

We have thought about this. In fact, this is the theory that Dr. Michel has been adhering to for the past year; I have been concerned more with the actual movement of larvae. I am not sure of the temperature gradients at various times of the year, at different levels, but maybe some of our geological colleagues could comment on this.

THE SIGNIFICANCE OF WINTER SURVIVAL OF FREE-LIVING STAGES ON
THE EPIDEMIOLOGY OF NEMATODIASIS: ITS EFFECT IN CONNECTION
WITH SET-STOCKING AND ALTERNATE GRAZING WITH SHEEP AND CATTLE

O. Helle

Institut for Indremedisin I, Norges Veterinærhøgskole,
Boks 8146 Dep., Oslo 1, Norway.

INTRODUCTION

The following gastro-intestinal nematodes are found in
cattle in Norway; *Ostertagia ostertagi, O. lyrate, Nematodirus
helvetianus, N. battus, Cooperia oncophora, C. mcmasteri* and *Trichuris* sp:
species of the same genera also occur in Norwegian sheep. The
grazing period for cattle is usually 4 - 5 months and parasites
which are pasture transmitted must either survive winter as
free-living stages on the pasture or in carrier animals. The
free-living stages of all the common species of cattle nematodes
are able to survive the winter in Norway, but with sheep the
free-living stages of some of the nematodes show poor winter
survival on the pasture. These include *Haemonchus contortus,
Trichostrongylus* spp, *Cooperia curticei, Bunostomum trigonocephalum* and
Oesophagostomum venulosum. Cattle can also be infected with species
of the genera *Haemonchus, Trichostrongylus, Bunostomum* and
Oesophagostomum, but the absence of these nematodes from cattle
in Norway may be due to the management system or to the
resistance of adult cattle against nematode infection.
Calves are usually raised separately from their dams, and
parasites which do not survive the winter on the pasture, have
little opportunity to infect calves. Cattle aged more than one
year generally have few gastro-intestinal parasites which
is reflected in low faecal egg counts. Lambs on the other
hand, are raised with the ewes, which may pass large numbers
of nematode eggs in the faeces in the spring. Nematodes which
are unable to survive the winter in the pasture, have a good
chance to be transmitted from adult sheep to the offspring
during the spring. The control of the nematodes which are
unable to survive the winter in the pasture is not difficult.
If sheep are treated with anthelmintics in winter time and are

turned out on pasture without nematode eggs in the faeces, nematodes of the genera *Haemonchus*, *Trichostrongylus* etc. will disappear from the flock, and only the winter resistant species will remain. In such flocks, the nematode fauna of sheep parallels that of Norwegian cattle, with a dominance of *Ostertagia* spp., *Nematodirus* spp. and *Cooperia oncophora* (Helle, 1971).

MATERIAL AND METHODS

When sheep or cattle are kept on the same pasture for several consecutive years, it is difficult to control the winter resistant parasites. However, because sheep and cattle have different dominant species of nematodes, the following investigations were undertaken on the effect of different grazing systems on the occurrence of winter-resistant parasites in sheep and cattle in the following conditions:

1. Permanent sheep pasture, 10 ewes with twin lambs.

2. Permanent calf pasture, 12 calves, ½ - 1 year old.

3. Mixed grazing, 6 calves and 5 ewes with twins.

4. Alternate grazing, 12 calves and 10 ewes with twins, alternating every second year on two pastures.

The investigations were carried out from 1973 to 1978 and a preliminary report has been given (Oeveraas et al., 1977). From the first year onward the ewes were treated against nematodes in the spring before they went on pasture, and the lambs were treated in the beginning of August. Anthelmintic treatment of calves was not intended, but it became evident during the first two years that calves on permanent pasture, as well as on mixed grazing suffered from nematode infections. Consequently during the third year of the experiment the calves on permanent pasture were treated with thiabendazole 20 and 40 days after the beginning of grazing. From the fourth year onward fenbendazole was used for calves on permanent pasture as well as on pasture with mixed grazing. This treatment resulted in a reasonable control of the nematodes.

RESULTS

In calves on alternate grazings only negligible numbers
of eggs of the common cattle nematodes were found, despite the
fact that no anthelmintic treatment was given. The calves were
in good condition. Thus, the overwintered sheep nematodes were
of no importance for the calves. However, calves could be
infected to some degree with *Nematodirus battus* and they could
thus recontaminate the pasture to result in *N. battus* infection
in lambs the following spring. With this exception, the
alternate grazing system also provided satisfactory control of
the nematodes of sheep. On all the sheep pastures, treatment
had to be carried out against *Nematodirus battus*.

CONCLUSION

The influence of the different grazing systems on the
weight gain revealed that the alternate grazing system was the
most successful for the calves. Mixed grazing showed no
advantage compared with permanent grazing. In lambs the best
weight gain occurred on mixed grazing. This was perhaps due
to the tendency of sheep to select the best plants when grazing
in competition with the calves. The alternate grazing system
was less superior to permanent grazing in lambs than in calves.

REFERENCES

Helle, O., 1971. The effect on sheep parasites of grazing in alternate
    years by sheep and cattle. A comparison with set-stocking, and the
    use of anthelmintics with these grazing managements. Acta. vet.
    scand. (Suppl.) 33, 59 pp.
Oeveraas, J., Pestalozzi, M., Helle, O., Nedkvitne, J.J. and Matre, T.,
    1977. Mixed Grazing Research in Norway. Rep. Europ. Ass. Anim.
    Prod. 28th Ann. Meet. Brussels 1977.

DISCUSSION

J.F. Michel *(UK)*

It has always seemed to me that, in these alternate
grazing systems, the short-term effect will be the emergence
species common to both hosts, that they will become dominant,
and then, only subsequently, will we see a return of those with
a limited host range and they, perhaps, become more host tolerant.

R.J. Thomas *(UK)*

Can you confirm that *Nematodirus battus* was, in fact, picked
up and transmitted by the calves. Did you find *N. battus* eggs
in the calf faeces?

O. Helle *(Norway)*

Yes, but in low numbers. The method used was the McMaster
technique. It is a rather crude method for cattle faeces.
However, in general, in the field in June, you could say that
the calves had a mean of 10 - 40 eggs/g.

R.J. Thomas

We have found that *N. battus* will survive over two years
with no sheep grazing pasture in the intervening year; in fact
with no grazing at all in the intervening year. We still get
a small *N. battus* peak coming up in the spring of the second
year. This appears to be due to eggs which do not reach the
third stage in the year in which they are shed. They then
develop further in the intervening year, coming up again in the
second year. I was not sure whether your *N. battus* are surviving
through two years in this way, or being transmitted by the
calves.

O. Helle

I cannot give a clear answer to this. However, if you
think of the calf faeces over a period, and ten calves being
a mean of 40 eggs/g. as a total, that is a substantial number

of eggs being introduced to the pasture. It is not reasonable
to conclude that this increase could occur due to eggs carried
over for two winters.

J. Eckert (Switzerland)

I would like to comment on haémonchosis control. We
also have indications that overwinter survival of *Haemonchus*
larvae may be limited. We thought that if we treated all the
animals in spring - the ewes and the lambs - that we might be
able to prevent haemonchosis in an intensive sheep farm. But,
surprisingly, this was not possible. This means that, under
our conditions, although survival of *Haemonchus* larvae is
limited, the number is still sufficient to induce new infections
in a farm. I would like to ask if, with only one treatment,
can you completely prevent haemonchosis, or *Haemonchus* infection,
in the following year's flock of sheep?

O. Helle

It depends on what you mean by 'complete'. I would not
like to say 100%, but we have made a lot of observations on
Haemonchus. First, I used tracer lambs and never found *Haemonchus*
in them (these were tracers for winter survival). Generally,
Haemonchus disappeared completely. There is a winter survival
of some of the *Trichostrongylus* species, but this is very limited,
and after one, two or three years they disappear. And to Dr.
Michel: on a pasture grazed permanently by sheep, pure sheep
strain of parasites, mainly *Ostertagia circumcincta* and *Nematodirus
battus* emerge. *Cooperia onchophora* disappears. But, in lambs,
grazed either together with cattle or in an alternate manner
Cooperia onchophora also occurs in sheep. In cattle in such
circumstances it is *Ostertagia ostertagi, Nematodirus helvetianus*
and *Cooperia onchophora* which dominate. The situation might
change if we continued for a long period with sheep and cattle
on alternative grazing so, as Dr. Michel suggested, we might
find some adaptation. Our studies were for a short duration
of three years.

J.F. Michel

Would Dr. Connan like to comment on the survival of *Haemonchus* on pasture.

R.M. Connan   *(UK)*

Only to say that my own results agree with those of Dr. Helle. In one particular flock there were outbreaks of haemonchosis in both ewes and lambs. Each summer they lost sheep over a period of ten years. Then, the owner started to treat animals during the hardest period in winter. From then on, though *Haemonchus* has not disappeared from the farm, it is present in very small numbers. The original parasite underwent arrest but now the *Haemonchus* on the farm does not arrest at all. It does just survive at very small levels overwinter on the pasture; I expect there are one or two worms for the following year.

J. Armour

What were the relative stocking rates of the sheep and cattle in the mixed grazing - per acre or per hectare?

O. Helle

I do not have the exact figures. There would be something like 6 calves and 5 ewes plus 10 lambs in a 1 acre field.

J. Armour

On the basis of animal units that is a disproportionate number of calves, which would favour the development of parasitism in the calves. We have had very good results with mixed grazing but we are using half that number of calves in relation to the number of ewes. You are favouring the transmission of cattle parasites with that number of calves.

O. Helle

I would just like to make a small comment on *Haemonchus* as we are discussing this. In Norway the summer climate is a limiting factor. We find it on the lowlands, in the eastern country, and it follows the coast. However, going northwards, 50% of the northern part of the country is free of *Haemonchus* and the parasite is also absent from mountain grazing. In Sweden, *Haemonchus* is found only in the western parts and not in the drier eastern parts.

WINTER OSTERTAGIASIS IN SWEDISH CATTLE

Olle Nilsson
Swedish Laboratory Services Ltd., Kristianstad, Sweden

ABSTRACT

Young cattle on permanent pastures in Sweden are exposed to substantial numbers of Ostertagia spp. *larvae in the autumn, and these are inhibited at the fourth larval stage. Nevertheless, Type II ostertagiasis is regarded as an uncommon disease. One explanation for this may be that the condition has been overlooked hitherto because the resumption of development of the worms starts in May when the animals are at grass again.*

P. Nansen, R.J. Jørgensen, E.J.L. Soulsby (eds), Epidemiology and Control of Nematodiasis in Cattle.
Copyright © 1981 ECSC, EEC, EAEC, Brussels – Luxembourg. All rights reserved.

INTRODUCTION

The epidemiological pattern of bovine ostertagiasis in Sweden corresponds to the situation seen in other European countries. Infective larvae overwinter on the pastures, the larval contamination is reduced during spring and early summer to a very low level in July. Recontamination results in a rise in larval contamination in August and September (Nilsson and Sorelius, 1973).

Permanent pastures are frequently in consecutive use in Sweden and grazing cattle are exposed to substantial numbers of infective *Ostertagia* larvae in the autumn. It is estimated that 900 000 young cattle were grazing on grass in 1978. In spite of this situation the Type II ostertagiasis syndrome is seldom reported by veterinary practitioners.

This presentation provides a picture of the actual situation. The basic data were obtained in collaboration with the Department of Cattle and Sheep Disease, Faculty of Veterinary Medicine, Swedish University of Agricultural Sciences, Uppsala, Sweden. Details have been published elsewhere (Olsson, 1977; Olsson et al., 1978; Olsson and Holtenius, 1980) and relevant extracts of these results are combined with results of our own investigations in southern Sweden since 1974.

MATERIAL AND METHODS

Abomasa from slaughtered normal young cattle were collected at the abattoirs in Uppsala and Kristianstad. Abomasa from emergency slaughtered animals are also included (Kristianstad).

Tracer calves were used for estimating the degree of larvae inhibition successively during the autumn. The animals were under conditions which precluded further infection after grazing to allow maturition of hyperbiotic larvae. All parasitological examinations were performed in accordance with commonly adopted standard methods.

RESULTS

It was shown by tracer calves that ingested larvae were inhibited at the fourth larval stage to a slight degree as early as in August. As the autumn progressed the proportion of inhibited larvae increased to the extent that more than 90% of the total worm population was inhibited. The degree of inhibition was independent of the previous exposure of animals to larvae and the numbers of parasites that had become established (Table 1).

TABLE 1

THE INCIDENCE OF INHIBITED *OSTERTAGIA* LARVAE IN ABOMASA OF TRACER CALVES IN CORRELATION TO THE GRAZING PERIOD

Out on grass	Housed	Inhibition percent	
		Average	Range
May	End of August	33	26 - 48
	End of September	86	70 - 92
	End of October	96	84 - 98
August	End of August	7	4 - 15
	End of September	57	43 - 68
	End of October	93	78 - 97

About half the number of abomasa, which were examined from October to April, harboured a low number of worms. About 5% of the animals had substantial numbers of worms (Table 2).

TABLE 2

DISTRIBUTION OF THE NUMBERS OF *OSTERTAGIA* IN 167 ABOMASA OF NORMALLY SLAUGHTERED YOUNG CATTLE FROM OCTOBER UNTIL APRIL

No. *Ostertagia*	No. abomasa	Percent
< 10 000	98	59
10 000 - 30 000	34	20
30 000 - 100 000	26	16
>100 000	9	5

During the period October - April, approximately 94% of the total worm population were fourth stage larvae. In a few abomasa with a low number of worms (<1 000) the population of fourth stage larvae was less than 50%. Of 22 emergency slaughtered young cattle, one was sent in because of anorexia and malnutrition in April 1974. A total of 716 000 worms were recovered from it and 89% of the worms were fourth stage larvae.

The resumed development of arrested larvae in grazing animals started in May. In 21 abomasa, which were examined from May 1 to May 21, about 60% of the total worm population were fourth stage larvae. This figure decreased to about 35% (average of 14 abomasa) from the end of May to the beginning of July.

DISCUSSION

It was shown that the proportion of inhibited fourth larval stages increases successively during late summer and autumn to reach about the 90% level in October. This situation persists until April the following year. About 5% of the animals examined harboured more than 100 000 worms. It is surprising to find such a low number of heavily infected animals in view of the potential herbage contamination. This may be explained by the fact that autumn-born bull calves are over-represented in the slaughterhouse material and these animals are normally slaughtered at 18 months of age and are often given supplementary feed in the autumn when there is a shortage of grass. This would tend to decrease the number of larvae acquired by an animal.

Maturation of larvae starts in May, i.e. at the earliest about 7 months after the onset of hypobiosis. This period of dormancy is longer in Sweden than for example in England (Michel et al., 1976). Thus, the worms seem to be adapted to the existing climate and the management, a situation which favours the survival of their progeny. Until this situation became known, our observation of Type II ostertagia syndrome was focused on the housing period and the real significance of the disease may have been overlooked.

The practical consequences of these findings are that the potential risks for Type II ostertagiasis would probably occur in May when the animals return to grass. With the management systems of Sweden, about 500 000 heifers are the main risk group and these animals are out on grass without supplementary feeding until late autumn. Olsson (1978) has described clinical cases of Type II ostertagiasis in heifers on a dairy farm near Stockholm and he has discussed the importance of the disease.

The question arises whether or not the selected material which was abomasa from well-fattened and clinically normal animals, satisfactorily represents the actual situation. One of 22 emergency slaughtered calves suffered from obvious Type II ostertagiasis. Since the start of this investigation the practitioners and many farmers in southern Sweden were asked to report suspected cases of parasitic disorders in young cattle during the winter period. To date Type II ostertagiasis has been confirmed in five herds in February and March (Svelab, Kristianstad). Three of these herds had Charolais or Hereford suckling calves and the affected animals were approximately one year old. However, the morbidity rate was low. The other two herds consisted of Swedish Friesian cattle and the young cattle were in a poor condition in March.

In several controlled weight gain trials, which have been performed every winter since 1975, young bull calves with a previous exposure to larvae maintained a normal weight gain up the end of the trials in April. On the other hand, it has been relatively easy to find animals in poor condition during the winter months for special trials and which at slaughter were heavily infected with worms in different stages of development and also had severe ostertagia lesions in the abomasum.

Development of arrested larvae thus occurs also at times other than in May and onwards, but a simultaneous maturation of large numbers of larvae appears to occur only in exceptional cases.

CONCLUSIONS

Inhibition of *Ostertagia* spp. larvae at the early fourth larval stage reaches 90% from October until April. Resumption of development commences in May. To a minor degree, more or less complete maturation can take place during the winter months but this is rare. Under the existing climatic and management conditions for heifer calves in Sweden, these animals are likely to suffer from Type II ostertagiasis.

REFERENCES

Michel, J.F., Lancaster, M.B. and Hong, C. 1976. Observations on the resumed development of arrested *Ostertagia ostertagi* in naturally infected yearling cattle. J. Comp. Path. 86, 73-80.

Nilsson, O. and Sorelius, L. 1973. Trichostrongylidinfektioner hos nötkreatur i Severige. Nord. Vet.-Med., 25, 65-78.

Olsson, G. 1977. Vinterostertagios i Sverige - en slaktmaterialstudie. Svensk Vet.-Tidn., 29, 361-365.

Olsson, G., Holtenius, P. and Haraldsson, I. 1978. Vinterostertagios - klinik och patologi. Svensk Vet. -Tidn., 30, 453-459.

Olsson, G. and Holtenius, P. 1980. Studies on the Epidemiology of *Ostertagia ostertagi* in Calves. Nord. Vet.-Med., 32, 28-37.

DISCUSSION

J.F. Michel *(UK)*

I was interested in your comments on the value of yarding because, in the United Kingdom, we feel that the subject is still somewhat open and there are vague plans for another medium-sized collaborative effort.

J. Armour *(UK)*

I would like to comment on a situation that I met a couple of weeks ago. I was asked to investigate a problem thought to be winter ostertagiasis or Type II in the herd of the Hannah Dairy Research Institute. The agriculturists who work there do not appear to recognise that worms exist in cattle. The animals are never dosed and there was a classical case of Type II ostertagiasis. The other animals were reputed to be doing perfectly well. The animals were on the highest possible quality silage and the mean daily weight gain of the animals was 0.19 kg/d. Parasitism was not suspected because diarrhoea had not been evident.

This is a common situation met with in south-west Scotland and which may be occurring in the northern part of Sweden. Too many people believe that in the diagnosis of parasitic disease, diarrhoea is an essential clinical sign which must be present before it is reasonable to make a diagnosis of parasitism.

GENERAL DISCUSSION

H.J. Over *(The Netherlands)*

I would like to consider the involvement of earthworms in the spread of larvae and/or eggs of *trichostrongyles* into soil. It is unlikely that earthworms are the only invertebrates concerned. In fact it is probable that many invertebrates assist and this will depend on the nature and structure of the soil.

J.F. Michel *(UK)*

Would someone like to speculate about what form investigations on this topic might take?

H.J. Over

A study of this role of particle size of the soil and the penetration and retention of larvae related to this would be most useful.

J. Eckert *(Switzerland)*

I would like to ask Dr. Raynaud whether fewer tracer animals may be of significance when put on a large area. What we are measuring is the infection risk. As long as we assume that the food intake is similar in the tracer animals, this measurement of the infection risk is independent of the size of the area in which the animals are grazing. I would like to know what risk exists for some of the calves grazing on a large area compared to when the animals are put on a small area and highly overstocked. We have information on the infection risk which indicates that it does not depend on the area on which the animals are grazing. It is comparable with the grazing area which the other animals have.

J.-P. Raynaud *(France)*

In your work the initial contamination is in the pasture around the home? Animals start with a few weeks in the home pasture, and it is there that the initial contamination of the calves starts. Then the animals are moved to the alpage. With the Limousin calf, for example, when you have ten calves in ten hectares, can you really put out tracers? We know, we have tried and it is impossible, because the tracer is so different from the normal animal, they are killed by the normal. What could be the system to control either the pasture or the availability of the larvae, in such a cow/calf system where you have ten animals per ten hectares? It is an extensive area. This compares to your system in alpage which is also a very extensive system.

J.F. Michel

There are two elements here. One is the question of area; I suppose the thought there was that there would be gross inequalities in the distribution of worms, so that if you had a large area some calves, especially if they had a different grazing pattern, would not be grazing where the calves which you are trying to monitor were grazing. The other point was the practical difficulty of using a tracer calf as a measure of what is happening to the single suckled calf. I suppose the only answer is to use a single suckled calf as a tracer.

J.-P. Raynaud

Yes, the principals.

J.F. Michel

No, not the principals. To have tracer calves, not as hand reared calves, but to have a cow and calf.

R.J. Jørgensen (Denmark)

I have a question for Professor Eckert on the over-wintering of lungworm larvae in Switzerland. You believe that overwintering of larvae in the lungs of animals is the most important. Can you be sure that larvae do not overwinter, or do you think that overwintering in the animal is the most important thing? It is my experience that lungworm larvae

survive freezing very well, and the drop in larvae on the
pasture which takes place in spring occurs before animals are
turned out (here in Denmark) and during the first weeks there
on pasture.

J. Eckert

Our statements are based on the following studies.
Several years ago we distributed faecal samples with lungworm
larvae in the midlands and hilly areas, and we could not
recover any larvae after the winter months. I cannot recall
the exact data but we could not find living larvae after some
months - the samples were distributed in autumn.

The second experiment was done on a pasture which in the
previous year was heavily contaminated with clinical cases of
Dictyocaulasis, The following spring we turned out some tracer
animals and they did not pick up any lungworm infections.
These results may now be interpreted differently in view of
the paper, which we heard this morning, concerning the
probability that lungworm larvae may survive in the soil. This
could be the explanation why tracer animals, which had been
grazed for about 14 days in spring, were not infected. However,
our impression was that overwinter survival of larvae is not
important, and similar results were obtained in Austria. On
the other hand, we could isolate inhibited larvae from the
lungs of cattle during winter time.

R.J. Jørgensen

I do not think you should give up this idea, because
overwintering lungworm infection means sufficient larvae are
picked up perhaps by a single animal, these then produce a
patent infection.

J.F. Michel

I think there is great individual variation, with respect
to *Dictyocaulus* infection.

H.-J. Bürger *(FRG)*

I would like to quote results obtained by Mr. Bunke. He placed a dozen tracer calves, in spring, on pastures which had been contaminated with *Dictyocaulus* larvae the previous autumn. The animals were put out in May, and by the first few days of June, we could not find a single lungworm in any of these calves. We purposely restricted the animals to those areas of the pastures where most of the larvae would probably have been - and the animals had to graze this part of the pasture closely. No *Dictyocaulus* was found in any of these tracer animals in spring.

J. Eckert

We distributed faecal samples and examined them until the end of April. We could not find larvae at this time. We used tracer animals and, one group was grazed from the 3rd of May until the 24th May and these animals had trichostrongylids but not lungworms. Other animals of the group remained on the same pasture until the end of September and still there was no lungworm infection at all. However, these animals picked up fairly high numbers of trichostrongylids. On this evidence we concluded that overwintering of *Dictyocaulus* larvae may be negligible under our conditions in Switzerland.

G. Urquhart *(UK)*

I would like to refer to the question of whether over-wintered lungworm larvae mature gradually in the spring. Some twenty years ago in an abattoir survey of animals which had died in the first and second year of life, we found the incidence of infection was roughly 30%; about 10, 20 or 30 lungworms per animal. There was a gradual increase in the number of lungs with adult lungworms of the order of 10, 14, 18 and 25 worms per set of lungs. One got the impression that each month there was a larger number of adult lungworms than previously. This would suggest that lungworm larvae do mature and adults commence excreting larvae.

J.F. Michel

Would anyone like to take up Dr. Bürger's suggestion
that the mid-season increase in the pasture contamination with
trichostrongyle larvae should be predictable? I was wondering
whether he also thinks that the rate of decline in the pasture
infestation in the spring is predictable? I would like to
ask if these things are, in fact, capable of being forecast and
whether there would be any practical value in doing so?

H.-J. Bürger

My data do not indicate that the decline in spring is
predictable. We have shown previously that the number of
larvae present on pastures in autumn is correlated to the
number on the pastures in the spring. We compared the data of
September/early October with those in March and early April.
However, I cannot say that the decline in spring is predictable.
The first increase during mid-summer might be predictable,
since the rise of the larval counts occurred at the same time
on a variety of pastures.

There is a practical use of prediction insofar as we
want an answer to the question which is often put to us by
farmers, as well as veterinary practitioners, namely, can we
delay the movement of the calves to other pastures - and of
the heifers and bulls during the second year as well - to late
July or early August? I think we can now say yes! But still
we are not certain about this.

J.F. Michel

Does anyone else have strong feelings about the usefulness
of forecasting?

H.J. Over

Looking at Dr. Bürger's data, to forecast for fall and
spring is very reliable. But when spring comes you see these
larval counts come back anyhow, so it makes no sense to say it

is forecasting - it is like forecasting spring, it will come
with grass growth!

J.F. Michel

Yes, with grass growth. So grass growth is predictable,
and it is variable from year to year.

H.J. Over

I would like to ask Dr. Bürger whether the fields he
described were in one locality?

H.-J. Bürger

Yes, the pastures which I showed you were in one
locality - one, two, three beside the other, in all 1½ km
from one end of the farm to the other.

However, in the other study, showing the increase during
September, those were different fields, and were about 15 km
away from the first group.

H.J. Over

That bears on the point of the summer prediction. You
mentioned the occurrence of a thunderstorm in August; it fell
on all three pastures; one obviously reacted and the others
did not. I don't think you can use this in relation to fore-
casts.

J. Armour (UK)

I wish to explain a situation that we have in two
different parts of Scotland. In the Edinburgh area (East
Scotland) Ostertagiasis often is not observed. However in the
West it occurs annually. In 1977/78, the rainfall increased
markedly in the East of Scotland; it showed quite a different
pattern. Normally this area has a rainfall not dissimilar to
the southeast of England (perhaps marginally more). However,
for two years there were 10 - 15 inches of rain more than usual

and Ostertagiasis was common in East Scotland. Were there to be a good prediction formula it would be very useful because, in many years, in many parts of Scotland there is very little need to take any control measure.

R.M. Connan *(UK)*

Are you talking about Type 1 or Type 2 Ostertagiasis?

J. Armour

Type 1.

R.M. Connan

We see Ostertagiasis in our area (Cambridgeshire).

J. Armour

However, in Linlithgow and Fife (and so on) the disease is reputed not to occur.

R.J. Thomas *(UK)*

With regard to the overwintering of larvae and their decline in spring, I think the number of larvae that over-winter is more important than the rate of decline. I think the rate of decline is steady and depending when spring arrives, there is a proportion of larvae surviving. The important factor is the number of overwintering larvae which constitute the starting point. Olleranshaw has suggested that one can predict this from the weather conditions of the previous autumn. This may be useful.

J.F. Michel

If the decline in larval populations in the spring depends on grass growth then is there any need for sophisticated forecasting techniques?

H.-J. Bürger

At this point I would like to mention the work of the Copenhagen people who demonstrated some of the consequences of larval survival. They put the animals out to pasture at different times of the year, which would include periods when larval populations had declined.

N. Downey *(Ireland)*

I would like to ask Dr. Bürger if he noticed, in years where he got a late season increase in pasture infection, if this was followed by more overwintering infection.

H.J. Bürger

The results were equivocal. I do not think the number of larvae which overwinter depends on the number in the mid-summer increase. The mid-summer increase can end up with even lower numbers, for example in situations with two or three dry years; in these the larval counts decreased after an early peak in July or August, while it increased in other years which were particularly wet during late September and October. I cannot see from my data any correlation between the mid-summer increase and the overwintering of larvae.

N. Downey *(Ireland)*

Even if the increase is late? Recently we have had very warm late summers and one would have expected more development and survival over winter.

R.J. Jørgensen

The Danish experiments indicate clearly that the climatic conditions in spring are most important in relation to the number of overwintered larvae. This is assessed by the number of larvae acquired by grazing calves. The Danish farmer will turn his animals out when there is a period of warm weather and provided there is sufficient herbage, therefore it is a question of the air temperature.

SESSION 4

CONTROL I

Chairman: N.E. Downey

VACCINATION OR TACTICAL TREATMENT WITH LEVAMISOLE AGAINST LUNGWORM

L. Pouplard and M. Pecheur

Faculty of Veterinary Medicine, 45 rue des Veterinaires,
B-1070 Brussels, Belgium

ABSTRACT

In a study on 30 young calves, the use of Dictyocaulus viviparus vaccine is compared with an early administration of Levamisole. The results indicate that even when close supervision is maintained, vaccination remains indispensable as part of a general strategic control programme against parasitism in young cattle.

INTRODUCTION

Parasitic bronchitis and gastro-intestinal trichostrongylosis are responsible for the more important parasitic disease
problems in Belgium and a strategy for control of these infections of young grazing cattle has been advocated for several years
The following timetable for prophylactic measures is offered to
cattle breeders:

Mid-March	first dose of parasitic bronchitis vaccine
Mid-April	(a) second dose of vaccine, and
	(b) treatment of pastures with calcium cyanamide
Early May	turning out all animals to pasture
Mid-June	first strategic anthelmintic treatment
Mid-July	(a) second strategic anthelmintic treatment, and
	(b) change of pasture to a non-contaminated
	plot, or one previously treated with cyanamide
End of October	housing of cattle with final anthelmintic treatment.

If coughing occurs earlier in the year, the first strategic
anthelmintic treatment can be administered sooner.

The question remains, however, as to whether parasitic
bronchitis vaccination still has a place in such a programme,
in view of the highly effective anthelmintics which are now
available. In fact, since an anthelmintic drug is available
that is active against the *Dictyocaulus* species when used as early
as the sixth week after infection, it might be considered that
dosing at such a time would be sufficient to control lungworm
infections. An early disappearance of the infection after such
a treatment could help animals build sufficient immunity to
resist new infections. In fact, this prophylactic method was
in current practice when no vaccines were available, and also
when anthelmintic drugs, such as diethylcarbamazine, had only

a limited anthelmintic action. Diethylcarbamazine is known to
be effective only against immature forms, but when used during
the pre-patent phase it effectively prevented *Dictyocaulus*
infections while helping to establish a certain degree of
immunity. With the availability of more active anthelmintic
agents, such as levamisole, this method of prophylaxis perhaps
could be even more effective. This raises an important question:
is vaccination needed? Would an early anthelmintic treatment
be preferable? What are the economic aspects of this?

MATERIAL AND METHODS

Thirty young calves of 200 kg maximum body weight were
purchased in March and April, 1979. Of these, six calves were
infected in early April with 60 third stage larvae (L3) of
Dictyocaulus viviparus per kg of liveweight to produce carriers
which would create pasture contamination. Twelve calves were
vaccinated against parasitic bronchitis by the conventional
method and twelve unvaccinated calves were designated for early
treatment. The contaminating calves were pastured April 28 on
Plots C and D of a 4 ha pasture, divided as in the diagram
below, with an opening in the fence between the two plots.

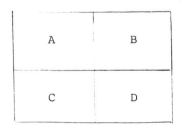

On May 7, 1979, the two groups of twelve calves each
were grazed together on the plots so as to be challenged with
a comparable initial parasitic infection. On June 6, the
carrier animals were withdrawn from pasture, and the two 12-calf
groups were again divided. Those vaccinated were pastured on
Plot D, and the others on Plot C. The fence between both plots

was then closed. Faeces samples were examined from individual animals at weekly intervals to determine the anthelmintic treatment time, and also to make a continuous estimate of the degree of infection. On July 20, the two groups were moved to new grazing plots: vaccinated calves were moved to Plot B, while non-vaccinated animals went over to Plot A. On August 20, both groups were moved back to their initial plots, and from then on they were moved from one plot to the other to allow proper grass growth. Clinical observations were closed October 1.

RESULTS

The carrier animals contaminated their respective plots satisfactorily, since faecal examination showed levels consistently above 200 larvae/g. One month after being turned out to pasture (i.e. at the time the two groups of 12 calves each were separated), four of the non-vaccinated animals already were passing *Dictyocaulus* larvae in their faeces and by June 13 all animals of this group were passing larvae. Typical clinical signs of parasitic bronchitis then appeared and levamisole treatment was given July 3 (i.e. eight weeks after the animals had been turned out to grass).

The vaccinated calves started to pass larvae one week later than the non-vaccinated animals. The faecal larval counts remained extremely low throughout the whole season except in one animal which had to be treated with levamisole on July 20 (Figure 1). Clinical signs remained severe and persisted in the non-vaccinated animals while they were absent or of short duration in the vaccinated group. The faecal larval counts of the two groups are shown in Figure 2.

Weight gains were rather similar in both groups, but growth was slightly better in the vaccinated animals, whose average starting weight had been 16.9 kg below that of the controls. Average weight of the non-vaccinated group was 162.8 kg on May 7, and 257.6 kg on September 24, i.e. a 94.8 kg weight gain. For the same dates, live weight averages were

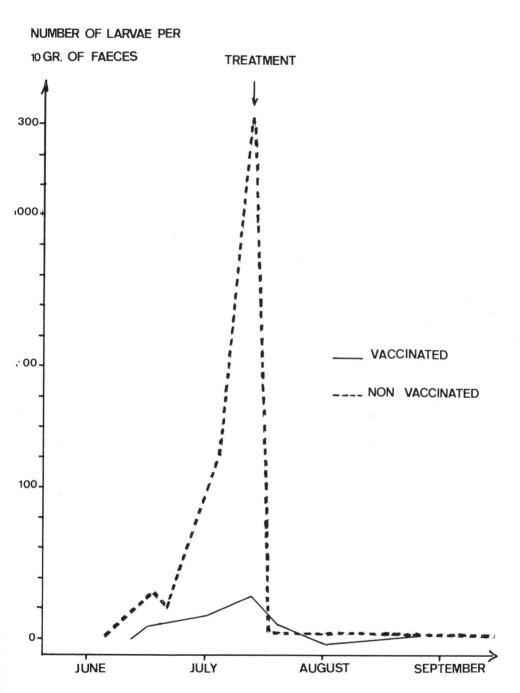

Fig. 1   Faecal larval counts of vaccinated and non-vaccinated groups.

318

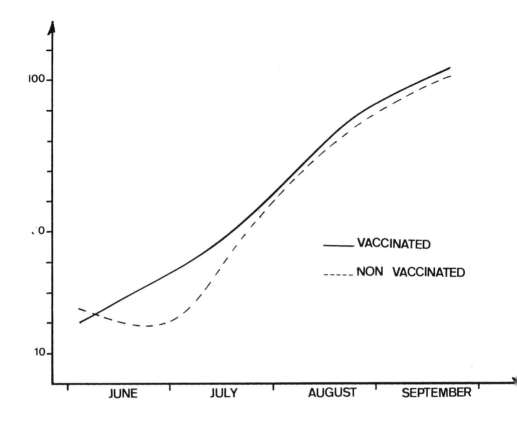

Fig. 2.   Weight increase in kg in vaccinated and non-vaccinated groups.

145.9 kg and 242.0 kg respectively in the vaccinated group,
i.e. 96.1 kg weight gain. The average live weight of non-
vaccinated animals had gone down from 186.8 kg on June 6 to
182.3 kg on July 3, i.e. a loss of 4.5 kg, during the month
prior to anthelmintic treatment. In comparison, during the
same time, in vaccinated animals live weight of the vaccinated
animals had increased from 165.9 kg to 181.0 kg, a weight gain
of 15.1 kg.

DISCUSSION

Vaccination afforded effective protection when the animals
were subjected to severe infection. Vaccine protection was

broken to a minor extent only in a single animal of the group. Though unvaccinated animals were treated effectively with levamisole, they suffered considerable weight loss during the critical period even though early and effective action had been assured by the close observation of animals during the study. Under practical field circumstances such close supervision would not have been possible and it is unlikely that anthelmintic therapy would have been administered in time. Hence weight loss would have been far greater than was demonstrated in this study.

The experience of Duncan et al. (1979) supports these observations. These workers compared the behaviour of seven vaccinated calves with that of seven non-vaccinated calves when subjected to natural parasitic infection with overwintered larvae. The seven vaccinated calves survived, and clinical signs were light and of short duration. In addition, larval extretion in the faeces was low. In contrast, three of the unvaccinated calved died, the clinical signs were persistent and severe, and pasture larval contamination was marked. The authors concluded that parasitic bronchitis cannot be prevented by tactical use of the anthelmintic agents designed to control bovine ostertagiosis, and only vaccination can successfully solve this problem.

CONCLUSIONS

The strategic use of anthelmintic regimens can provide effective control of gastro-intestinal trichostrongylosis. The primary reason for this is that parasitic development follows a similar pattern from year to year, irrespective of weather conditions. Thus reliable predictions can be based on this consistent pattern and prophylactic programmes can be devised. In contrast, predicting the time of year when parasitic bronchitis will appear is much more difficult. Therefore, strategic anthelmintic regimens, effective against *Dictyocaulus*, may well be improperly timed, for it is impossible to know accurately

320

the degree of bovine infection unless faecal examinations are
performed regularly. Under practical field conditions, such
regular examinations cannot be undertaken. Hence, vaccination
against parasitic bronchitis remains indispensable as part of
a general strategic plan against parasitism in young cattle.

REFERENCES

Duncan, J., Armour, J., Bairden, K., Urquhart, G. and Jørgensen, R. 1979.
     Studies on the epidemiology of bovine parasitic bronchitis.
     The Vet. Rec. 104, 274.
Pouplard, L. and Pecheur, M. 1974. Lutte stratégique contre les verminoses
     du bétail. Comptes rendus de recherches IRSIA, 38, 1-153.
Pouplard, L. and Pecheur, M. 1977. Bekämpfung der Wurmkrankheiten von
     Weidevieh. Hohenheimer Arbeiten, 87, 1-64.
Pouplard, L. 1979. Gehen sie die Wurmbrut strategisch an Deutsche
     Schwarzbunte, 2, 40-42.

DISCUSSION

F.H.M. Borgsteede *(The Netherlands)*

Can you explain the compensatory growth of the un-vaccin-
ated group, where they reached almost the same weightgain level
by the end of the season? Also, do you think that trichostrongyles may play a role in this? You say that the growth
of the vaccinated group was satisfactory, but they had a growth
rate of 15 kg per month, which means 500 g/d and I would not
say that is very satisfactory.

L. Pouplard *(Belgium)*

I cannot explain the small difference because our trial
was only concerned with whether to vaccinate or not. However,
there was also a heavy trichostrongylid infection. Perhaps
we will have to change our plans next year. We need to apply
a prophylactic plan with a treatment of six weeks or twelve
weeks, etc. We did not do that in this study because our aim
only was to compare the vaccinated and the unvaccinated animals.
Both groups suffered from trichostrongylidosis, and this infection was not considered in the present study. If we were to do
a new trial, we would compare the two methods with vaccination
and no vaccination, but we would use a strategic treatment also.
But here our goal was just to compare vaccination or not with
an early treatment of levamisole.

J-P. Raynaud *(France)*

Some experiments we have done in France may explain the
compensatory growth. When you have a permanent pasture and
two comparable groups of animals, by about July or August
the animals, when they become very sick, do not eat at all.
So this is a time for the grass to grow. However, the protected
animals still eat the grass. When the animals clinically
recover, they are faced with a very good high pasture which
allows them to compensate readily. This is not an explanation,
it is just an observation.

H.-J. Bürger *(FRG)*

It happened to us recently, that the first indication of parasitic gastro-enteritis occurring was when the grass was growing better on the pasture of the group that ultimately fell sick. These animals apparently did not eat less than those that were later unaffected, but there was more grass on this particular paddock for some time. On the next inspection some of the animals had diarrhoea. This may well contribute to compensatory growth.

J. Armour *(UK)*

I would like to ask Professor Pouplard if he examined the lungs of the animals. Did you compare the pathology?

L. Pouplard

No, we are still using the animals in the experiment. They are overwintering and we are going to compare the weight-gains after wintering in the barn.

J. Armour

I was thinking of the pathological changes of the two different groups. The pathological changes in the lungs of the vaccinates, which have been under challenge, and those which have been treated and then, perhaps, exposed to some re-infection

L. Pouplard

Yes, there was re-infection, and our first idea was to kill the animals, but we decided to look at the weightgain problem of animals, comparing those in animals with and without clinical signs. We want to check the difference after a period in the barn. Many farmers say there is a bad case of lungworm after one season in the barn.

J. Eckert *(Switzerland)*

You recommend treatment in June and July, and then the animals remain on the same pasture?

L. Pouplard

No. If possible the farmer will change the pasture around the middle of July. If possible it is best to put the animal on another pasture where they normally make hay and leave it there until slaughter in October.

J. Eckert

But if they stay on the same pasture, is it sufficient to treat them the last time in July?

L. Pouplard

Usually, yes. Not always. We could give more treatment but we had to find a system where the cost was not too high. But normally, yes; we have to be very careful.

TREATMENT OF CATTLE NEMATODIASIS WITH ®PANACUR*

D. Düwel

Hoechst AG, Helminthologie, Postfach 80 03 20,
D-9230 Frankfurt/M. 80, Federal Republic of Germany.

ABSTRACT

The data on investigations with fenbendazole (FBZ) a vermifugal anthelminthic are summarised. FBZ is well tolerated up to 267 - 400 times the oral therapeutic does of 5 - 7.5 mg/kg. Pharmacokinetic data demonstrate a short half-life for the compound in serum and milk; residues in tissues are extremely small. The mode of action has been demonstrated to be a combination of a disorder of the energy metabolism and neurotoxis effects.

The spectrum of activity of FBZ covers practically all the economically important nematodes of the gastro-intestinal tract and lungs of cattle; FBZ is effective against both adult and immature nematodes including the inhibited stages of Ostertagia and other nematodes. In addition, it has an ovicidal and larvicidal activity. The weightgains and the increase in milk output which result after FBZ treatment emphasise the advantage of treatment with FBZ.

*) Registered trade mark of Hoechst AG, Frankfurt/M; generic name: fenbendazole; chemical name: methyl-[5-(phenyl-thio)-benzimidazole-2-carbamat].

P. Nansen, R.J. Jørgensen, E.J.L. Soulsby (eds), Epidemiology and Control of Nematodiasis in Cattle.

INTRODUCTION

Helminth infection in cattle, depending on the severity of infection, interferes with production, for example, by the depression of weightgain; there may be loss of weight in severe infections and death may occur in very severe infections. Anthelmintics and appropriate accompanying measures are economic necessities for productive livestock in the majority of countries of the world.

A broad spectrum of activity is demanded of modern anthelmintics and several new anthelmintics belong to the benzimidazole series. The compounds have brought an improvement in efficacy and a reduction of the therapeutic dose required and, at the same time, have provided a better tolerability, i.e. a widening of the chemotherapeutic index. An example of such development is fenbendazole, the active principle of 'Panacur'.

The modern criteria used for evaluation of an anthelmintic include general and special tolerance (for example, teratogenic side effects and influence on fertility) and in addition residue characteristics, ovicidal and/or larvicidal activities, as well as the action against so-called problem parasitoses.

TOLERANCE

Fenbendazole was found to be nontoxic after single and repeated administration. LD_{50} values are not available for laboratory and domestic animals because the quantity of the active principle to be administered is too great. Thus bovines tolerate more than 2 000 mg fenbendazole/kg body weight, which is 267 - 400 times the therapeutic dose (Düwel, 1976, 1977; James, 1979).

No reactions of intolerance have been observed in numerous controlled field trials, in special tests, or after several years' practical use in many countries, under various climatic and feeding conditions. This clinical evidence is in agreement with the finding that fenbendazole, apart from its anthelmintic action, has no untoward pharmacological effect on the central nervous system or the autonomous nervous system (Düwel, 1977).

In contrast to other anthelmintics (including some recent ones) there is no evidence of fenbendazole having teratogenic or fertility-inhibiting properties. For example, repeated administration of fenbendazole in a therapeutic dose, or a single dose amounting to several times the therapeutic dose, did not cause teratogenic damage in calves or the offspring of other domestic animals (Becker, 1975; Tiefenbach, 1976). The insemination index or the sperm quality of bulls treated with fenbendazole were not adversely affected (Krause et al., 1975).

TABLE 1

TEST FOR TOLERANCE OF SINGLE OR REPEATED ORAL DOSES OF FENBENDAZOLE IN LABORATORY AND TARGET ANIMALS

Animal species	Duration of experiment (days)	Maximum tolerated dose (mg/kg body weight)
Rat	1	> 10 000*
	30	2 500
	90	1 600[2,3]
Rabbit	1	< 3 200*
Dog	1	> 500[3]
	30	80
	90	125
Sheep	1	> 5 000*
	30	15
Cattle	1	> 2 000[3]
Pig	1	> 5 000*
Horse	1	> 1 000[3]

*) The maximum amount that was possible to administer

2) In some animals the dosage increased to 2 500 mg/kg body weight from the 61st day onwards.

3) Higher dosages not tested.

METABOLISM AND PHARMACOKINETICS

The metabolism and pharmacokinetics of fenbendazole have been extensively investigated (Figure 1). Fenbendazole is absorbed only to a limited extent and is then excreted in the faeces and in the urine, mainly in the form of metabolites (Christ et al., 1974; Düwel et al., 1975; Düwel, 1977). The half-life for elimination from the blood varies from 10 to approximately 28 h, depending on the animal species. After treatment of bovines with 7.5 mg FBZ/kg the elimination half-lives are 13 and 14 h for serum and milk, respectively. Residues in edible tissues (muscle, fat, organs) are extremely small (Düwel, 1976, 1977). Twelve cattle were given 10 mg FBZ/kg, and 15 sheep and 12 pigs were given the therapeutic dose of 5 mg/kg orally. They were slaughtered 2, 5, 7 or 14 days later. Some sheep were also slaughtered 21 days later. Tissues were examined for residual amounts of the drug and the maximum drug residues that were present in animals killed two days after treatment are shown below:

	Cattle	Sheep	Pigs
Meat	0.47 ppm	0.27 ppm	0.24 ppm
Fat	1.31 ppm (5th day)	0.86 ppm	0.24 ppm
Liver	8.4 ppm	4.4 ppm	0.76 ppm
Kidney	1.04 ppm	0.69 ppm	0.62 ppm

In cattle, the tissue concentrations fell below the detectable limit from the 5th day in kidney, from the 7th day in fat and muscle and from the 14th day in the liver. In sheep, fenbendazole was no longer detectable from the 5th day in kidney, from the 14th day in muscle and fat and from the 21st day in the liver. In pigs, there was no residue in kidneys and muscle on the 5th day, or in fat on the 7th day after treatment. However, residues in concentrations almost beyond the detectable limit were still present in the liver on the 14th day.

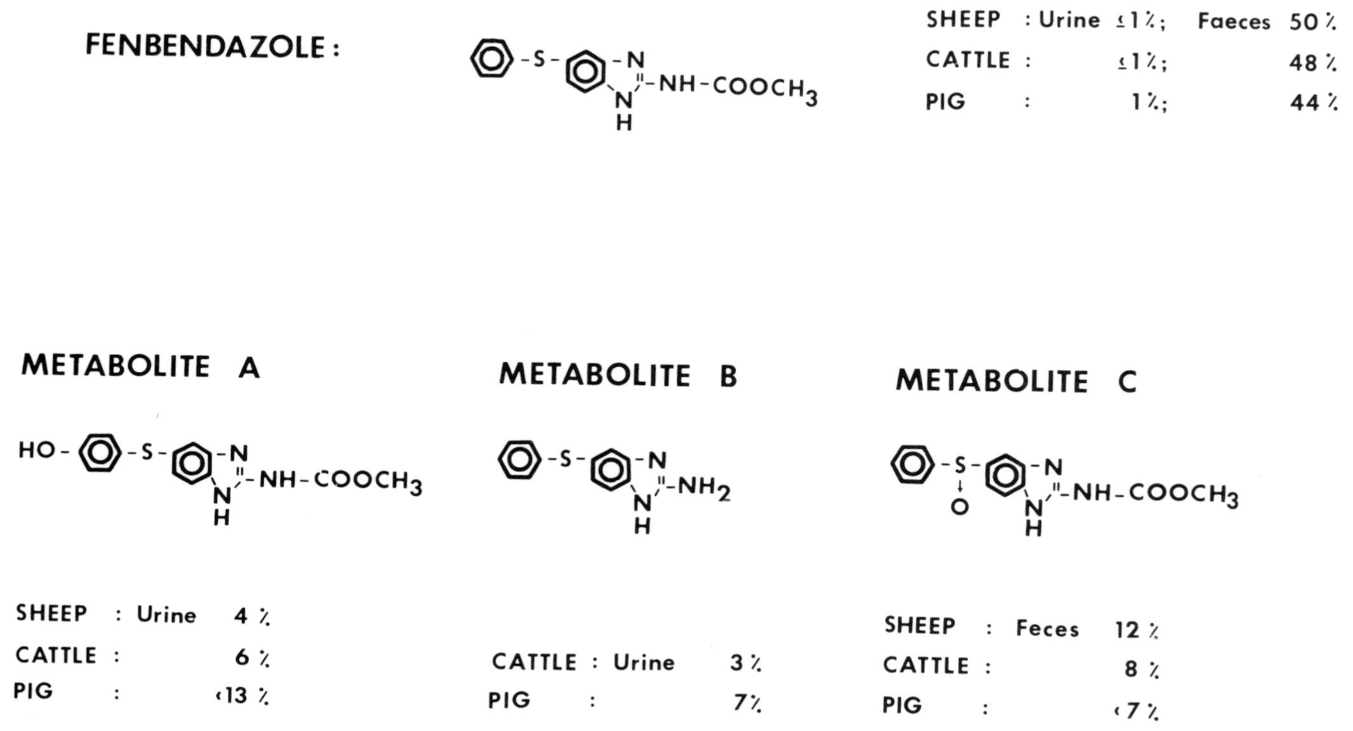

Fig. 1.   Metabolism of fenbendazole.

TABLE 2

PHARMACOKINETIC DATA OF FENBENDAZOLE (FLUOROMETRIC METHOD: DETECTABLE LIMIT 0.05 PPM)

Animal species	Dose mg/kg b.w. orally	Appearance of maximum levels (hrs after administration)	Maximum concentration (ppm)	Duration of detectable levels (hrs)	Mean elimination half-life (hrs)
Rabbit (serum)	50 100	30 48	2.6 3.6	78 78	15 21
Pig (serum)	5	6-12	0.45	48	10
Sheep (serum)	5	6-24	0.40	96	26
Cattle (serum)	7.5 10	24-30 24-30	1.10 1.60	102 120	13 14
Cattle Milk	7.5 10	30 54	0.35 0.55	96 96	14
Goat Milk	5	30	0.30	54	

These low residues are accompanied by good tolerance characteristics. As a result, the acceptable daily intake values set for man are relatively high, so that no withdrawal times have been fixed in the Federal Republic of Germany or in many other countries. This applies also to the milk of lactating cows (and of sheep and goats) (Becker, 1976). Further, the milk of treated cows does not pose any technological problems in cheese production (Heeschen et al., 1979).

MODE OF ACTION

The mode of action is a disorder of the energy metabolism accompanied by neurotoxis effects. The incorporation of glucose into the glycogen molecule and the degradation of endogenous glycogen are inhibited in nematodes. This leads to starvation of the parasite due to exhaustion of its energy reserves (Düwel, 1976). In the course of these and other disturbances in the energy metabolism (Prichard et al., 1978a, 1978b) there

TABLE 3

PHARMACOKINETIC STUDIES WITH ^{14}C-FENBENDAZOLE (DETECTABLE LIMIT 0.01 PPM)

Animal species	Dose mg/kg b.w. orally	Appearance of maximum levels (hrs after administration)	Maximum concentration (ppm)	Mean elimination half-life (hrs)	Excretion via urine	Excretion via faeces	Drug concentration in liver: ppm (days after administration)
Rat (blood)	10	5-7	0.19	6	7%	predominant	
Rabbit (blood)	10	8	0.90	13	21%	predominant	
Dog (blood)	10	6-24	0.04-0.4	15	7%	predominant	
Pig (blood)	5	4.5	0.86	7.4	33%	predominant	0.26 (7)
Sheep (blood)	5	31-55	0.24-0.32	28	7%	> 90%	2.7 (7)
Cattle (blood)	5	28-30	0.52	15	14%	77%	1.4 (15)
Cattle (milk)	5	8-22	0.59	14			

is disruption of cytoplasmic microtubules in the intestinal
epithelium of nematodes and in the tegumental cells of cestodes
(Friedman et al., 1978; Ireland et al., 1979; Düwel et al., 1978).
Finally, a neurotoxic effect has been detected also which results
in a transient paralysis of the parasite (Düwel, 1976). Fenbendazole should therefore be classed as a vermifugal anthelmintic,
with the worms dying at a later stage. However, I am of the
opinion that the mode of action is somewhat like a jig-saw
puzzle with many pieces still missing to complete the full
picture.

ANTHELMINTIC ACTIVITY

The spectrum of activity of fenbendazole in bovines for all
practical purposes covers all the important nematodes of the
abomasum, and small and large intestine, as well as those of the
lungs. These parasites are eliminated by a dose of 5 - 7.5 mg
FBZ/kg body weight.

Additionally, the drug is active against *Chabertia, Strongyloides* and *Neoascaris*. The high efficacy against immature and adult
nematodes, noted under experimental conditions, has been confirmed in numerous field trials (Düwel, 1979).

Fenbendazole, in a single dose of 7.5 mg/kg orally, is
effective against inhibited 4th stage larvae of *Ostertagia
ostertagi*. These are deeply embedded in the mucous membrane of
the abomasum and, hitherto, it has not been possible to achieve
a therapeutic effect with other anthelmintic compounds. These
developmental stages are responsible for winter ostertagiasis
or ostertagiasis type II. The efficacy of fenbendazole against
such developmental stages was reported first by Anderson et al.,
1975, 1977, in Australia, and later, in Europe, Duncan et al.
(1976) confirmed the results. Laboratory experiments and field
trials in other parts of the world confirm the efficacy against
ostertagiasis type II (e.g. Nagle, 1977; LeStang et al., 1978;
Callinan et al., 1979; Williams et al., 1979). A few investigations report the effect of fenbendazole as variable or

inadequate on developmental stages (Elliott, 1977; Lancaster et al., 1977; Inderbitzin et al., 1978). There has not yet been any satisfactory explanation for this variation, but it is possible that the metabolism of hypobiotic stages varies, depending on the age of infection or due to influences of the host animal, or this metabolism, possibly influenced by internal or external conditions, is subject to flucuations.

TABLE 4

ANTHELMINTIC EFFICACY OF FENBENDAZOLE IN CATTLE

Nematode/genus (location of adult worms)	Stage of development	Percent reduction in worm burden
Haemonchus (abomasum)	immature mature	98.1 - 100 100
Ostertagia (abomasum)	immature mature	92.1 - 100 90 - 100
Trichostrongylus (abomasum, small intestine)	immature mature	100 100
Cooperia (small intestine)	immature mature	100 99.9 - 100
Nematodirus (small intestine)	immature mature	100 > 95 - 100
Bunostomum (small intestine)	immature mature	100 100
Oesophagostomum (large intestine)	immature mature	100 100
Capillaria (caecum, colon)	immature mature	100 100
Trichuris (caecum, colon)	immature mature	100 100
Dictyocaulus viviparus (lung)	immature mature	99 - 100 100

In addition, technical or experimental conditions, such as artificial or natural infection, age and weight of the treated animals, time of treatment and rate of passage of fenbendazole through the rumen, may be factors which have an influence of efficacy. Studies in Scotland, using naturally infected cattle, have shown that fenbendazole has a powerful anthelmintic effect on the inhibited larval stages of *Ostertagia*, independently of whether the infective larvae (L_3) were exposed for a prolonged period to 'cool conditions' on pasture or not (Duncan et al., 1978).

PHARMACOLOGICAL ACTION

Fenbendazole first causes paralysis of the worms which subsequently leads to the death of the worms, the time taken depending on the amount of the dosing absorbed by the worms. It is possible that the anatomical location of the inhibited stages, being deeply embedded in the mucous membrane, render elimination difficult after fenbendazole treatment. This can be especially so when fenbendazole levels either are too low or are of too short duration; for example, when the rumen loses its function as a reservoir due to a change in the ruminal pH, in the rate of rumen emptying, etc. Under such circumstances there might be no elimination of inhibited stages during the period of this paralysis. However, the times hitherto selected for autopsy during the tests may be too short for the dead stages to have been removed by the cellular systems of the host. The data of Snider et al. (1980) on the therapy of ostertagiasis type II with fenbendazole or albendazole, lends support to this hypothesis. The study found that the burden of early 4th stage larvae (EL_4) was reduced by 94 - 99% after fenbendazole treatment and of the stages remaining in the animals up to 80% were dead. There were no dead stages in the untreated controls. An experiment with 16 bullocks to confirm the results of Snider et al. (1980) showed, following treatment with fenbendazole, a general efficacy of 93 - 97% against inhibited *Ostertagia* stages, however all the inhibited stages which remained in the animal were alive. Nevertheless, this must be considered to have limited value since the number of inhibited larval stages per animal, on average, was 3 300 EL_4 (600 - 10 800) and this is considered to be very low (Düwel et al., 1980).

However, generally, fenbendazole achieves a high degree of effectiveness against hypobiotic stages such that good weight gains in clinically infected animals are attainable during the winter months following treatment.

Fenbendazole has been reported to have an effect on the gastro-intestinal nematodes of cattle (Lancaster et al., 1977; Duncan et al., 1978) and also on inhibited stages of *Dictyocaulus viviparus* in cattle (Inderbitzin et al., 1978; Pfeiffer, 1978). A similar effect on inhibited stages in sheep has been reported by Thomas (1978).

OVICIDAL/LARVICIDAL ACTIVITY

The ovicidal and larvicidal activity of fenbendazole, which is demonstrable as early as a few hours after administration of the therapeutic dose, is of epidemiological importance. Studies in cattle artificially infected with different nematodes, have shown that a reduction in egg output started 22 - 24 h after treatment, and from 36 h after treatment eggs were no longer detectable by faecal examination. An absence of egg output lasted for up to 4 weeks after treatment. However, larvicidal activity was evident as early as 8 h after treatment and larvae no longer developed in faecal cultures. This effect was evident with all nematodes examined in the trial: *O. ostertagi*, *H. contortus*, *T. axei*, *Cooperia* spp., *N. helvetianus* and *Oe. radiatum* (Düwel, 1979).

The ovicidal activity of fenbendazole was manifested not only by the lack of larval development, but also was evident by morphological changes in the blastomeres of the egg. This suggests that the eggs were damaged in the uterus of the worms by fenbendazole. Examples of such damage to eggs of *Ostertagia* and *Nematodirus* are presented in Figures 2a and 2b (Kirsch, 1976).

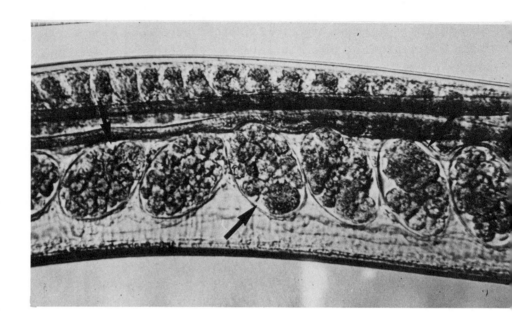

Fig. 2a.   Ovicidal activity of fenbendazole. Morphological alterations
            of *Ostertagia* eggs in the uterus after FBZ treatment.

ECONOMIC ASPECTS

    The profitability of treatment of cattle with fenbendazole
has been investigated in a number of trials. After allowances
had been made for husbandry methods and feeding procedures in
different countries, additional weight gains occurred in treated
animals as compared to non-treated controls. Following three
treatments with fenbendazole during the period July to November,
treated animals gained 58 kg more in weight than controls in a
trial in Germany (n = 14 + 14). The cattle were kept under
observation for 11 months (Figure 3)(Düwel, 1976). In New
Zealand, trials were conducted under varying farm and feed
conditions. Groups of 28 - 30 cattle were treated and weighed
three times at intervals of 4 weeks and the trial was concluded
4 weeks after the last treatment. The worm burden (as measured
by faecal egg output) was low. Nevertheless, there were distinct
differences between untreated and treated animals in the majority
of cases as is shown in Figure 4. In some groups weight loss

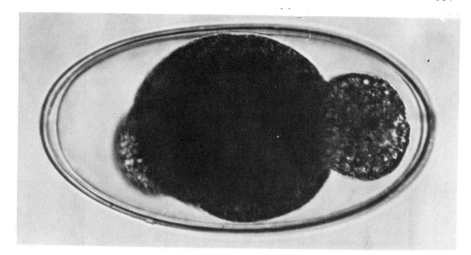

A.

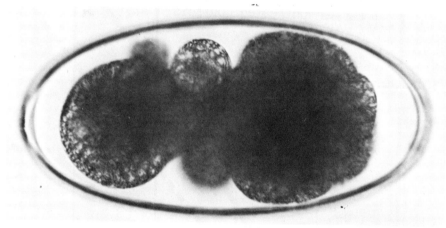

B.

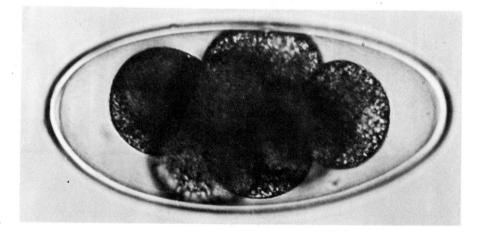

C.

Fig. 2b.   Ovicidal activity of fenbendazole. Morphological alterations
(A, B) of *Nematodirus* eggs, isolated from faeces of FBZ treated
animal in comparison to normal development (C).

338

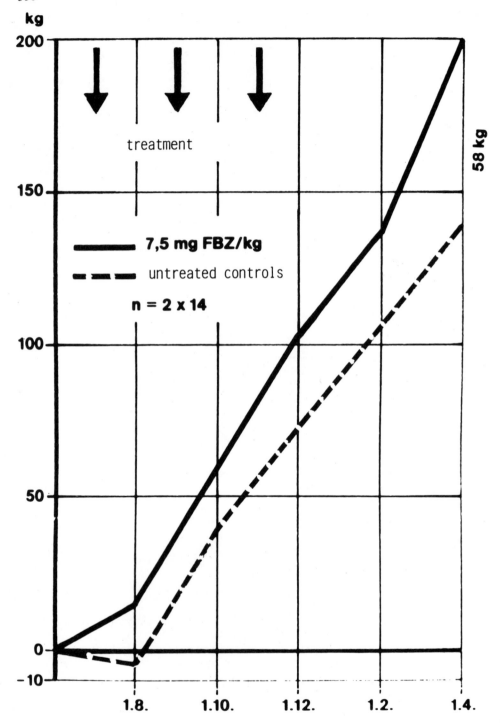

Fig. 3.   Weight gains in cattle within 10 months.

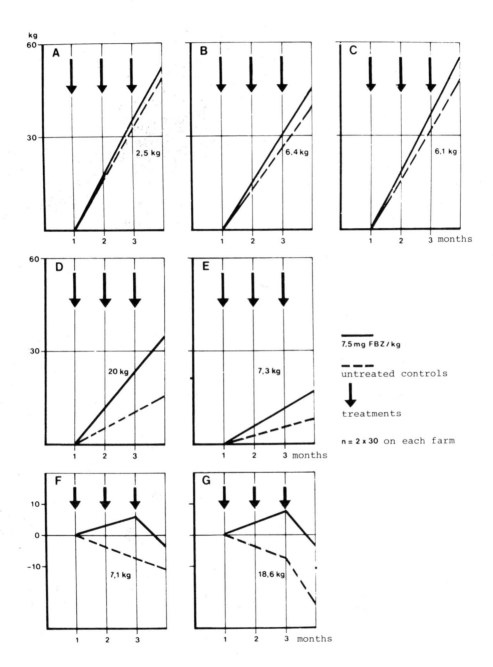

Fig. 4.   Weight gains in cattle within 3 months on 7 different farms in
New Zealand.

occurred because of feed shortage in the third months of the trial. However, even under the conditions, weight losses were less in treated animals than in untreated controls (Tiefenbach, 1980).

Subclinical helminth infection of dairy cows is reputed to affect adversely the milk output. In four trials conducted so far, it was found that the milk output was increased following treatment with fenbendazole. In a study in England, eight herds were treated in which *Ostertagia* infection had been detected in cows on pasture. Treatment with fenbendazole shortly before calving resulted in an average increase in milk output during the subsequent lactation period of 173 kg per cow compared to the previous lactation period, and compared also to untreated controls, with heifers an increased milk output as high as 526 kg per animal, compared to controls, was detected (McBeath et al., 1979).

The treatment of cows during the descending part of the lactation curve, showed increased outputs of 0.17 and 0.25 l/cow/d in favour of the treated animals, 2 - 6 weeks after fenbendazole treatment (Barger, 1979). In a further study, an increase in the milk quantity by approximately 3 - 4% and an increase in the milk fat by 7 - 8%, compared to the controls, was detected within a period of 6 weeks and 3 months after treatment with fenbendazole and thiabendazole, respectively (Tiefenbach, 1980).

REFERENCES

Anderson, N., 1975. Control strategies for *Ostertagia* infections of beef
cattle. CSIRO-Division of Animal Health, Annual Report, pp. 76-77.

Anderson, N., 1977. The efficiency of levamisole, thiabendazole and fenbendazole against naturally acquired infections of *Ostertagia ostertagi*
in cattle. Res. Vet. Sci. 23, 298-302.

Barger, J.A., 1979. Milk production of grazing dairy cattle after a single
anthelmintic treatment. Austr. Vet. J. 55, 68-70.

Becker, W., 1975. Die Anwendung von Panacur bei trächtigen Tieren. Second
European Multicolloquy of Parasitology, Trogir/Yugoslavia, pp. 105-106.

Becker, W., 1976. Die Bewertung von Rückständen nach Anwendung von Panacur.
Berl. Münch. tierärztl. Wschr. 89, 453-456.

Callinan, A.P.L. and Cummins, L.J., 1979. Efficacy of anthelmintics against
cattle nematodes. Austr. Vet. J. 55, 370-373.

Christ, O., Kellner, H.-M. and Klöpffer, G., 1974. Studies on the pharmacokinetics and metabolism with fenbendazole - a new anthelmintic.
Proc. 3rd Int. Congr. Parasit., Munich. 3, 1448-1449.

Duncan, J.L., Armour, J., Bairden, K., Jennings, J.W. and Urquhart, G.M.,
1976. The successful removal of inhibited 4th stage *Ostertagia
ostertagi* larvae by fenbendazole. Vet. Rec. 98, 342.

Duncan, J.L., Armour, J. and Bairden, K., 1978. Autumn and winter fenbendazole treatment against inhibited 4th stage *Ostertagia ostertagi* larvae
in cattle. Vet. Rec. 103, 211-213.

Düwel, D., Hajdú, P. and Damm, D., 1975. Zur Pharmakokinetik von Fenbendazol.
Ber. Münch. tierärztl. Wschr. 88, 131-134.

Düwel, D., 1976. Panacur - die Entwicklung eines neuen Breitband-Anthelminthikums. Die Blauen Hefte Nr. 55, 189-203.

Düwel, D., 1977. Fenbendazole II. Biological properties and activity.
Pesticide Sci. 8, 550-555.

Düwel, D. and Schleich, H., 1978. *In vivo* Untersuchungen zur Wirkungsweise
von Fenbendazol. Zbl. Vet. Med. B. 25, 800-805.

Düwel, D., 1979. Zur oviziden und larviziden Wirksamkeit von Panacur. Die
Blauen Hefte Nr. 59, 441-452.

Düwel, D., 1979. Panacur - Summary and evaluation of the worldwide published
investigations. Published by Hoechst AG, Frankfurt/M., pp. 90.

342

Düwel, D. and Kirsch, R., 1980. Laborexperimentelle Untersuchungen mit Panacur. Die Blauen Hefte Nr. 61 (in press).

Elliott, D.C., 1977. The effect of fenbendazole in removing inhibited early-4th-stage *Ostertagia ostertagi* from yearling cattle. New Zealand Vet. J. 25, 145-147.

Friedman, P.A. and Platzer, E.G., 1978. Interaction of anthelmintic benzimidazoles and benzimidazole derivatives with bovine brain tubulin. Biochem. Biophys. Acta 544, 605-614.

Heeschen, W., Kaiser, M., Hamann, J. and Blüthgen, A., 1979. Zum Einfluss einer Panacur-Behandlung auf die Molkereitauglichkeit der Milch. Tierärztl. Umschau 34, 45-48.

Inderbitzin, F. and Eckert, J., 1978. Die Wirkung von Fenbendazol (Panacur) gegen gehemmte Stadien von *Dictyocaulus viviparus* und *Ostertagia ostertagi* bei Kälbern. Berl. Münch. tierärztl. Wschr. 91, 395-399.

Ireland, Chr. M., Gull, K., Gutteridge, W.E. and Pogson, Ch. J., 1979. The interaction of benzimidazole carbamates with mammalian microtubule protein. Biochem. Pharmacol. 28, 2680-2682.

James, R., 1979. Zur Prüfung von Panacur in Australien. Die Blauen Hefte Nr. 59, 465-474.

Kirsch, R., 1976. Morphologische Veränderungen an Trichostrongyliden-Eiren nach Fenbendazol-Behandlung. Z. Parasitenkd. 50, 223.

Krause, D., Reinhard, H.J., Köhler, W. and Tiefenbach, B., 1975. Untersuchungen uber die Wirkung des Anthelminthikums Fenbendazol auf die Spermaqualität von Besamungsbullen. Dtsch. tierärztl. Wschr. 82, 231-233.

Lancaster, M.B. and Hong, C., 1977. Action of fenbendazole on arrested 4th stage larvae of *Ostertagia ostertagi*. Vet. Rec. 101, 81-82.

McBeath, D.G., Dean, S.P. and Preston, N.K., 1979. The effect of a preparturient fenbendazole treatment on lactation yield in dairy cows. Vet. Rec. 105, 507-509.

Nagle, E.J., 1977. Aspects of intensive beef production from grassland. Thesis, The National University of Ireland, Dublin., pp. 97.

Pfeiffer, H. 1978. Zur Wirksamkeit von Fenbendazol nach wiederholter Verabreichung niedriger Dosen gegen entwicklungsgehemmte Rinderlungenwürmer. Wiener tierärztl. Wschr. 65, 343-346.

Prichard, R.K., Donald, A.D., Dash, K.M. and Hennessy, D.R., 1978a. Factors involved in the relative anthelmintic tolerance of arrested 4th stage larvae of *Ostertagia ostertagi*. Vet. Rec. 102, 382.

Pritchard, R.K., Hennessy, D.R. and Steel, J.W., 1978. Prolonged administration: a new concept for increasing the spectrum and effectiveness of anthelmintics. Vet. Parasitology, 4, 309-315.

Snider III, T.G. and Williams, J.C., 1980. Recovery of dead early-4th-stage
Ostertagia ostertagi following benzimidazole administration. Vet. Rec.
106, 34.

LeStang, J.-P., Hubert, J. and Kerbouef, D., 1978. Etude de l'efficacite
du fenbendazole dans le traitement de l'ostertagiose bovine de pretype
II. Rev. Méd. Vét. 129, 1355-1369.

Thomas, R.J., 1978. The efficacy of in-feed medication with fenbendazole
against gastro-intestinal nematodes of sheep, with particular reference
to inhibited larvae. Vet. Rec. 102, 394-397.

Tiefenbach, B., 1976. Panacur - weltweite klinische Prüfung eines neuen
Breitband-Anthelminthikums. Die Blauen Hefte Nr. 55, 204-218.

Tiefenbach, B., 1980. Ökonomische Aspekte einer anthelminthisch Behandlung
mit Panacur. Die Blauen Hefte Nr. 62 (in press)

Williams, J.C., Knox, J.W., Sheehan, D.S. and Fuselier, R.H., 1979. Activity
of fenbendazole against inhibited early 4th-stage larvae of *Ostertagia
ostertagi*. Am. J. Vet. Res. 40, 1087-1090.

DISCUSSION

J. Eckert *(Switzerland)*

 Apparently, there is some unexplained variation in the
activity of fenbendazole against inhibited stages. Some experiments indicate that the use of small doses, over a period, may
be superior to a single treatment. What are the recent recommendations about this? Should we treat the animals once only,
or would it be better to treat them for some days with lower
doses?

D. Düwel *(FRG)*

 I have not heard of any trials where inhibited larvae of
Ostertagia have been treated with repeated small doses with
resulting high efficacy. However, in the case of inhibited
lungworm larval stages, repeated treatments with low doses
gave better results than a single treatment. The same occurs
with other parasites e.g. *Trichinella* or *Trichuris*. We have done
some laboratory investigations and have found that after a
single treatment of 7.5 mg we achieve a satisfactory basic serum
level of the drug.

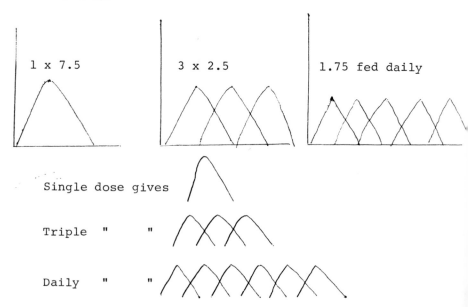

1 x 7.5   3 x 2.5   1.75 fed daily

Single dose gives

Triple   "   "

Daily   "   "

However, if we treat the animal three times with lower doses, we have peak levels repeated (as in the diagram); or if we treat for 5 - 7 days with 1 mg/kg, we would have a permanent serum level of fenbendazole and hence would have a therapeutic influence over a longer period. Thus we might have a higher efficacy, especially in problem parasites. However, it may not be possible to do repeated treatments in all cases because this needs a lot of manpower. It might be possible to treat with medicated feed, e.g. with licks or blocks, as is common in Britain, or with pellets.

R.M. Connan *(UK)*

Williams and his co-worker investigated the efficacy of fenbendazole and albendazole against arrested larvae. Nine and 11 days after treatment they still found dead and dying worms in the mucosae. My experience in sheep suggests that the drug is removed very quickly. This suggests that the worms die slowly or, alternatively, the dead worms are not digested. Is this a factor in the differences in susceptibility of arrested larvae or not to anthelmintics?

D. Düwel

I cannot answer this, I only know that the situation in sheep is completely different from cattle. In sheep the larvae are not so deeply embedded in the mucosa as they are in cattle. Of course we were surprised by the finding of Williams too. We repeated the work but we did not find dead larvae in the mucosa.

R.M. Connan

I was hoping that somebody might tell us about their experiences with the phenomenon.

J. Armour *(UK)*

We always used to keep animals for seven days before slaughter. We have not observed the phenomenon described by Williams. However, based on Williams' data, animals are now kept for 14 days after treatment before slaughter.

D. Düwel

In his first trial, Anderson slaughtered 2 days after administration of fenbendazole and he found no efficacy against inhibited stages. He repeated the trial, slaughtering at 7 - 9 days after treatment. Then he had a good efficacy of more than 80% or 90%.

J. Euzeby *(France)*

I would like to ask some questions about larvicidal and ovicidal activity. What about the action on eggs of *Moniezia?*

D. Düwel

None.

J. Euzeby

It is important because the drug is able to immobilise the worm, but it does not kill the eggs and one may have plenty of eggs spread on the pastures.

D. Düwel

After treatment of *Moniezia* in sheep, and cattle too, it is very difficult to collect segments of the tapeworms because the segments are destroyed during the passage in the gut. But we never have collected faeces and looked for the eggs of *Moniezia* spp.

J. Euzeby

What about the ovicidal activity in nematodes? Is it really an ovicidal activity or just an inhibition of egg-laying which will resume later on?

D. Düwel

No, it is a real ovicidal effect. We can observe the same effect on eggs isolated from worms four hours after treatment.

J. Euzeby

    When you make up a culture in which larval development is inhibited, are these cultures made up from the faeces of animals which have been treated?

D. Düwel

    No. We collect the eggs from faeces of treated animals and put them in another clean faecal culture.

O. Nilsson *(Sweden)*

    You referred to my comments this morning and I want to avoid a misunderstanding. I did not say that fenbendazole did not have activity against the worm. I said that when we used fenbendazole, in cattle in November, we did not see a better weightgain. To complete this I can give you the figure of the plasma pepsinogen level; it never exceeded one unit during the whole trial period, from the 4th November to the 14th April. That means that if an animal does not suffer clinically from the maturation of larvae, we cannot accept that lower weight-gains will occur.

D. Düwel

    Bearing this in mind, where we have made strategic treat-ment in northern Germany we have the best weightgains during the housing period. Just after housing there is a difference between treated and untreated controls of about 15 kg weight-gain, but later during the housing period a much larger differ-ence between treated and untreated animals is seen.

O. Nilsson

    Might it be a question of what is the intensity of the primary infection? Normally we have the highest primary infection in May, and the lower infection in October.

D. Düwel

    That may be the answer.

J.F. Michel *(UK)*

I thought I should add some information to what my colleagues, Hong and Lancaster, have been doing in the matter of the
efficacy against arrested *Ostertagia*. They have been looking to
confirm their previous results and to determine whether the
time at which infection is acquired is important and whether
or not the length of time that the worms were conditioned on
the pasture has some effect. Their conclusion is that the
failure of fenbendazole to kill arrested *Ostertagia*, which occurs
from time to time, is not related to these factors.

H. de Keyser *(Belgium)*

I would like to make one comment on the weightgain trials.
When you do weightgain trials is it not necessary to use twins,
because the heritability of weightgain is between 20% and 40%
in the same family of animals? Everyone is talking about
weightgain, but is it weightgain on the same amount of food,
or is it weightgain on *ad libitum* food?

D. Düwel

It is easier to answer with my second example. In New
Zealand there were no twins and all the animals were on pasture
and had the opportunity to take up different amounts of grass.
Therefore, perhaps it was not really a correct trial. In the
trial which I mentioned in northwest Germany we used twins,
but we know that twins do not always eat the same amount of
grass. However, during the wintertime in the housing period,
each animal was given food according to their weight plus a
little bit more. This means that we have a true weightgain
corresponding to the food intake conversion. More important
than the liveweight gain is weightgain between the comparison
of water loss of the fresh carcase weight and the cold carcase
weight - that means the shrinkage - and also the killing-out
percent. If you compare both groups there is a much greater
difference than the 58 kg mentioned.

A NEW METHOD OF CONTROL OF GASTRO-INTESTINAL PARASITES IN GRAZING CALVES

R.M. Jones

Parasitology Department, Pfizer Central Research,
Pfizer Limited, Sandwich, Kent, UK.

ABSTRACT

Control of parasitic gastro-enteritis (PGE) in grazing calves has relied mainly upon strategic therapeutic dosing or modification of pasture management practices, or a combination of both. These procedures, though effective, suffer from the practical disadvantage that the farmer is often unable to provide either the labour or clean pastures at the appropriate time and are consequently not properly applied. An alternative approach, which has been investigated over recent years, is the use of continuous anthelmintic medication during the first part of the grazing season to protect calves from overwintered infection on pasture and prevent the subsequent build-up of disease producing levels of pasture contamination. The practical application of this approach requires the combination of an anthelmintic which is effective at economic dosage levels and a reliable delivery system.

This paper describes the field testing of an intraruminal device (morantel sustained release bolus - MSRB) designed to release morantel tartrate continuously at effective dose levels for a period of about 60 days. Ten studies were conducted on commercial and experimental farms in England, France, Germany and Sweden during the 1978 grazing season to a common experimental design. The morantel sustained release bolus (MSRB) was administered to test calves at turnout in the spring.

The efficacy of the MSRB was assessed principally on comparisons of the weight gains over the grazing season between control treated animals and the incidence of clinical disease. Faecal egg counts provided a further assessment of anti-parasitic activity. Herbage larval counts and tracer calves were also used to measure the efficacy of the MSRB in reducing pasture larval contamination.

P. Nansen, R.J. Jørgensen, E.J.L. Soulsby (eds), Epidemiology and Control of Nematodiasis in Cattle.

The combined results show that the MSRB was consistently effective in controlling PGE on the trial farms where a moderate to severe parasite challenge occurred. Overall, 178 MSRB treated calves showed a mean weight gain advantage over their contemporary controls of 21.2 kg at the end of the grazing season on all sites. The number of acute clinical cases of PGE requiring therapeutic treatment was reduced from 62 to 5. Parasitological data show that this result was achieved by the MSRB preventing the mid-summer rise in pasture larval contamination and thus eliminating the detrimental effect of high parasite challenge in the latter part of the grazing season, and the data also show that the MSRB is a complete control mechanism for gastro-intestinal nematodes in calves.

INTRODUCTION

Current methods of control of parasitic gastro-enteritis
in grazing calves rely mainly on repeat therapeutic dosing with
anthelmintics and/or modification of pasture management to avoid
exposure to high levels of pasture infection. These procedures,
though effective, are not often properly applied since the farmer
is not able to provide labour for dosing or clean pasture at the
appropriate time.

An alternative approach has received attention over recent
years involving the administration of anthelmintics during the
first part of the grazing season, with the objective of preventing the propagation of parasites originating from overwintered
infection on pasture and thereby the mid-season rise in pasture
larval contamination. This method of control has been shown to
be feasible by Pott et al. (1974), using anthelmintic at two
weekly intervals in May and June, and by Downey et al. (1974),
using drinking water to deliver anthelmintics over a similar
period. Pott et al. (1979) also demonstrated the effectiveness
of low level morantel tartrate given in feed for the first 60
days of the grazing season.

Practical drawbacks to the use of these conventional
methods of anthelmintic medication in grazing bovines have
precluded the wide-spread application of early season anthelmintic treatment for the control of parasitic gastro-enteritis.
This paper describes field testing of a delivery system which
makes possible the convenient and reliable continuous medication
of grazing calves. The delivery system consists of an intra-
ruminal device (morantel sustained release bolus - MSRB) which
is designed to be administered orally to calves at the beginning
of the grazing season to give a continuous slow release of
morantel for a period of about 2 months. A summary report of the
results of a series of trials, conducted to evaluate the MSRB
in four European countries during the 1978 grazing season, is
presented.

MATERIAL AND METHODS

The present study involved 356 first season grazing calves in ten separate field trials conducted on farms in England, France, Germany and Sweden. The selected pastures had been grazed by cattle the previous year and were divided into two (Trial Farms 7, 8, 9 and 10) or four equal areas. Groups of at least 8 calves were set stocked on each pasture area for the whole of the grazing season (until October or November). Replicate groups were used where 32 or more calves were available, in an attempt to counteract variable pasture effects. The calves, which had not previously grazed, were randomised into groups on the basis of bodyweight, breed and sex just before turnout. Either two of four groups or one of two groups of calves were randomly selected to receive MSRB while the other groups remained as untreated controls. The MSRB was administered with a special gun, 1 - 11 days before turnout. The MSRB was designed to deliver morantel into the rumen continuously for about 60 days. It consisted of a cylindrical sintered poly-thene outer shell, 7.62 cm (3.0 inches) long and 2.54 cm (1.0 inch) in diameter, impregnated with cellulose acetate. The bolus contained an inner stainless steel sleeve which, in turn, contained holes of finite number and dimension to control the rate of drug release and to increase density; it was filled with a blend of morantel tartrate (9.0 g of base), polyethylene glycol 400, and sodium metaphosphate. The density of the bolus was 2.4 g/ml.

Bodyweights of the trial calves were recorded at monthly intervals and faecal samples taken for egg counts by the McMaster technique every two or four weeks. Each animal was checked with a metal detector at regular intervals to confirm retention of the MSRB.

Herbage samples for larval counts were taken from each pasture area every two weeks, commencing four to six weeks before the proposed turnout date. The numbers of infective larvae were calculated on the basis of weight of herbage, dried to a constant moisture level at 50°C.

One worm-free tracer calf was introduced into each pasture area every four weeks from June until October. The tracer calves were allowed to graze for two weeks, and were then removed and housed for three weeks prior to slaughter for worm counts.

The abomasum and small intestine were examined separately for worms and counts were carried out by standard methods. The abomasal mucosa was subjected to peptic digestion for recovery of immature stages.

On Trial Farms 9 and 10, a proportion of the trial animals were also slaughtered for worm counts at the end of the grazing season.

RESULTS

Pasture larval counts and faecal egg counts from Trial Farm 5, located in south east Kent, England, are shown in Figure 1. This illustrates, in graphical form, the classical epidemiological pattern in the control calves. The overwintered pasture larval infection was declining when the calves were turned out in May. Excretion of eggs in the faeces commenced about four weeks after turnout, which led to a rapid rise in pasture larval contamination in July and the herbage counts remained high for the rest of the grazing season. In contrast to this, there was no significant egg deposition in the MSRB treated animals and there was no equivalent mid-summer rise in pasture larval counts. However, there was a small rise in the pasture larval concentration at the end of the grazing season.

Figure 2 illustrates the severe check in weight gain in the control animals from the end of July onwards, which coincided with the rise in the level of concentration of the pasture larvae on Trial Farm 5. In contrast, the treated calves

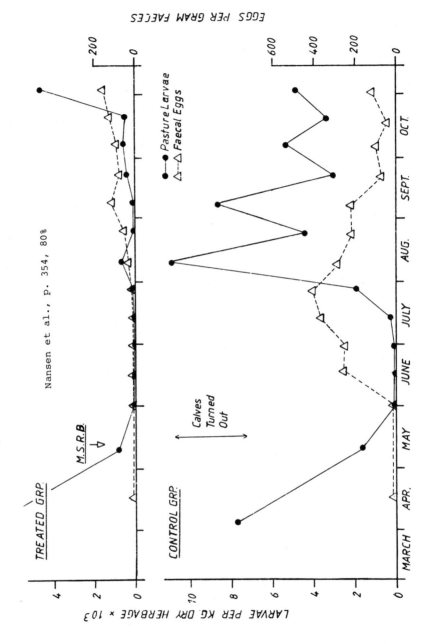

Fig 1: Mean pasture larval counts and mean faecal egg counts of MSRB treated and untreated calves – Trial Farm 5.

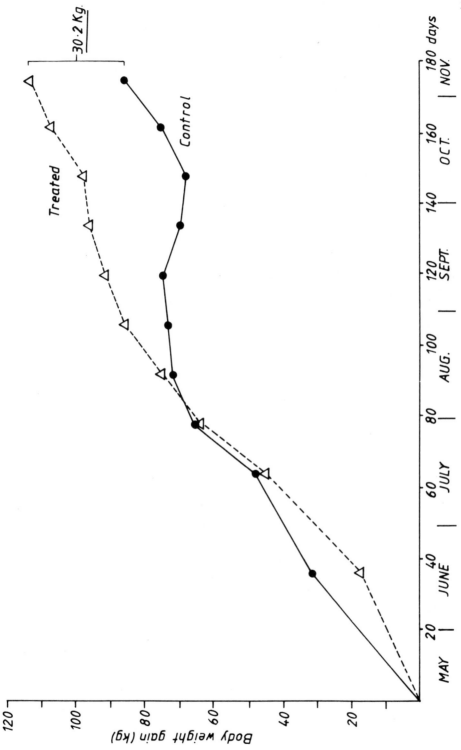

Fig 2: Liveweight gain of MSRB treated and untreated calves - Trial Farm 5.

continued to grow at their previous rate and, at the end of
the grazing season, had a weight gain advantage of 30.2 kg
over the control animals.

Data summarising the clinical findings and performance
of all the trial animals are shown in Table 1. A study of
the mean weight gain advantage of the MSRB treated animals over
the controls indicates the remarkable consistency of the response
irrespective of the geographical area in which individual trials
were carried out. In seven out of the ten trial farms, the mean
weight gain of the MSRB treated calves showed a significant
advantage over the control animals at the end of the grazing
season.

Clinical outbreaks of parasitic gastro-enteritis occurred
on four farms (three in the UK and one in France) as a result
of exposure to high levels of infection in the late summer
and autumn. A total of 62 cases requiring therapeutic treatment occurred in controls, but only 5 on one site in France in
MSRB treated animals.

Worm burdens in tracer calves from Trial Farm 4 are shown
in Figure 3. Worm burdens were largely *Ostertagia*; *Cooperia* were
also recovered consistently, but represented only a maximum of
11% of the total worm burden (in September). The control tracer
calves demonstrated an increasing total worm count from June
to October. Worm counts in the tracers which grazed with the
MSRB treated animals were similar to controls in the initial
stages but were much lower at the end of the grazing season.
Figure 3 also shows that 4th stage worms were not found in
significant numbers until September. In control tracers their
proportion increased from 8% in September to 54% in October,
when the 4th stage *Ostertagia* burden was 36 730. The highest
proportion in the MSRB treated tracers was 13% in October, but
this represented a worm burden of only 410.

At the end of the grazing season on Trial Farms 9 and 10,
two calves from each group, which had been paired for initial

TABLE 1

SUMMARY OF CLINICAL AND PERFORMANCE DATA

Trial Farm	Location	Animals per treatment	Number of clinical cases of parasitic gastro-enteritis requiring therapeutic treatment		Mean weight gain advantage MSRB over control at the end of the grazing season (kg)	Significance
			MSRB	CONTROL		
1	Norfolk, UK	17	0	17	18.2	$P < 0.01$
2	Norfolk, UK	18	0	2	13.4	$P < 0.05$
3	Kent, UK	24	0	7	17.1	$P < 0.05$
4	Kent, UK	31	0	0	36.5	$P < 0.001$
5	Kent, UK	20	0	0	30.2	$P < 0.001$
6	Eure, France	20	5	36	13.3	$P < 0.01$
7	Niedersachsen, Germany	12	0	0	12.0	–
8	Niedersachsen, Germany	13	0	0	12.0	–
9	Skaraborg, Sweden	12	0	0	32.5	$P < 0.01$
10	Skaraborg, Sweden	11	0	0	9.5	–
Overall		178	5	62	21.2	$P < 0.01$

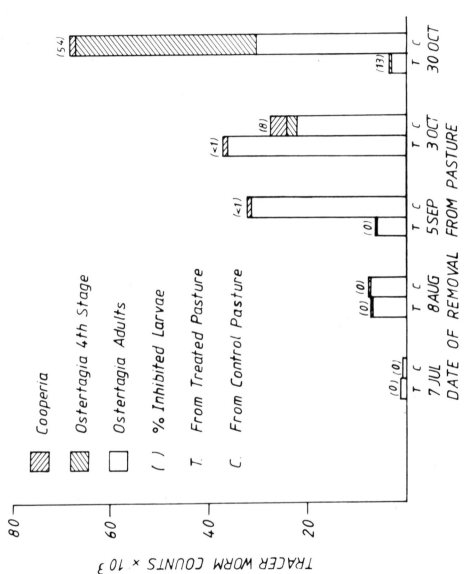

Fig 3: Worm counts in tracer calves grazing with control animals (C) and with MSRB treated animals (T) – Trial Farm 4.

bodyweight, were slaughtered for worm counts and the results are summarised in Table 2. Mean burdens of inhibited *Ostertagia* larvae (pretype II infection) were 66 500 in controls, compared with 9 800 in MSRB treated animals - a reduction of 85%.

DISCUSSION

Judged on clinical and performance data, the MSRB given at turnout in the spring was highly and consistently effective in controlling parasitic gastro-enteritis in calves over the entire grazing season in this series of studies conducted in different geographical areas under variable climatic conditions. Moderate to severe clinical disease (diarrhoea and weight loss) occurred in control animals during the latter part of the grazing season on four trial farms - three in the UK and one in France. Therapeutic anthelmintic treatment was required to check the progress of the disease outbreaks. A total of 62 treatments were given to controls compared to 5 (in the French trial) to the MSRB treated calves.

Average weight gains over the grazing season were greater in the MSRB treated calves than in controls in all ten trials. In Trial 7 the weight gain advantage was statistically significant. Overall, 178 MSRB treated calves showed a statistically significant weight gain advantage over their contemporary controls of 21.2 kg (P <0.01) at the end of the grazing season.

The parasitological findings demonstrated that this result was achieved by the MSRB preventing significant build-up of contamination of pasture with infective larvae. The epidemiological pattern illustrated by the sequence of events in controls was similar on all farms, differing only in the timing of the mid-summer rise of pasture larvae. The pattern followed that previously described for various regions in the UK by a number of workers (Michel, 1966; Michel and Lancaster, 1970; Armour, 1970; Pott et al., 1978, 1979) and is exemplified by Trial Farm 5 (Figure 1). The calves were infected by acquisition of overwintered infective larvae soon after turnout and began to

TABLE 2

WORM COUNTS IN TRIAL CALVES AT TERMINATION – TRIAL FARMS 9 AND 10

	Number of calves	Ostertagia			Cooperia			Nematodirus	Total
		Adults	5th Stage	4th Stage	Adults	5th Stage	4th Stage		
Control	4	39 000	5 025	66 500	850	550	5 225	225	117 375
MSRB	4	3 525	750	9 800	6 075	2 025	9 150	275	28 975

excrete worm eggs in the faeces 3 - 4 weeks later. Increasing deposition of eggs was followed by a sudden and substantial rise in pasture larval levels in July which then remained high for the rest of the grazing season. Exposure to these high parasitic levels on pasture after July resulted in a severe check in weight gain (Figure 2).

In contrast, although the MSRB treated calves were exposed to a similar level of pasture infection at the beginning of the season, egg deposition was insignificant and there was no equivalent of the mid-summer rise in pasture larval contamination which occurred in controls. Consequently, the treated calves were not exposed to a high parasite challenge and continued to gain weight at a consistent rate throughout the grazing season.

The sudden increase in larval concentration at the end of the grazing season on pasture grazed by MSRB treated animals, which can be seen in Figure 1, was an unexpected, but common, phenomenon in the trials. This contamination may have originated from a population of worms which was passaged through the grazing calves after the MSRB was exhausted, indicating that the period of morantel release was less than required to allow overwintered larvae to decline below a threshold level. The exceptionally mild autumn in Europe in 1978 would have favoured the late translation of eggs to infective larvae. If this explanation is correct, then prolonging the period of release would be predicted to prevent this late larval contamination. However, the possibility cannot be excluded that it arose from another source suggested by Bairden et al. (1979), when overwintered eggs or larvae survive for long periods in the soil and become available as infective larvae at a later stage than larvae overwintering on herbage.

A further benefit, which accrues from the early season use of the MSRB, is a reduction in burdens of inhibited *Ostertagia* larvae (pretype II infection) at the end of the grazing season. Typical tracer data (Figure 3) show that there is a reduction,

362

not only in the total number of inhibition-prone larvae acquired
but also in the proportion of larvae which become inhibited.
One possible explanation for this phenomenon is that the MSRB
delays the appearance of larvae on pasture and therefore shortens
the period available for conditioning by the climatic factors
which are believed to play a part in inducing inhibition. Whatever the mechanism, the net result is lowered burdens of
inhibited *Ostertagia* larvae (Table 2) and a reduced risk of
type II Ostertagiasis during the following winter.

These combined results show that the morantel sustained
release device, given at turnout in the spring, is highly
effective in controlling parasitic gastro-enteritis in calves
and in improving their productivity. It provides, for the first
time, a convenient and reliable means of control without the
need to handle or move the animals after turnout. Additionally,
it reduces the risk of type II Ostertagiasis during the following
winter.

ACKNOWLEDGEMENTS

Dr. D.S. Dresback of our Pharmaceutical Research and
Development Department designed and developed the MSRB to the
stage of practical utility described in these trials.

The study in France was in collaboration with Dr. J.-P.
Raynaud and Mr. J.P. Le Stang, the studies in Germany were in
collaboration with Dr. H.J. Bürger, and the studies in Sweden
were in collaboration with Dr. S. Tolling and Dr. M. Törnquist.
This paper is published with the permission of the Research
Director, Pfizer Central Research.

REFERENCES

Armour, J., 1970. Bovine Ostertagiasis: A Review. Vet. Rec. 86, 184-189.

Bairden, K., Parkins, J.J. and Armour, J., 1979. Bovine Ostertagiasis: A changing epidemiological pattern? Vet. Rec., 105, 33-35.

Downey, N.E., O'Shea, J. and Spillane, T.A., 1974. Preliminary observations on the use of low-level medication in calves' drinking water as a means of endoparasite control. Irish Vet. J., 28, 221-222.

Michel, J.F., 1966. The epidemiology and control of parasitic gastro-enteritis in calves. Publikation der IV Internationalen Tagung der Welt-gesellschaft für Buiatrik, Zürich, 272-287.

Michel, J.F. and Lancaster, M.B., 1970. Experiments on the control of parasitic gastro-enteritis in calves. J. Helminthol., 44, 107-140.

Pott, J.M., Jones, R.M. and Cornwell, R.L., 1974. Control of bovine parasitic gastro-enteritis by reduction of pasture larval levels. Proc. 3rd Int. Congr. Parasitol., Munich, Vol. 2, 747.

Pott, J.M., Jones, R.M. and Cornwell, R.L., 1978. Observations on Parasitic Gastro-enteritis and Bronchitis in grazing calves : untreated calves. Int. J. Parasitol., 8, 331-339.

Pott, J.M., Jones, R.M. and Cornwell, R.L., 1979. Observations on Parasitic Gastro-enteritis and Bronchitis in grazing calves : effect of low level feed incorporation of morantel in early season. Int. J. Parasitol., 9, 153-157.

DISCUSSION

N. Downey *(Ireland)*

Dr. Jones has given us plenty of food for thought, because what he has talked about is an innovation and, like all innovations, it will no doubt provoke a lot of comment and, perhaps, controversy. I would like to start, if I may, by saying that not all other slow-dose delivery systems are necessarily ineffective or unreliable. For example, we feel that our method is quite reliable.

J. Euzeby *(France)*

What is the amount of Morantel released each day?

R.M. Jones *(UK)*

150 mg of base per day.

J.F. Michel *(UK)*

One must welcome this innovation. If the control of oestertagiasis is to be based on the routine use of drugs alone, then the first half of the season is the more rational time to give them than the second half of the season. However, I wonder if anyone would give an opinion on whether this low-dosage use of anthelmintics does not introduce a danger of speeding the arrival of drug resistance.

R.M. Jones

One has to be conscious of the risk of development of resistance, but I am confident and comfortable about the possibility of this development having an economic impact over the next few years compared with the benefits of such a mechanism to control disease. There is no reported resistance to anthelmintics for cattle parasites. There is no case where resistance to Morantel has arisen as a result of field use. The parasites of cattle, which we are trying to control under temperate conditions, have a long generation time.

There are only two, sometimes three, generations in a season. Because of the long generation time the chances of resistant helminths being selected quickly are that much more reduced. We have been unable, so far, to induce any tolerance in the laboratory - using the device against *Ostertagia* and *Cooperia* - and we have been unable to see any change in the susceptibility

E.J.L. Soulsby *(UK)*

Could you tell us what the device is? How long is it retained and in what proportion of cattle is it rejected? And is this a major problem?

R.M. Jones

During these trials we had about a 6% regurgitation rate during the actual active life of the device. In fact the results presented make allowances for this and incorporate that; we have not taken out the animal that regurgitates the device. If one or two animals lose the device and are not protected, it does not matter in terms of the overall contamination of the pasture since this is a herd situation. The paper reports a prototype device that we were testing in 1978; we have developed the device since. In trials in 1979, we reduced the regurgitation rate to approximately 1%. The device is an intra-ruminal device which sits in the reticulum; it is much the size and shape of the magnesium bolus. It is, in fact, a reservoir of Morantel; the Morantel is released through a membrane. Since it is the property of my pharmaceutical colleagues, who developed it in the USA it would not be proper for me to tell you much more about it, but I have given you the principle of the device. However, as a final reply to Professor Soulsby, after it is empty then its density changes; sometimes it is regurgitated, other times it remains *in situ*. We have had as many as eight devices in animals for two years.

J. Eckert *(Switzerland)*

Do you have any information on the immune status of these animals which have been treated? How large were the worm numbers? Do they develop an immunity after this treatment?

J.M. Jones

We have followed the 1978 studies through to 1979, looking at the growth through the winter and then by returning LAD treated animals to infested pastures the following year. We have demonstrated in two studies that there is no difference in the immune status. Animals are being sufficiently infected; we are not eliminating all worms, but we are keeping them below the level which is critical as far as production performance is concerned.

J. Armour *(UK)*

Concerning the control of 'nematodiasis' in calves, what about lungworms?

J.M. Jones

Control of lungworm by this technique is much more difficult because of the unpredictability of lungworm disease rather than the fact that the device would not be effective. Morantel is ineffective therapeutically against established lungworms. Given continuously in low level, Morantel is prophylactic against ingested third stage larvae so that, during the active period of release from the device it will also control lungworm. We have yet to find a way of using it to get seasonal control; that is the difference. The device will control lungworm while it is releasing drug but to achieve seasonal control, as we can with the parasitic gastro-enteritis, we have got to work out the relationships between the timing of the device and the epidemiology.

J. Armour
_____

The tracer calf technique gives so much information in terms of the structure of the wormburden, possible onset of resistance and the seasonal inhibition.

R.M. Jones
_____

Our objective was to compare pasture larval infectivity and my comments relate to that objective. I agree with the point you are making that you get much more information from the tracer worm count technique about inhibition rate and measuring the actual infection rate.

J. Eckert
_____

Did you make a total calculation of the costs of both techniques also in terms of labour costs? Did you compare these?

R.M. Jones
_____

I have not done this yet. My immediate analysis of this is that the tracer worm technique will end up being very much more expensive, even when you put in the labour costs.

E.J.L. Soulsby
_____

The recovery time was over the spring and summer. The larval recovery technique emphasises larvae that are infective and that will mature when they get into the animal. Later in the year presumably there will be some ageing pats containing larvae that are senile. Do you think that your correlation would still hold when larvae of increasing age are found on the herbage?

R.M. Jones
_____

That is difficult to answer. We measured into October and November and the correlations were still pretty much on the straight line. Absolute qualitative comparison is not being made and we are just showing that the comparative trends that we measure by both techniques, are interchangeable.

SOME REMARKS AND CONTROL METHODS OF GASTRO-INTESTINAL NEMATODIASIS IN CATTLE IN PIEDMONT, ITALY

E. Vigliani

Istituto Zooprofilattico Sperimentale,
Del Piemonte e Della Liguria, Torino, Italy.

ABSTRACT

The present report of investigations carried out from January to September 1977 describes the methods used in diagnostic and investigation work on gastro-intestinal nematodes affecting cattle in Piedmont. Based on post mortem examinations, all cattle were found infected. Trichostrongylidae were prevalent in cattle from flat and hilly areas while Oesophagostomum prevailed in the mountains.

INTRODUCTION

A report to establish the distribution of gastro-intestinal nematodes of cattle would be of interest for the regional economy of Piedmont.

In 1969, Balbo carried out a helmintological survey on nemotodes in the province of Cuneo. The present report includes the whole area of Piedmont and includes observations on seasonal fluctuations in the different infections.

There are approximately 1 million bovines in Piedmont, about 700 000 are found in the province of Cuneo, and hence the data presented come mostly from animals of that zone.

MATERIAL AND METHODS

Seventy abomasa and intestines from 15 - 18 months old grazing cattle were examined. The intestinal parts were ligated, put in separate containers and opened. They were washed with 5% formalin to kill and fix the parasites.

A sediment was obtained and removed to one litre beakers where a second sedimentation was performed. The sediment was examined for parasites in Petri dishes on a dark background. Due to the small size of parasites of the abomasum, and small intestine, the examination was carried out in daylight, and with only small portions of sediment at the time. Parasites were kept in Raillet's solution, and identification was carried out on male specimens which were cleared in lactophenol, and mounted in gum arabic.

RESULTS

The following percentage infections were observed:

Cattle infected by *Ostertagia* sp.   100%

  "   "   " *Cooperia* sp.   21%

  "   "   " *Trychostrongylus axei*   59%

  "   "   " *Haemonchus* sp.   58%

  "   "   " *Nematodirus* sp.   29%

  "   "   " *Bunostomum phlebotomum*   14%

  "   "   " *Oesophagostomum radiatum*   65%

  "   "   " *Trichuris discolor*   13%

The frequency of the parasitic genera in the various provinces is shown in Table 1, and the seasonal distribution is shown in Figure 1.

TABLE 1

FREQUENCY OF PARASITE GENERA IN THE PROVINCES OF PIEDMONT

	Cuneo	Torino	Vercelli	Asti	Alessandria	Novara
Ostertagia	+++	++	++	+	++	+
Cooperia	++	+	+	+	+	+
Trichostrongylus	++	++	++	+	+	+
Haemoncus	++	++	+	+	+	
Nematodirus	++	++			+	
Bunostomum	+	+		+		
Oesophagostomum	+++	++	+			+
Trichuris	+	+	+			

The number of parasites was comparatively low in spring but high in June, July and August. Only *Bunostomum* and *Nematodirus* deviated from this pattern.

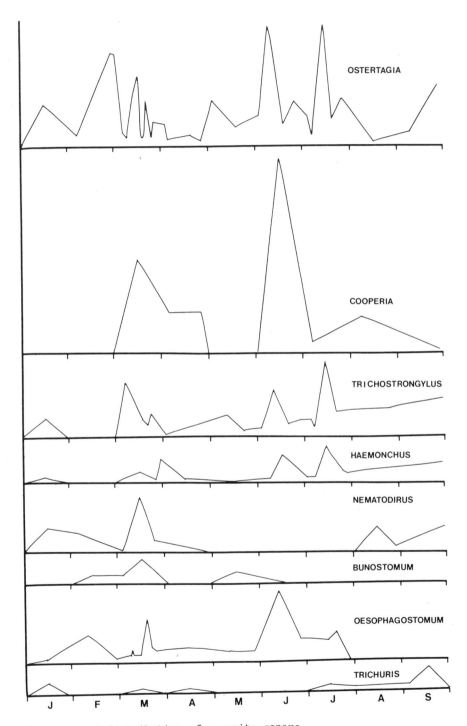

Fig. 1. Seasonal distribution of parasite genera.

DISCUSSION

All the animals examined were found infected by a single or more than one species of nematodes. The number of parasites found was often low. Young animals were more heavily infected than adult cattle. The highest number of parasites were found in abomasa, fewer worms were found in the large intestines and the lowest numbers were recovered from the small intestines.

We have been unable to provide an explanation for the increase in parasite numbers during the month of March, an increase which is comparatively high, although it does not reach that of the summer months.

The geographic distribution of the various genera was of interest. Thus the Trichostrongylidae were especially prevalent in flat and hilly zones, while *Oesophagostomum* was found predominantly in the mountains, and in zones near the mountains.

We conclude that gastro-intestinal parasitism is a significant infection in Piedmont cattle, and that the distribution of the parasites is almost identical to that reported in a previous survey.

REFERENCES

Balbo, T., 1969. Diagnosi sperimentale della strongilosi dei bovini e
        diffusione dei relativi strongili nella provincia di Cuneo. Atti
        del convegno su 'Le strongilosi gastro-intestinali dei bovini in
        Piemonte', Cinzano.
Balbo, T., 1973. Indagini sulla situazione parassitologica nei nammiferi
        del Parco Nazionale del Gran Paradiso. Parassitologia 15.
Casarosa, L., 1977. Parassitologia degli animali domestici, C.G. Edizioni
        Medico scientifiche.
Euzeby, J., 1958. Diagnostic expérimental des elimintoses animals, Vigot
        Freres ed.
Noble, E.R. and Noble, G.A., 1961. Parasitology. The biology of animal
        parasites.
Sobrero, L., 1974. Guida sperimentale allo studio della parassitologia
        veterinaria, Cacucci Editore, Bari.
Soulsby, E.J.L., 1968. Helminths,Arthropods and Protozoa of Domestic
        Animals, 4th ed., Bailliére, Tindall Ltd.
Yorke, W. and Maplestone, P.P., 1962. The nematode parasites of verte-
        brates. Hafner, New York.

DISCUSSION

H.J. Over *(The Netherlands)*

You suggested that Oesophogostomum was more numerous in the mountainous areas than it is in the flat regions.

E. Vigliani *(Italy)*

Yes. It is prevalent in mountains.

H.J. Over

Have you any suggestions on what the reason for this might be?

E. Vigliani

I do not know! This is the first time we have investigated it.

D. Barth *(FRG)*

Looking at your tables and graphs, it is quite obvious that the peak levels of all genera are in March and then in June and July. Can you give an explanation of where the parasites in March are coming from? Also, perhaps you can give an explanation of the grazing system in this area. Are animals on pasture in winter?

E. Vigliani

In winter, no. It is not possible for the studies to continue in the winter. We begin in January and cease in September.

J.F. Michel *(UK)*

What age group is represented here?

E. Vigliani

The animals are 18 months and over.

E.J.L. Soulsby *(UK)*

With the burdens you have observed, do you consider these to be of economic significance?

E. Vigliani

There is sometimes a small influence with clinical symptoms but no obvious effect on production performance.

E.J.L. Soulsby

You have no information?

E. Vigliani

Yes, I have information, but there is a very small effect.

SESSION 4

CONTROL II

Chairman: J. Euzeby

SOME OBSERVATIONS ON THE CONTROL OF TRICHOSTRONGYLOSIS IN CALVES IN THE FIELD

J. Jansen and G.K. van Meurs

Institute of Veterinary Parasitology and Parasitic Diseases,
Department of Herd Health and Ambulatory Clinic,
State University of Utrecht, The Netherlands.

ABSTRACT

Control systems for the prevention of trichostrongylosis in calves in Utrecht are based mainly on avoiding the over-wintered larval infections on the grass and the mid-summer increase of infective larvae on the pasture. The systems consist mainly of providing advice about the use and change of pastures and the use of anthelmintic treatments.

The correct application of preventive programmes is hampered, however, many times by various factors such as unpredictable dry weather, farm management systems, and the unwillingness of some farmers to cooperate.

P. Nansen, R.J. Jørgensen, E.J.L. Soulsby (eds), Epidemiology and Control of Nematodiasis in Cattle.

INTRODUCTION

For about six years we have been visiting farms to obtain
better information about the problems associated with
trichostrongylid infections in calves and the possibilities of
preventing trichostrongylosis and the consequent loss in
production. We use the visits for teaching students
experience of parasitological problems under practical
circumstances, while at the same time we advise the farmers
about the correct use of pastures and treatments with anthelmint.

MATERIAL AND METHODS

The observations were made on commercial farms in the
province of Utrecht.

When we suspect that there might be a trichostrongylosis
problem we ascertain the history of the situation, inspect the
animals and make faecal examinations. The history taking
includes questions about numbers of cows, heifers, calves etc.,
number of hectares, disease incidence, grazing history, number
and times of anthelmintic treatments, feeding regime etc.
Frequently, it is very difficult to ascertain the exact
grazing history because many farmers do not keep a detailed
record of the use of their land. At our request some farmers
are now using a 'pasture-calendar' as a form of record which is
easily maintained. It is necessary usually to question
repeatedly about treatments in order to get a true picture
of the situation. The inspection of the calves includes
noting the clinical signs of trichostrongylosis and the age
and feeding regimen are taken into account when the condition
of the animals is. judged. Estimation of the liveweight of the
calves is done by use of a measuring tape. Faecal examinations,
usually are done on pooled samples from groups of calves. A
diagnosis is based largely on the history and the clinical
examination rather than on the results of the faecal examination

The control systems which are recommended for the prevention of trichostrongylosis are based on avoiding, 1. the over-wintered larval infection on the grass and, 2. the mid-summer increase of infective larvae on the pasture. Depending on the local situation, control measures can include: turning out of calves on pasture without infection history, turning out later than normal or onto mown pasture, changing pasture, use of anthelmintic treatments, alternate grazing of cattle and sheep and combinations of these measures.

RESULTS

We have found that it is relatively easy to draw up a theoretical prophylactic programme, when the number of cows, calves, hectares and so on is known. For example the programme may consist of turning out the calves late, changing the pasture in July and if required, combining this with anthelmintic treatment, and for the rest of the grazing season providing regular changes to mown pastures. In practice, however, the execution of a programme may be hampered by various factors associated with the management practiced by the farmer or with unpredictable weather conditions.

Nethertheless, a good start can be achieved if, at least, a safe pasture (e.g. a pasture not used for young cattle in the previous grazing season or mown early in the present season), is chosen for use as the first pasture. There is a strong tendency in our country to turn the calves out late, e.g. at the end of May or even in June and to change pasture some five weeks later in July. Moreover, in contrast to some decades ago, there is more silage made than hay and farmers have the possibilities to turn out calves onto mown pastures from the second half of May. However, even with these circumstances or even later in summer a preventive scheme can be wrecked because of an unexpected low yield of grass in periods of drought.

Additional difficulties to those caused by dry weather are the following: farm management has changed radically during a few decades, in that about twice as many cows are kept on farms than before, and hence twice the number of calves are born and reared; of the calves born 30 - 35% are reared on the farm and this led to a high grazing density. At the same time the main parturition period has been extended considerably from the three or four months in winter and early spring as was the situation in the past, to the greater part of the year, from early autumn into the following summer. Therefore, many farmers now are grazing two, sometimes three, different age-groups of calves, each group needing its own preventive programme. A further point is that on farms with an intensified management system there has been a reduction of man-power and consequently farmers do not have enough time or personnel to inspect all groups of animals regularly or to pay sufficient attention to disorders or to individual animals. Moreover, many farmers, in these circumstances, are more concerned with the producing animals rather than for the future producers or young stock. Frequently we observe that a preventive scheme is performed exactly as recommended for the oldest age-group animals but groups of calves may be neglected.

Special problems may arise in making a preventive programme when dairy cows are milked indoors. In that case pastures near the farm buildings are reserved for the milking cows and cannot be used for the calves. The calves may then be grazed at some distance which implies more time and work especially if the calves need to be fed concentrates. The factors reduce the possibilities for changing pastures. The opposite situation occurs on farms concerned with cheese-making. Here the whey is fed to the calves, and for this the calves have to be at hand near the farm, and often they are kept on the same pasture every year, which favours outbreaks of ostertagiasis. Some farmers, who find it impossible to cope with these problems, place their calves with specialised rearing farmers whose concern is to rear calves of several owners up to pregnant heifers.

Little can be done by way of advice and prevention programmes on farms owned by farmers who do not recognise that their calves are failing to grow well due to trichostrongylid infections or do not consider their animals to be in a poor condition.

CONCLUSIONS

Controlling trichostrongylosis in the field needs preventive programmes designed for each farm. The success of preventive programmes is higher on farms where there is no obvious clinical problem and on which advising is easy. On farms with minor clinical problems and skilful farmers the success rate is also high, but on farms with an unsuitable management system or owned by non-cooperative or incapable farmers, efforts to introduce preventive programmes have had minimal success.

DISCUSSION

R.M. Jones (UK)

I would like to make a comment rather than put a question. I can confirm, certainly in my own experience, that the frequency with which the control programmes - particularly sophisticated control programmes - are implemented properly is very, very rare indeed. Farmers have so many problems in providing pasture at the right time, and labour at the right time, that the control programmes are not implemented correctly. I would like to support Dr. Jansen; this is my experience in the United Kingdom.

J.F. Michel (UK)

Surely it is only a reflection of the lack of care and thought which has been devoted to drawing up control programmes, if in practice they prove to be unworkable. I think that we have been extremely remiss, as a group, in making recommendations without really working out what the agricultural implications are. We rush in without an adequate understanding of the needs of the particular farm enterprise, and I think that it is in this situation that a great deal of work requires to be done.

J. Jansen (The Netherlands)

This is quite true, and maybe I can explain as to what we do at the Ambulatory Clinic. It is part of our educational system to send students to the farms to examine the problems; this is to let the students see what the problems are and how difficult it might be to do anything about them. They have had lectures on epidemiology, on clinical conditions, or prophylaxis, on preventive programmes and on therapy, etc. Now they see the problem in the natural context and in this way they can also see how difficult it is in practice.

J.-P. Raynaud *(France)*

I would like to make a comment on the late turning-out of calves. This is a practical aspect because the farmers, for various reasons, prefer turning out later - as late as possible. Then, the choice is about the pasture. In principle the pastures are cut before grazing. However, I have seen occasions where the pasture is cut and the grass given fresh to the animals, which are kept indoors. So there are many possibilities for the infection of animals.

J. Armour *(UK)*

I agree with Dr. Jansen. The big problem is getting the message across to the farmer and getting the whole message across. Last year on the early morning farmers' programme on the BBC, a leading UK veterinarian was advising farmers, 'Now it is mid-July - dose your cattle'. There was no question of giving advice on moving them; that was an example of half the message getting across.

J.F. Michel

The point I was making was not that we are not getting the message across, but that we have not got a saleable message - we have got a half-baked message.

J. Armour

No, I would not agree. I think we have got a saleable message.

J.F. Michel

No! When we say, for example, that half the message is 'dose in July' and you might say that the whole message, for the sake of argument, is to move as well. We have not really considered where he is going to move to, what are the agricultural implications of doing so and how can it be arranged to do it every year.

J. Armour

But I have always maintained that it is an individual farm problem. This is what Dr. Jansen is doing; he is educating the population who are advising on farms.

H.J. Over *(The Netherlands)*

I think Dr. Foldager might come into this because yesterday he was talking about change of pasture in the middle of the season.

J. Foldager *(Denmark)*

Yes, and I might make a comment in connection with this discussion. In Denmark we have extension agents. The extension agents collaborate very closely with the research workers. This means there is close contact between research and the field situations. During the last two years we have instructed farmers how to implement the results of research. However, we have also found that the extension agents are needed to provide an understanding of what it is all about. One might report research results but if one cannot provide a simple solution to a problem the extension agents are not going to advise the farmers satisfactorily - particularly about moving the cattle. I have heard the comment several times, 'I cannot get the farmer to move'. Now the extension agents are reporting that they can now get the farmers to move their animals. When the programme was first presented it looked very complicated and it looked as if one had to move animals a long distance. Then we explained that you take the original area and divide it into one third and two thirds; for the first period of the grazing season animals are on one third of the area, and after that they are moved to the other side of the fence - still within the same field - and they never return to the original third. Grass is cut for silage or hay on the non-grazed part of the field.

N. Downey *(Ireland)*

I would like to quote Dr. Michel on this. Very often the
recommendations are not all that practical. For instance you
could not sell the idea of late turn out of calves in spring
to Irish farmers. There are climatic, husbandry and, perhaps,
even sociological reasons for this.

J. Armour

Another incalculable factor is that if the information
is free it is often not heeded - if it is paid for, farmers
listen to it.

COORDINATED RESEARCH PROGRAMME ON CONTROL OF OSTERTAGIASIS IN GRAZING CALVES IN DENMARK

[1]J. Foldager, [1]Kr. Sejrsen, [2]P. Nansen, [2]R.J. Jørgensen, [3]Sv.Aa. Henriksen and [2]J.W. Hansen

[1]National Institute of Animal Science, 25 Rolighedsvej, DK-1958 Copenhagen V., Denmark
[2]Royal Veterinary and Agricultural University, 13 Bülowsvej, DK-1870 Copenhagen V., Denmark
[3]State Veterinary Serum Laboratory, 27 Bülowsvej, DK-1870 Copenhagen V., Denmark

INTRODUCTION

A coordinated research programme on ostertagiasis in calves at pasture was initiated in 1974. The participating institutions are: National Institute of Animal Science, Royal Veterinary and Agricultural University and the State Veterinary Serum Laboratory.

EXPERIMENTAL METHODS

Since 1974 the coordinated research group has conducted 17 factorial experiments with a total of 568 calves at pasture. The calves were from 1.1 to 11.2 months old at the beginning of the experiments, and they were subjected to the following independent variables:

Variable one	Variable two
Anthelmintic treatments or Date of turning out or Stocking rate *	Paddock change mid-July

The presentation will be limited to a discussion of daily gains in relation to control methods. Only selected supporting parasitological data or other evidence will be mentioned.

P. Nansen, R.J. Jørgensen, E.J.L. Soulsby (eds), Epidemiology and Control of Nematodiasis in Cattle.

Details of control methods used in the three main groups of experiments and their effects will be presented jointly. The method of calf handling and measurements were common in all trials.

Stocking rate

In all subgroups the stocking rate, from turning out in spring to mid-July, was twice as great as the stocking rate from mid-July to turning in in autumn. This was due to the seasonal variation in grass production under Danish conditions in that approximately 2/3rds of the grass production of grazed paddocks takes place during the spring (Figure 1). Therefore, the general outline of calf handling was as shown in Figure 2.

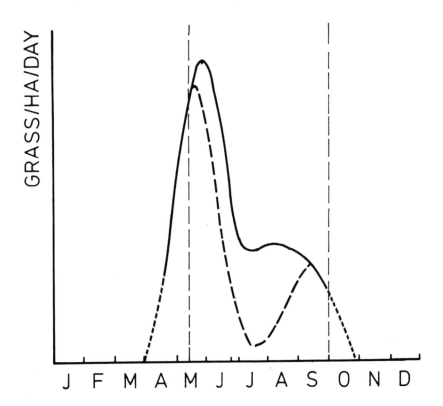

Fig. 1: Seasonal variation in grass production. ——— Normal year; ------- Dry year. (From Østergaard, 1977).

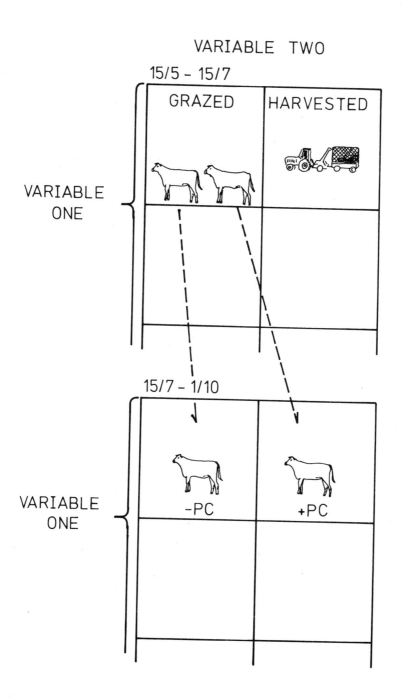

Fig. 2: Outline of calf handling. PC = paddock change mid-July

From turning out in spring to mid-July all calves on
control methods in variable one were grazing one half of the
total paddock area. The remaining one half of the paddock area
was harvested, and the calves did not have access to it.

From mid-July to turning in in autumn one half of the
calves remained in the initial paddock, and the other one half
of the calves were moved to the harvested area. This method
introduced the control methods in variable two and adjustments
of stocking rates.

Measurements

The dependent variables studied, which may be divided
into general and special measurements, are listed in Table 1.

TABLE 1

REPEATED MEASUREMENTS

General	Special
Field:	Field:
L_3 contamination of grass	L_3 distribution in grass
Grass quantity	Grass yield
Grass quality	Grass digestibility
Temperature	
Rainfall	
Animal:	Animal:
Live weight	Grass intake
EPG faeces	Grazing behaviour
Serum pepsinogen	Performance during winter
Serum albumin	
Clinical condition	

Average daily gains were calculated for the periods before
and after paddock change in mid-July. Infective larvae on
herbage, eggs in faeces, serum pepsinogen etc., were determined
by procedures which have been described previously.

RESULTS

L$_3$-contamination of grass

The seasonal variation in L$_3$-contamination of grass has been described for England (Michel, 1968), Sweden (Nilsson and Sorelius, 1973) and Denmark (Henriksen et al., 1974, 1975). The pattern of variation is identical in the three countries, but the time of decline in spring and the later increase in the summer are delayed approximately two weeks in Sweden compared to Denmark, and in Denmark compared to England, respectively. This may be explained by the difference in the climatic conditions at the geographical latitudes. However, the number of L$_3$ on grass is also affected by local climatic conditions. These are some of the reasons for separate analysis and experiments in distinct geographical regions.

During each year of the Danish research group programme one group of calves, on each of the farms, grazed the initial paddock throughout the summer without the use of the control methods listed under variable one. Studies with these groups (Figures 3 and 4) revealed that during dry summers (1975, 1976) the L$_3$-contamination was markedly lower than in normal summers, and the increase generally occurring in mid-July was delayed to mid or late August.

Anthelmintic* treatment and paddock changes

Experimental: the effect of anthelmintic treatment schemes and paddock changes were studied in 7 trials, and the following anthelmintic treatment schemes were tested:

1X: treated on the date of paddock change;

2X: treated 20 days after turn out and on the date of paddock change;

BX: bi-weekly treatment from date of turn out to date of paddock change;

* Fenbendazole (Panacur) was used in all but one experiment.

AX: bi-weekly treatment from date of paddock change to date of turn in; and

7X: treated every three weeks throughout the grazing season.

At least one of the anthelmintic treatment schemes and untreated control were included in each experiment and the calves were either maintained in the same paddock throughout the season (-PC), or moved to a clean paddock mid-July (+PC).

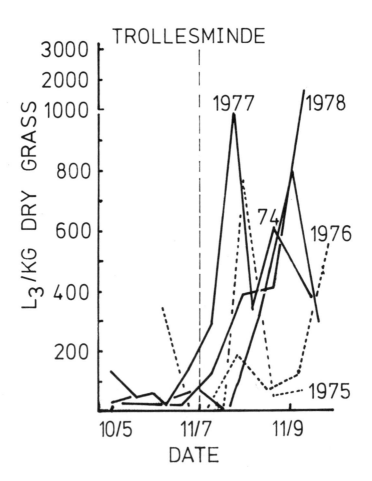

Fig. 3: Seasonal variation in L_3-contamination at farm one. (Trollesminde experimental farm).

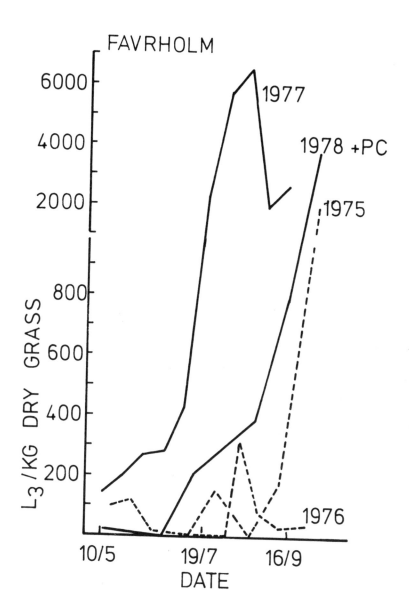

Fig. 4: Seasonal variation in L_3-contamination at farm two. (Favrholm experimental farm). PC = paddock change on June 30.

Trial U15 was conducted in a dry year, but the paddocks were irrigated. Therefore, this trial is considered to belong to the group of experiments conducted in normal years. In 1978 the spring was dry and the late summer was very wet.

The dates of turn out were between May 9 and 18. The date of paddock change was between July 9 and 13, except the trial in 1978 in which paddock change was on June 30 due to a lack of grass.

The average initial stocking rate was 16.7 animals/ha - or 2.7 t live weight/ha - and this is comparable to the medium stocking rate to be discussed later.

Daily gains before paddock change (Table 2) were not affected by variable one or variable two in any of the experiments except one. The significant interaction in trial U23 cannot be explained.

In all trials in normal years the daily gain after paddock change (Table 2) was higher in calves moved to a harvested paddock in mid-July than in those kept in the initial paddock throughout the summer. Similar results were obtained in dry years, but the differences were only significant in one of three trials. All anthelmintic treatment schemes tended to increase daily gains, but only in three trials were the increases significant and, in these, anthelmintic treatments were repeated either throughout the entire summer or after paddock change. The interaction between variables was not significant in any of the trials.

Substantiating measurements: the daily gains in relation to control methods in this group of experiments may be substantiated by trial U30.

In paddocks grazed throughout the summer L_3-contamination of grass (Figure 5) was increasing after the paddock change. However, the increasing trend was broken by anthelmintic treat-

ments. In paddocks with zero grazing to mid-July, the number
of L_3 was maintained at a low level throughout the summer period.
Similar results were obtained for L_3 in grass around faecal
droppings, but the level of contamination was higher.

TABLE 2

DAILY GAIN IN EXPERIMENTS ON ANTHELMINTIC TREATMENT AND PADDOCK CHANGE IN
CALVES AT PASTURE, g/d.

Exp. No.	Anthelmintic treatment							Paddock change			Trt XPC[A]
	OX	1X	2X	BX	AX	7X	Signi-ficance	−	+	Signi-ficance	
Before date of paddock change:											
Normal years											
U8	626	−	+42[B]	−	−	−21	NS	−	−	NS	NS
U15	376	−	+33	−	−	−	NS	−	−	NS	NS
U23	232	−	−	+54	+90	−	NS	−	−	NS	*
U30	213	−	−	−	+53	−	NS	−	−	NS	NS
Dry years											
U9	384	−	+102	−	−	−	*	372	+69[C]	*	NS
U11	424	+60	−	−	−	−	NS	−	−	NS	NS
U14	629	+16	−	−	−	−	NS	−	−	NS	NS
After date of paddock change:											
Normal years											
U8	364	−	+161	−	−	+251	**	221	+561	***	NS
U15	153	−	+17	−	−	−	NS	42	+238	***	NS
U23	337	−	−	−5	+103	−	NS	308	+123	***	NS
U30	303	−	−	−	+125	−	*	232	+268	***	NS
Dry years											
U9	391	−	+91	−	−	−	*	406	+96[D]	*	NS
U11	399	−25	−	−	−	−	NS	364	+45	NS	NS
U14	429	+71	−	−	−	−	NS	500	−71	NS	NS

[A] Paddock change

[B] Numbers with a sign are deviations

[C] Extended area: +120 g/d

[D] Extended area: −5 g/d

NS Not significant, *$P \leq 0.05$, **$P \leq 0.01$, ***$P \leq 0.001$

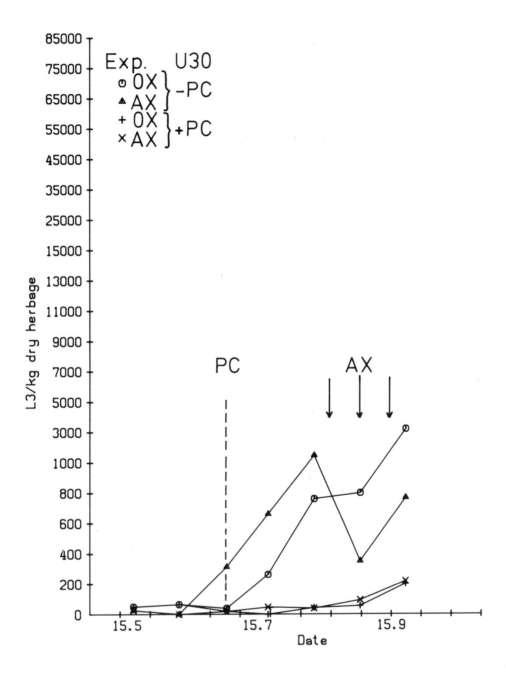

Fig. 5: Example of L_3-contamination of grass in an experiment on anthelmintic treatment (AX vs OX) and paddock change (+PC).

In all groups serum pepsinogen levels (Figure 6) increased throughout the trial. However, the rate of increase was less in treated than in untreated groups, and it was less in groups moved to a harvested paddock in July than in groups maintained in the initial paddocks all summer.

The trends in live weight gain (Figure 7) are in agreement with the results for L_3-contamination of grass and serum pepsinogen levels.

Date of turning out and paddock change

Experimental: the influence of date of turning out and paddock change was examined in three trials of which only one was conducted in a climatically normal year. In trial 1, half the calves were turned out to pasture at the normal time (i.e. between May 11 and 14) and the other one half was turned out late (i.e. between June 11 and 26), which is after the first cutting of pasture. From the dates of turning out to mid-July, the calves grazed one half of the paddock area and the remainder was harvested. Within date of turning out, one half of the calves was moved to the harvested area in mid-July, and the other one half was maintained on the initial paddocks. In one trial a group of calves was also turned out late to paddocks that had been grazed from normal turn out to late June by successive groups of parasite-free calves moved from the pasture after two weeks grazing.

The initial stocking rates averaged 19.2 animals/ha or 2.7 t live weight/ha. This is comparable to normal stocking rates.

Daily gains before paddock change (Table 3) were affected by the date of turning out. However, the differences are attributable to the daily gains in the period from late turning out to the time of paddock change, whereas no significant differences occurred during the period from normal turning out to late turning out.

400

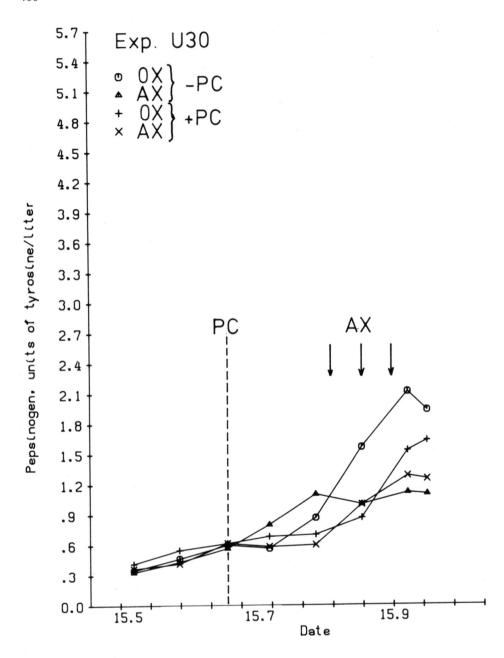

Fig. 6: Example of serum pepsinogen in an experiment on anthelmintic treatment (AX vs OX) and paddock change (±PC).

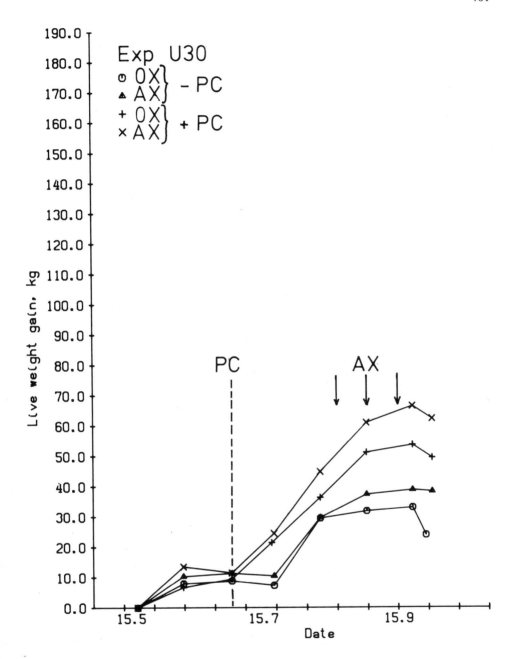

Fig. 7: Example of live weight gains in an experiment on anthelmintic treatment (AX vs OX) and paddock change (±PC).

TABLE 3

DAILY GAIN IN EXPERIMENTS ON DATE AT PASTURE AND PADDOCK CHANGE IN CALVES
AT PASTURE, g/d

Exp. no.	Date at pasture			Paddock change				Trt. XPC[C]
	N	L	Signi-ficance	−	+	+G[D]	Signi-ficance	
Before date of paddock change:								
Normal year								
U21	399	+67[E]	B	374	+117	−	*	NS
Dry years								
U10	761	−166	**	720	−43	−3	NS	NS
U13	157	+259	**	228	+116	−	B	NS
After date of paddock change:								
Normal year								
U21	247	+226	***	314	+92	−	***	A
Dry years								
U10	227	+168	**	237	+143	−9	**	NS
U13	195	−160	**	116	−2	−	NS	NS

[C] Paddock change

[D] To a paddock grazed during spring

NS Not significant, [B]$P \leq 0.25$, [A]$P \leq 0.10$, *$P \leq 0.05$, **$P \leq 0.01$, ***$P \leq 0.001$

[E] Numbers with a sign are deviations

After a paddock change in mid-July, the daily gains
(Table 3) were affected by both variables, and in the experiment
in a normal year the interaction approached significance. In
dry years the effect of turning out calves late were conflicting
and might be attributed to the quantity of grass. In the normal
year, daily gains after paddock change were the same for calves
turned out late, whether or not they were moved in mid-July,
and in calves turned out at the normal time and moved to a clean
paddock in mid-July. Gains in these three groups were higher
than in calves turned out at the normal time and maintained in
the initial paddock. Calves moved to a previously grazed paddock
had gains similar to those kept in the initial paddock all summer.

Stocking rate and paddock change

Experimental: the effect of stocking rate and paddock change were tested in six experiments. The initial stocking rates were:

Low:	1.9 - 2.1 t live weight/ha
Medium:	2.7 - 3.1 t live weight/ha
High:	3.6 - 4.2 t live weight/ha

Within trials fertilisation per ha of pasture was the same at all stocking rates.

The calves were turned out to pasture between May 11 and 18 and they grazed one half of the area designated to each stocking rate. The other half of the area was harvested. Between July 12 and 17, half of the calves within each initial stocking rate were moved to the harvested area. This introduced variable two and, simultaneously, the initial stocking rates were halved. In one experiment (U29) the method of paddock change was applied in all groups and, instead of the stocking rates, were combined with low and high nitrogen application. The nitrogen levels were 100 vs 0 kg N/ha after paddock change.

All three stocking rates were compared in three trials, medium and high were tested in two trials and, finally, low and high stocking rates were used in one trial.

Daily gains before paddock change (Table 4) tended to decrease as stocking rates increased, and this trend was significant in one trial.

After the date of paddock change (Table 4) the effects of both stocking rate and paddock change were highly significant in all trials, except that conducted in a dry year. Furthermore, the interaction between variable one and two approached significance in all but two trials. The daily gain decreased approximately linearly at increasing stocking rate, but the rate of decrease was least in groups moved to a harvested paddock in mid-July.

TABLE 4

DAILY GAIN IN EXPERIMENTS ON STOCKING RATE AND PADDOCK CHANGE IN CALVES AT PASTURE, g/d

Exp. no.	PC^C	Stocking rate				Paddock change			Trt X PC
		L	M	H	Significance	−	+	Significance	
Before date of paddock change:									
Normal years									
U15	±	589	−	376	**	−	−	NS	NS
U20	±	+32^E	402	−117	A	−	−	NS	NS
U22	±	−	760	−38	NS	−	−	NS	NS
U29	±	−	−	246	−	−	246	−	−
U31	±	−	486	−92	B	−	−	A	NS
Dry year									
U12		+258	294	−298	***	−	−	NS	NS
After date of paddock change:									
Normal years									
U15	±	410	−	153	***	170	393	***	NS
U20	−	+463	50	−66	***	−	−	***	A
	+	+124	585	−96		−	−		
U22	−	−	671	−176	***	−	−	*	*
	+	−	889	−394		−	−		
U29	±	+211	599	−103	***	−	−	NS^D	NS
U31	−		540	−512	***	−	−	***	***
	+		836	−243		−	−		
Dry year									
U12	±	+46	471	+74	NS	−	−	B	NS

^{C} Paddock change

^{D} Level of fertiliser application

NS Not significant, ^{B}P ≤0.25, ^{A}P ≤0.10, *P ≤0.05, **P ≤0.01, ***P ≤0.001

^{E} Numbers with a sign are deviations

The level of nitrogen application during late summer did
not affect the performance of the calves, but whether this is
an exception has not been confirmed. The trial was conducted
in 1978 and the late summer percipitation was exceptionally
high.

Substantiating measurements: the daily gains in relation
to the control methods in this group of trials may be substantiated by trial U31 as an example.

The L_3-contamination (Figure 8) increased after the date
of paddock change and the increase was larger at high than
medium stocking rate. Furthermore, the increase was generally
greater in paddocks grazed throughout the summer than in those
with zero grazing to mid-July.

The serum pepsinogen levels (Figure 9) increased throughout the summer. However, after the time of paddock change the
increase was larger in calves at the high than at the medium
stocking rate, and this difference was larger in calves kept
in the initial paddock all summer than in those moved to a
harvested area in mid-July.

In this experiment it was demonstrated very clearly that
the gain (Figure 10) was highest in calves which had the least
increase in serum pepsinogen during the summer season. This
suggests that animals at high stocking rates acquire significantly higher parasite burdens, especially when they are kept
in the same field all summer.

Paddock change

In 1975 the feasibility of paddock change was tested in
five trials on private farms. The daily gains (Table 5) tended
to be highest in calves moved to a harvested paddock in mid-July,
but the difference was only significant in one trial. However,
this may in part be due to the low rainfall that particular
year and also that calves were turned out rather late (mid-June).

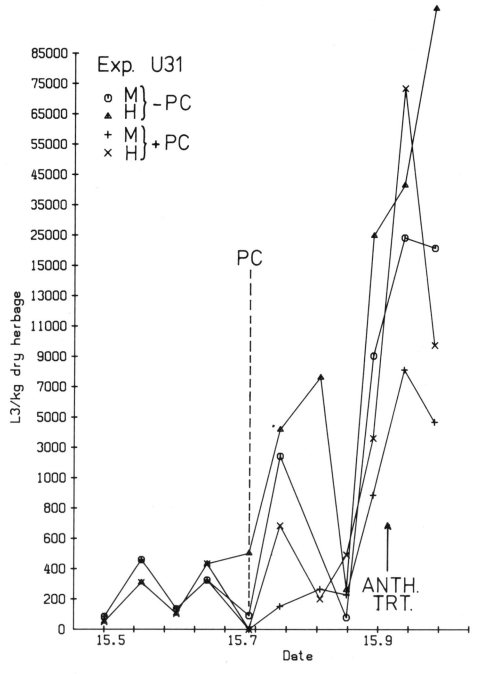

Fig. 8: Example of L_3-contamination of grass in an experiment on medium (M) and high (H) stocking rates and paddock change (±PC).

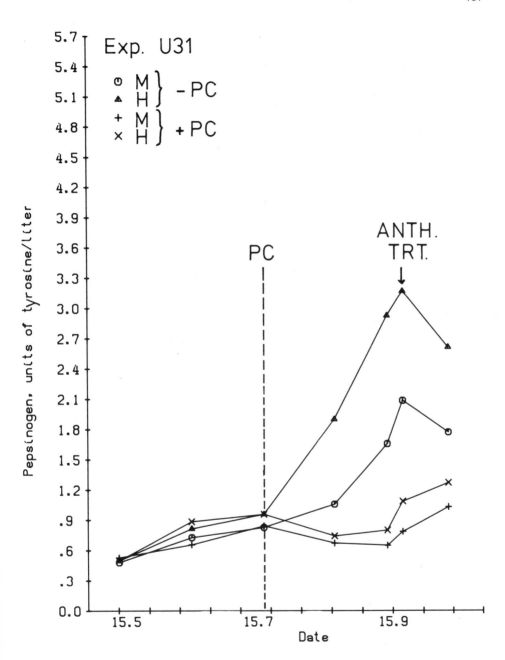

Fig. 9: Example of serum pepsinogen in an experiment on medium (M) and high (H) stocking rates and paddock change (±PC).

408

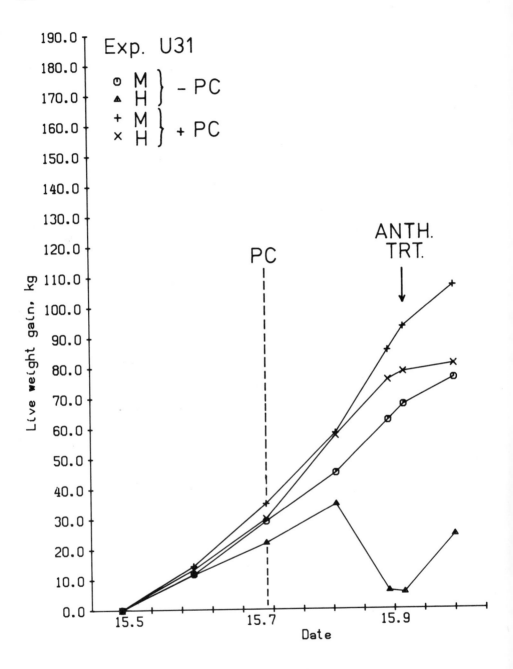

Fig. 10: Example of live weight gains in an experiment on medium (M) and high (H) stocking rates and paddock change (±PC).

TABLE 5

DAILY GAIN IN EXPERIMENTS ON PADDOCK CHANGE IN CALVES AT PASTURE, g/d

| Exp. no. | Before date of PC[C] | After date of PC | | Significance of PC | |
		-PC	+PC[E]	Before PC	After PC
H34	496	-47	+236	NS	*
H63	403	-19	+117	A	A
H521	444	89	+90	B	NS
H522	141	71	+115	NS	NS
H523	242	270	-47	NS	NS

NS Not significant

[B] P≤0.25, [A] P≤0.10, *P≤0.05

[C] Paddock change

[D] Actual gain

[E] Deviation

Animal performance during winter

The performance of animals during the winter following summer experiments were analysed in 6 experiments. In three trials the control methods during summer were anthelmintic treatments, in two trials it was date of turning out, and in one trial it was stocking rate. In all experiments these control methods were tested with or without paddock change in mid-July. In one trial (U21), one half of the animals within subgroups during summer were treated during winter, and the other half were untreated.

Daily gains during the winter period (Table 6) tended to be lowest in those groups which had the highest gains during summer. This may be expected due to differences in the stage of development at the end of the summer. However, the animals never fully compensated during the winter.

TABLE 6

DAILY GAIN DURING THE WINTER PERIOD IN HEIFERS AT PASTURE DURING THE PREVIOUS SUMMER, g/d

Exp. no.	Treatments during summer grazing										Trt. during winter		Significant of treatments [C]						
	Anthelmintic				Date of turn out		Stocking rate		Paddock change		Anthelmintic								
	OX	2X	AX	7X	N	L	M	H	-	+	-	+	T	P	TxP	M	TxM	PxM	TxPxM
U8	731	-	-48[D]	-16	-	-	-	-	730	-41	-	-	NS	NS	NS	-	-	-	-
U9	797	-36	-	-	-	-	-	-	780	+16	-	-	NS	NS	NS	-	-	-	-
U10	-	-	-	-	1029	+25	-	-	1072	-56	-	-	NS	NS	NS	-	-	-	-
U21	-	-	-	-	708	-22	-	-	701	-8	705	-15	NS	NS	**	NS	NS	NS	B
U30	701	-	+34	-	-	-	-	-	752	-68	-	-	*	***	NS	-	-	-	-
U31	-	-	-	-	-	-	581	+41	641	-79	-	-	NS	A	NS	-	-	-	-

NS Not significant, [B]P≤0.25, [A]P≤0.10, *P≤0.05, **P≤0.01, ***P≤0.001

[C] T = factor one during summer, P = paddock change at pasture, M = anthelmintic treatment in winter

[D] numbers with a sign are deviations

CONCLUSION

The experiments showed that daily gains were increased in calves at pasture when principles for control of ostertagiasis were applied. This is substantiated by parasitological measurements such as herbage larvae counts and serum pepsinogen levels. The efficiency of the various control methods under Danish conditions may be ranked as follows: paddock change in mid-July > turning out delayed to mid-June ≥ repeated anthelmintic treatments. However, the daily gains to be expected will depend not only upon these methods, but also on stocking rate and local climatic conditions.

Finally, animals with low daily gains at pasture due to ostertagiasis did not make full compensation during the winter period, and anthelmintic treatments during the winter had no beneficial effects.

ACKNOWLEDGEMENT

The studies were part of a joint Nordic project (NKJ No. 36) on gastro-intestinal nematodes of cattle, supported in Denmark by the Danish Agricultural and Veterinary Research Council (Grant No. 533/8).

REFERNECES

Henriksen, Sv.Aa., 1974. Parasitologiske graesmarksundersøgelser i Danmark. Proc. 12th Nord. Vet. Congr. Reykjavik 1974.

Henriksen, Sv.As., 1975. Løbe-tarmstrongylider hos kvaeg - II. En oversigt med saerlig henblik på *Ostertagia ostertagi*. Dansk Vet. Tidsskr. 58, 833-842.

Michel, J.F., 1968. The control of stomach-worm infection in young cattle. J. Br. Grassl. Soc. 23, 165-173.

Nilsson, O. and Sorelius, L., 1973. Trichostrongylideinfektioner hos nöt-kreatur i Sverige. Nord. Vet. Med., 25, 65-78.

Østergaard, V., 1977. Kan indtjeningen i husdyrbruget øges ved etablering af markvandingsanlaeg. Tidsskr. for Landokonomi 3.

THE USE OF ANTHELMINTIC GIVEN AT CONTINUOUS LOW DOSAGE IN DRINKING WATER TO CONTROL NEMATODIASIS IN CALVES

N.E. Downey and J. O'Shea

The Agricultural Institute, Dunsinea,
Castleknock, Co. Dublin, Ireland

ABSTRACT

A number of anthelmintic compounds were found to suppress the faecal output of trichostrongylid eggs or Dictyocaulus viviparus *larvae or both when administered at various low dosage levels via the drinking water to artificially infected calves maintained indoors. Under grazing conditions, morantel, levamisole and oxfendazole administered in this fashion to calves during May, June and early July suppressed egg output and this was reflected later in greatly reduced levels of infection on the herbage and in the calves. Calves receiving this system of parasite control achieved excellent liveweight gains. From clinical observations and liveweight data, animals that had undergone the treatment as calves in their first grazing season did not seem to be unduly susceptible to trichostrongylid infection in their second grazing season. Preliminary studies showed that the anthelmintics thiophanate and phenothiazine, administered in the drinking water at low daily dosage, had marked ovicidal and possibly larvicidal effects.*

P. Nansen, R.J. Jørgensen, E.J.L. Soulsby (eds), Epidemiology and Control of Nematodiasis in Cattle.
Copyright © 1981 ECSC, EEC, EAEC, Brussels – Luxembourg. All rights reserved.

INTRODUCTION

Downey, O'Shea and Spillane (1974), Downey and O'Shea (1977) and Downey and O'Shea (1978) have reported that continuous administration of anthelmintics at low daily dosage in drinking water suppressed the faecal output of trichostrongylid eggs by calves. The objective of this procedure is to limit parasitic contamination of herbage early in the grazing season and thus prevent the increase in infection which commonly occurs on the sward in the post-July period (Michel, 1969; Downey, 1973; Bürger, 1974). Preliminary findings (Downey and O'Shea, 1977) showed that the method might be adapted also to the control of *Dictyocaulus viviparus* infection.

The present communication describes a series of validation experiments in which the method was tested under controlled indoor conditions, using various anthelmintics. Grazing trials were designed to test the method for parasitic control under practical conditions, to evaluate its effect on calf production and on resistance of the host to re-infection. Preliminary studies were conducted on the ovicidal effects of the anthelmintics thiophanate and phenothiazine.

MATERIALS AND METHODS

Animals

Artificially reared male Friesian calves were used, except in studies of ovicidal effects when the calves were males of the Jersey breed. For indoor validation studies, the animals were housed throughout, while for grazing studies, they were housed until required. In these circumstances accidental nematode infection was unlikely and it was not detected on faecal examination. Calves for grazing experiments were born in spring and in experiments 1 - 4 (see later), they were undergoing their first season at pasture.

Medication

The anthelmintic to be evaluated was added to the drinking water at a concentration estimated to supply each calf with a low daily dosage. In early experiments the entire water supply for the treated groups contained anthelmintic. In later work, anthelmintic was added to an amount of water estimated to be the calves' minimum daily consumption, requirement in excess of this being supplied as untreated water (see O'Shea and Downey, these proceedings). The calves were weighed at the beginning of the experiment and at weekly intervals thereafter, and the dose rate computed according to the group's mean live-weight at each weighing.

Validation studies

A series of indoor experiments was conducted over several years. Various anthelmintic compounds were evaluated for their capacity, when given as already described, to suppress the faecal output of trichostrongylid eggs and *D. viviparus* larvae. Groups of calves received trickle infections with *O. ostertagi*, *C. oncophora* and *D. viviparus* according to schedules in Table 1. Calves were randomly assigned to treated and control groups each of 4 or 6 calves. Treated groups received medication (Table 3) in the drinking water, beginning on the first day of infection and each experiment was of approximately 8 to 10 weeks duration. Individual faeces samples were examined at weekly or twice-weekly intervals for trichostrongylid eggs (Parfitt, 1958) and *D. viviparus* larvae (Parfitt, 1955), the results being expressed as eggs per g of faeces (epg) and larvae per g (lpg) respectively.

Grazing experiments

For these experiments (designated 1 to 4), grazing began at the beginning of May and ended in October/November. The calves grazed in a paddock system, but were essentially set-stocked, each group remaining throughout in a separate area of pasture. The stocking rate was approximately 3 - 4 calves per acre. In experiment 1, residual pasture infection with

TABLE 1

ARTIFICIAL INFECTION SCHEDULES ADOPTED FOR INDOOR VALIDATION EXPERIMENTS

Experiment	Trichostrongylids (*O. ostertagia* + *C. oncophora*) Ave. No. L_3/calf	*D. viviparus* Ave. No. L_3/calf
A	–	2 662
B	19 000 over 18 days	2 484 over 10 days
C_1	8 100 over 21 days	1 020 over 10 days
C_2	–	2 100 over 5 days
D	10 000 over 20 days	1 500 over 10 days

O. ostertagi and *C. oncophora* was simulated by giving each calf 500
third stage larvae (l_3) of each species every day for the first
6 weeks. In all other grazing experiments, calves were exposed
throughout to natural infection. Calves were randomly assigned
to treated and control groups, random assignment being restricted by initial liveweight. Treated groups received their anthelmintic medication in the drinking water from the day of turnout until the first or second week in July. Experiment 3 was
exceptional in that medication (oxfendazole) was given to one
group intermittently, i.e., 1 week in 3 from May to the beginning
of July and then reintroduced for 5 days in early August.
Additional medication with DEC to control parasitic bronchitis
was given as shown in Table 2. In experiment 3, 2 groups of
calves were given levamisole at 7.5 mg/kg in mid-July and
immediately moved to 'clean' pasture consisting of ungrazed
silage aftermath (see Table 2). Herbage larval counts (Parfitt,
1955) and calves' faecal egg counts were determined at weekly
intervals. Blood samples for plasma pepsinogen determinations
(Ross et al., 1967) were taken from calves in certain groups
at 2-week intervals in the latter part of the grazing season.
Parasitological data were not monitored in Experiment 4, the

objective of which was to assess calf production using this system of worm control. Calves were weighed at weekly intervals both to monitor their growth rate and to enable dosages to be computed.

The treatments imposed in the grazing experiment are shown in Table 2.

Effect on host resistance

Two groups, each consisting of 8 yearling cattle that had undergone the system of medication in calfhood, were grazed in separate adjoining areas (Plots A and B) of a pasture which had a history of heavy trichostrongylid infection the previous year. One group was put into Plot A at the end of April. Plot B was stocked with calves from April to mid-July, whereupon the calves were replaced by the second group of yearlings. The groups were reduced to 4 yearlings each early in September, as there was then insufficient herbage for the larger number. The 2 groups were faeces sampled regularly for epg counts. Liveweight gains were recorded and the animals were carefully observed for symptoms of nematodiasis.

Ovicidal effect

In an experiment to test this effect with thiophanate, groups of calves were given trickle infections consisting of a mixture of *O. ostertagi* and *C. oncophora*. For a preliminary study with phenothiazine, pairs ¿ calves were given monospecies infections consisting of either *O. ostertagi* or *C. oncophora*. The anthelmintics were administered in the drinking water as shown in Tables 7 and 8, beginning with the first inoculation of infective larvae. To determine ovicidal effect, eggs were obtained by salt flotation using 3 g faecal samples from each animal. The eggs were washed and then examined for embryo formation after incubating them in shallow water for 24 hours at $27^{\circ}C$. As a further test of ovicidal and possibly larvicidal effect, the faeces of each animal were mixed with vermiculite, kept moist and incubated at $27^{\circ}C$. For an experiment involving

TABLE 2

GROUPING AND TREATMENTS FOR GRAZING EXPERIMENTS 1 TO 4. (THE TERM 'CONVENTIONAL' DENOTES FULL THERAPEUTIC DOSES OF ANTHELMINTIC AT THE TIMES SHOWN)

Exp. No.	Group	No. of animals	Medication via drinking water* anthelmintic	daily dose (mg/kg)	Other worm control procedures
1	1	12	morantel	1.9	DEC:† periodic therapeutic doses to control 'husk'
	2	12	morantel	4.3	As for group 1
	3	12	levamisole	3.7	As for group 1
	4 (conventional)	12	–	–	(i) As for group 1 (ii) Banminth-D: therapeutic doses July, August, September
	5 (control)	12	–	–	As for group 1
2	1	14	levamisole DEC	3 10	–
	2	14	oxfendazole DEC	1 10	–
	3 (conventional)	14	–	–	levamisole (7.5 mg/kg): June, July, August, October
	4 (control)	14	–	–	levamisole (7.5 mg/kg): October

TABLE 2 (Continued)

Exp. No.	Group	No. of Animals	Medication via drinking water*		Other worm control procedures
			anthelmintic	daily dose (mg/kg)	
3	1	8	levamisole / DEC	3 / 10	—
	2	8	oxfendazole+ / DEC	1 / 10	—
	3 (control)	8	—	—	levamisole (7.5 mg/kg): September 1, 20
	4	7	levamisole	3)	(i) moved to aftermath, July 12 (ii) levamisole (7.5 mg/kg): July 12, September 1, 20
	5	7	—	)	—
4	1	15	levamisole / DEC	3 / 10	—
	2 (control)	15	—	—	levamisole (7.5 mg/kg): July, August, September

† DEC = diethylcarbamazine citrite

* Medication lasted from turn-out (beginning of May) until early July except for DEC which was given from late July onwards, continuously in experiment 2 and during every third week in experiments 3 and 4.

+ Oxfendazole given during every third week (May to early July) and again for 5 days in early August.

the use of the anthelmintic thiophanate, incubation was carried out for 9 days to estimate the number of eggs giving rise to third stage larvae (l_3). When phenothiazine was being tested for these effects, faecal cultures were examined at 2, 5 and 9 days to ascertain numbers of larvae developing to first (l_1), second (l_2) and l_3 stages respectively. Early in this latter experiment, portions of the same culture were examined at each of the 3 stages, but for later determinations, 100 g of faeces per animal was divided into 3 equal portions, each being incubated and examined separately at the intervals stated.

TABLE 3

ACCUMULATED TRICHOSTRONGYLID EGG COUNTS (epg) AND *D. viviparus* LARVAL COUNTS (lpg) IN FAECES* OF ARTIFICIALLY INFECTED CALVES, MAINTAINED INDOORS, TREATED GROUPS HAVING ACCESS TO VARIOUS ANTHELMINTICS AT LOW DAILY DOSAGES IN THE DRINKING WATER (SUMMARY OF 5 EXPERIMENTS)

Anthelmintic	Daily dose (mg/kg)	Trichostrongylid		*D. viviparus*	
		Treated	Control	Treated	Control
Levamisole	2.1	–	–	16.0)	80
	2.7	–	–	0.6)	
Morantel	1.6	1725)		31.0)	1010
	3.5	140)	7128	0.1)	
Levamisole	3.9	74)		0.1)	
Morantel + DEC+	1.4)	149)		0.0)	
	10.0)	)		)	
Morantel + DEC	2.0)	67)	2854	0.03)	33
	13.5)	)		)	
Oxfendazole	1.0	9)		0.0)	
DEC	12.0	–	–	0.4)	125
DEC	10.0	–	–	1.6)	
Thiophanate	7-14	502	3162	0.5	7

* Obtained by adding either egg or larval counts twice-weekly after first infection

+ DEC = diethylcarbamazine citrate

RESULTS

Table 3 shows that all the anthelmintic compounds administered at low daily dosages via the drinking water markedly

suppressed the faecal output of trichostrongylid eggs and
D. viviparus larvae in calves infected under artificial indoor
conditions. The results represent average reductions of 93 and
97 percent for eggs and larvae respectively.

GRAZING EXPERIMENT 1

Figure 1 shows that morantel administered to group 2 at
4.3 mg/kg daily in the manner described during May, June and
early July caused a marked suppression of trichostrongylid egg
output and that this was reflected later in a greatly reduced
level of herbage infection. This resulted in less infection
in the calves as denoted by their continuing low egg counts in
August, September and October compared with controls. Data
from groups 1, 3 and 4 (see Table 2) have been omitted from
Figure 1. Morantel administered at 1.9 mg/kg to group 1
appeared to delay rather than prevent a later increase in
herbage infection while results obtained with levamisole at
3.7 (group 3) were about equal to those seen with morantel at
4.3 mg/kg. Conventional therapy (group 4) reduced egg counts
considerably in the latter part of the grazing season.

Blood pepsinogen levels (Table 4) remained around normal
in groups 2 and 3, being somewhat lower in group 3. The levels
were significantly higher in controls (group 5) on all occasions
during August to early November, while group 1 showed an
increased level in October/November. The conventionally
treated animals showed levels of pepsinogen that were similar
to those of the controls.

GRAZING EXPERIMENT 2

Levamisole at 3 mg/kg and oxfendazole at 1 mg/kg daily in
the drinking water (groups 1 and 2) in early season were about
equally effective in suppressing calves' egg output, thereby
preventing the later massive increase in herbage infection seen
in the control plot (Figure 2). Groups 1 and 2 maintained quite
low egg counts, indicating that these animals acquired less

422

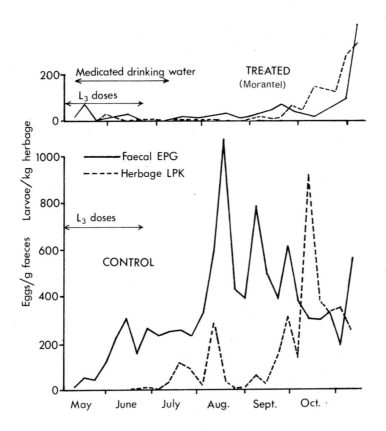

Fig. 1: Fluctuations in calves' faecal egg counts (epg) and in trichostrongyle herbage larval counts (lpk) in experiment 1: upper
graph for group 2, lower graph for group t (control).

infection than controls throughout the experiment. Data from
group 3 (see Table 2) are omitted from Figure 2. Egg counts of
animals in this group were reduced in late season after each
therapeutic dose of anthelmintic but, as in experiment 1, the
reduction in egg count was not reflected in reduced plasma
pepsinogen levels, which were similar to those of the controls
(Table 4). In contrast, pepsinogen levels in groups 1 and 2
were significantly lower than in the controls.

TABLE 4

MEAN PLASMA PEPSINOGEN LEVEL (i.u./l) OF CALVES IN 3 GRAZING EXPERIMENTS AND THEIR SIGNIFICANCE. (FOR DETAILS OF GROUP MEDICATION, SEE TABLE 2)

Exp.	Group	Medication	Aug.	Sept.	Oct.	Nov.
1	1	Morantel	0.3	0.5 0.5	0.9 1.3	1.9
	2	Morantel	0.3	0.5 0.4	0.9 1.1	1.1
	3	Levamisole	0.4	0.4 0.4	0.3 0.6	0.6
	4	Conventional*	0.7	1.7 1.2	1.6 2.9	2.0
	5	Control	1.2	1.5 1.3	1.8 1.7	1.8
	Significance			P < 0.001		P < 0.01
2	1	Levamisole	0.8 0.7	0.8 0.7	1.0	–
	2	Oxfendazole	0.8 0.6	0.7 1.5	1.0	–
	3	Conventional+	1.2 1.3	1.8 2.3	2.1	–
	4	Control	1.2 1.2	2.1 2.5	2.6	–
	Significance		P < 0.05	P < 0.001		
3	1	Levamisole	1.1 0.4	1.2 1.3	1.2	–
	2	Oxfendazole	0.8 0.4	1.0 0.7	1.1	–
	3	Control	2.2 2.0	3.7 3.1	3.9	–
	Significance		P < 0.01	P < 0.001		

* Recommended therapeutic doses of a mixture of morantel and DEC ('Banminth-D', Pfizer) in July, August and September

+ Levamisole at 7.5 mg/kg in July, August and October.

Note: all other anthelmintic medication given at low daily dosage via drinking water as shown in Table 2.

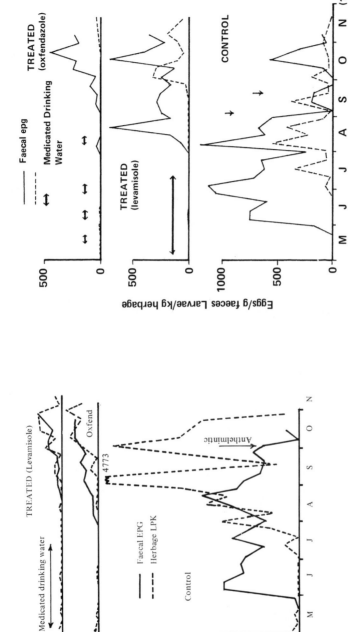

Fig. 3: Fluctuations in calves' faecal egg counts (epg) and in herbage trichostrongyle larval counts (lpk) in experiment 3: upper graph for group 2, middle graph for group 1 and lower graph for group 3 (control).

Fig. 2: Fluctuations in calves' faecal egg counts (epg) and in herbage trichostrongyle larval counts (lpk) in experiment 2: upper graph for group 1, middle graph for group 2 and lower graph for group 4 (control).

It was noted in experiments 1 and 2 that herbage infection increased somewhat at the end of the grazing season. This increase was accompanied by a rise in egg counts of calves and in experiment 2, 2 calves in group 2 (oxfendazole) but none in group 1 (levamisole) showed clinical signs of parasitic gastro-enteritis in October.

GRAZING EXPERIMENT 3

The results of experiment 3 (Figure 3) were rather similar to those of experiments 1 and 2. The re-introduction of oxfendazole medication (group 2) for 5 days in early August, however, eliminated the terminal rise in herbage infection level seen in the foregoing experiments. Plasma pepsinogen (Table 4) was consistently lower in calves of the 2 treated groups (1 and 2) than in the control (group 3), the differences (as with previous experiments) being highly significant. The treatments imposed on groups 1 and 2 caused highly significant ($P < 0.001$) increases in liveweight gain compared with the control group 3 (Table 5). Liveweight data related to groups 4 and 5 (Table 2) are included in Table 5 for completeness. These groups were mainly intended to provide epidemiological data and will not be considered in the present communication.

GRAZING EXPERIMENT 4

A single determination of plasma pepsinogen (on September 9) showed that calves in group 1, given levamisole at 3 mg/kg daily as already described, had a level of 1.5 i.u./l compared with 3.4 i.u./l for group 2 (control), the difference being highly significant ($P < 0.01$). Table 5 shows that group 1 gained significantly ($P < 0.001$) more weight than the control group.

The administration of DEC in the drinking water in experiments 2, 3 and 4 (see Table 2), was intended for the control of *D. viviparus* infection. In the event, infection with this parasite did not occur in significant amounts in any of these experiments.

426

TABLE 5

MEAN INITIAL WEIGHTS AND LIVEWEIGHT GAINS (KG), MAY TO OCTOBER, OF CALVES IN 2 GRAZING EXPERIMENTS AND THEIR SIGNIFICANCE

TREATMENT	EXPERIMENT 3						EXPERIMENT 4		
	Lev.+	Oxfen.+	Control	Lev.+ & Move	Move only	F-test	Lev.+	Control	F-test
No. of Animals	8	8	8	7	7		15	15	
Initial weight	81.5	80.8	83.1	81.1	79.0		98.5	97.5	
Daily gain	0.76	0.73	0.55	0.64	0.57	P < 0.001	0.73	0.55	P < 0.007

+ Levamisole and oxfendazole administered at low daily dosage via drinking water in early season.

TABLE 6

LIVEWEIGHT GAINS (KG) OF CATTLE IN THEIR 2ND GRAZING SEASON

GRAZING CONDITIONS	Initial weight	Daily weight gain July 17 - September 9	Daily gain whole season	Final weight
No. of animals	8	8	4	4
A. Set-stocked whole season (From April 4)	313.0	0.77	0.77	468.5
B. Following calves from July 17	324.8	0.82	0.73	469.0

EFFECT ON HOST RESISTANCE

The egg counts of both groups of yearlings remained low, no animal showed clinical signs of parasitic infection and all animals made good liveweight gains (Table 6).

OVICIDAL EFFECTS

Tables 7 and 8 show that both thiophanate and phenothiazine respectively were markedly ovicidal and possibly larvicidal when administered continuously in the drinking water at daily low dosage levels. It is also apparent from these preliminary studies that egg development was resumed when thiophanate was withdrawn for 3 days and phenothiazine for 4 days.

TABLE 7

OVICIDAL EFFECT OF THIOPHANATE IN CALVES' DRINKING WATER: % VIABLE EGGS IN FAECES (GROUP MEAN epg COUNTS IN PARENTHESIS)

Daily dose (mg/kg)	Days after initial infection with *Ostertagia* and *Cooperia*					
	49	52	56	60		63
5-10	8 (118)	48 (63)	20 (74)	2 (51)		94 (76)
					Drug off	
7-14	0 (28)	0 (15)	10 (4)	54 (1)		90 (2)
0 (Control)	80 (383)	99 (3000)	96 (220)	99 (360)	–	98 (420)

DISCUSSION

From the results of indoor validation studies and grazing experiments, it is evident that daily medication in the drinking water consisting of either levamisole at 3 mg/kg or oxfendazole at 1 mg/kg satisfactorily suppressed the faecal output of trichostrongylid eggs and *D. viviparus* larvae. (In more recent, unpublished studies, oxfendazole caused excellent egg suppression at a daily dose of 0.4 mg/kg). DEC administered similarly suppressed *D. viviparus* larval output at 10 mg/kg and

TABLE 8

OVICIDAL AND POSSIBLE LARVICIDAL EFFECT OF PHENOTHIAZINE (10 mg/kg DAILY) IN CALVES' DRINKING WATER: % VIABLE EGGS AND NUMBERS OF TRICHOSTRONGYLE LARVAE RECOVERED FROM FAECAL CULTURES

| WORM GENUS | TREATMENT | During drug administration (means of 4 determinations) | | | 4 days after drug withdrawal | |
		Animal No.	Eggs % viable	Larvae $(l_1 + l_2 + l_3)$ (X 10^2)	Eggs % viable	Larvae $(l_1 + l_2 + l_3)$ (X 10^2)
Ostertagia	medicated	21	0	0	87	7.7
		22	0	0	99	12.6
	Control	7	86	43.3	99	14.6
Cooperia	medicated	25	0	0	100	0.6
		85	0	0	100	49.2
	Control	12	89	60.4	98	36.8

suppression was enhanced by an admixture of morantel at 1.4
and 2.0 mg/kg.

Under grazing conditions (experiment 1), morantel was
considerably less effective at 1.9 than at 4.3 mg/kg daily.
This was surprising in view of the good results obtained indoors
with a daily dose of 1.6 mg/kg. The dosage rates applicable
to experiment 1 are average amounts for the whole period of
medication. Probably at the lower dose level the intake of
morantel was occasionally too low to induce adequate egg
suppression. The variation in drug intake was probably due to
the method of administration used in experiment 1, whereby the
estimated amount of anthelmintic required per day was added to
the entire daily water supply (see also paper by O'Shea and
Downey). Alternatively, or perhaps additionally to the low
drug intake, there may have been partial degradation of morantel
in the water, though as a precaution, the drinking trough was
shaded from direct sunlight. The higher dose level of administration presumably would have compensated for uneven drug
intake or for any loss of drug activity or both.

Bains and Dalton (1978) have reported that thiophanate
given at repeated daily doses of 5 or 10 mg/kg decreased egg
counts to low levels in calves artificially infected with
O. ostertagi and *C. oncophora*. In the present study a dosage
rate of 14 mg/kg daily in drinking water was found necessary to
induce a satisfactory suppression of egg output (Table 3), doses
of 5, 7 and 10 mg/kg having proved rather less effective.
Thiophanate also was shown to possess ovicidal activity and
this aspect will be considered later.

The increase in herbage infection that occurred towards
the end of the season, despite earlier suppression of egg
contamination, has already been referred to in relation to
experiments 1 and 2. Work is underway to investigate the
origins of this increase. Since it was prevented by reintro-
ducing anthelmintic for 5 days at the beginning of August and
from a consideration of the egg count patterns of groups 1 and

2 in experiment 2 (Figure 2), it seems that eggs deposited late in the season can make a substantial contribution to the population of infective larvae on the sward.

Calves subjected to this method of parasite control gained about 30 percent more weight over the grazing season than calves (Controls) which received respectively 2 and 3 therapeutic doses of anthelmintic (e.g. experiments 3 and 4). The average daily gain (0.74 kg) for this system would enable animals to reach or even exceed the modern growth targets that are considered essential for the production of 2-year-old beef or replacement heifers. As this rate of gain was achieved with set-stocking and with little or no supplementary feed, the system has considerable economic potential.

The good performance and absence of clinical signs shown by animals when they were exposed to parasitic infection in their second grazing season indicated that the low-level medication in the drinking water received as calves did not seriously reduce resistance to reinfection in the long term.

Both thiophanate and phenothiazine when given as described were strikingly ovicidal and possibly larvicidal, characteristics that must enhance the value of these compounds when used in this system of parasite control. The results, in particular the resurgence of egg development upon drug withdrawal, agree with those of Bains and Dalton (1978) regarding thiophanate and with those of Shum (1976) who studied low level dosage regimens with phenothiazine in sheep.

There is the possible danger that the giving of an anthelmintic repeatedly at low dosage might give rise to strains of worms that are resistant to the anthelmintic. Naturally such a risk, if it exists, would be common to any system involving low-dosage administration, such as, for example, medicated feed blocks or slow-release devices. On the other hand, should such resistance arise by a process of selection, it may well be more likely to result from using full therapeutic doses which would tend to select mainly resistant strains, whereas small doses, because of possibly reduced efficacy, may give rise to a mixed population of resistant and non-resistant individuals, so that the resistant ones do not necessarily become predominant. This would need to be tested experimentally. However, the compounds evaluated in the present investigations have been used at low doses in the same area since 1974 and no evidence of drug resistance has appeared so far.

Webb et al. (1979) reported that in Australia drug resistance was not a problem on farms where chemically unrelated anthelmintics were used in a regimen of drug rotation. In case drug resistance arises, therefore, such a rotation would be entirely feasible in the present system in which a number of compounds can be utilised.

ACKNOWLEDGEMENTS

The authors wish to thank Mr. R. Peacock of Allen & Hanburys Research Ltd., England, for supplying infective *D. viviparus* larvae used in indoor validation experiments, Mr. T.A. Spillane for pepsinogen determintions, Mr. J. Sherrington for statistical analysis and Mr. T. Kendrick for the text figures. The technical assistance of Messrs. A. Baldwin, M. O'Sullivan and J. Farrell is also gratefully acknowledged.

432

REFERENCES

Bains, D.M. and Dalton, S.E., 1978. Repeat dosing of ruminants over
limited periods with the anthelmintic thiophanate. Veterinary
Record, 103, 527-530.

Bürger, H.-J., 1974. Epidemiology and control of trichostrongyle
infections in cattle. Proceedings of IIIrd International Congress of
Parasitology, Munich. Vol. 2, p. 744-746.

Downey, N.E., 1973. Nematode parasite infection of calf pasture in
relation to the health and performance of grazing calves. Veterinary
Record, 93, 505-514.

Downey, N.E., O'Shea, J. and Spillane, T.A., 1974. Preliminary observations
on the use of low-level medication in calves' drinking water as a
means of parasite control. Irish Veterinary Journal, 28, 221-222.

Downey, N.E. and O'Shea, J., 1977. Calf parasite control by means of
low-level anthelmintic administered via the drinking water.
Veterinary Record, 100, 265-266.

Downey, N.E. and O'Shea, J., 1978. The control of nematode parasites in
calves through low-level anthelmintic in the drinking water. Proc.
IVth International Congress of Parasitology, Warsaw. Section C.
p. 170-171.

Michel, J.F., 1969. Observations on the epidemiology of parasitic gastro-
enteritis in calves. Journal of Helminthology, 43, 111-133.

Parfitt, J.W., 1955. Two techniques used for the detection and enumeration
of the larvae of Dictyocaulus viviparus in faeces and herbage.
Laboratory Practice, 4, 15-16.

Parfitt, J.W., 1958. A technique for the enumeration of helminth eggs and
protozoan cysts from farm animals in Britain. Laboratory Practice, 7,
353-355.

Ross, J.G., Purcell, D.A., Dow, C. and Todd, J.R., 1967. Experimental
infections of calves with Trichostrongylus axei; the course and
development of infection and lesions in low level infections. Research
in Veterinary Science, 8, 201-206.

Shum, K.L., 1976. The impact of prophylactic chemicals on trichostrongylid
parasitism in sheep. Ph.D. Thesis, University of Wisconsin-Madison.

Webb, R.F., McCully, C.H., Clarke, F.L., Greentree, P. and Honey, P., 1979.
The incidence of thiabendazole resistance in field populations of
Haemonchus contortus on the northern tableland of New South Wales.
Australian Veterinary Journal, 55, 422-426.

SOME PHYSICAL ASPECTS OF CONTINUOUS LOW DOSAGE OF ANTHELMINTICS VIA DRINKING WATER

J. O'Shea and N.E. Downey

The Agricultural Institute, Dunsinea,
Castleknock, Co. Dublin, Ireland.

ABSTRACT

Factors influencing the drinking behaviour of calves receiving continuous low level dosage of anthelmintic in the drinking water were studied. An indoor experiment is described which indicates a positive correlation between effectiveness of parasite control and level of water intake. Similar effects were observed under grazing conditions. Data are presented relating water intake to calf weight and rainfall for a variety of anthelmintic treatments.

To achieve consistent dose levels anthelmintics should be included only in the first 0.5 gallons*of liquid which calves consume daily. In grazing experiments, where this was carried out using both soluble and insoluble anthelmintics, no evidence of unpalatability was noticed. Observations are presented on the drinking behaviour of individual calves consuming phenothiazine from a common trough under these circumstances. Details are given of a proposed system for the automatic administration of anthelmintics in drinking water.

---

* 1 gallon = 4.544 litres

P. Nansen, R.J. Jørgensen, E.J.L. Soulsby (eds), Epidemiology and Control of Nematodiasis in Cattle.

INTRODUCTION

The administration of medicaments or nutrients to animals by their drinking water is not a new concept. Antibiotics and anthelmintics for instance are commonly given to pigs and poultry in this manner. Other examples include the use of pleuronics for bloat control, urea as a cattle protein supplement and magnesium salts to combat grass tetany.

Downey and O'Shea (1980 these proceedings) describe a series of experiments carried out to evaluate the use of anthelmintics given at continuous low dosage in drinking water to control nematodiasis in calves. In the present communication some of the associated physical and behavioural studies undertaken are described, together with details of a proposed automatic procedure for the medication of calf drinking water.

MATERIALS AND METHODS

Indoor feeding experiment 1.

This experiment had four groups, each of six calves (average weight 113 kg). Group 1 received 3.5 mg/kg daily of levamisole in the drinking water, group 2, 3.9 mg; group 3 received 1.6 mg/kg daily of morantel, while group 4 acted as control. All calves were given a trichostrongylid infection, mainly *Ostertagia ostertagi*, at a dose rate of 165 larvae/kg over 18 days and *D. viviparus* at 22 larvae/kg over 10 days. Group water intakes were recorded daily for the 49-day duration of the experiment. Animals were weighed weekly.

Indoor feeding experiment 2.

This experiment involved three groups, each of eight calves. Group 1 received phenothiazine at 10 mg/kg bodyweight daily; group 2, 5 mg and group 3 acted as control. Phenothiazine was suspended in 4 gallons of aerated water at a fixed time each morning. Calves had previously received trickle infections of

D. viviparus and either *O. ostertagi* or *C. onchophora*. A 5-day observation was carried out on the calves in group 1 to ascertain individual drinking behaviour.

Grazing experiment 1.

Twelve calves were administered morantel tartrate at a fixed concentration in the water during the grazing season. Group water intake was measured and records were kept of liveweight and rainfall changes. (For parasitological and other details see Downey et al. 1974).

Grazing experiment 2.

This was a 5-treatment experiment involving 12 calves per group. Parasitological and medication data are shown in the preceding communication (Table 2, Experiment 1, Downey and O'Shea, 1980, these proceedings). Group water intakes, individual liveweight gains and meteorological data were recorded.

Feasibility studies.

These refer to grazing experiments where calves were offered their daily dose of anthelmintic in amounts corresponding to 0.5 gallons of water per calf. When calves had consumed this amount they received untreated water *ad libitum*. The main observations carried out in these trials were concerned with palatability problems. Difficulties with insoluble drugs were also studied.

Design of dosing equipment.

A preliminary diagram of the dosing equipment is shown in Figure 1.

At a predetermined time each day, e.g. 9 a.m., a solenoid (A) would be activated to fill the tank with fresh water. On reaching a certain level the solenoid is cut off by means of the float switch (B). For insoluble anthelmintics the main mixer (C) would then be set in motion. This would be followed

436

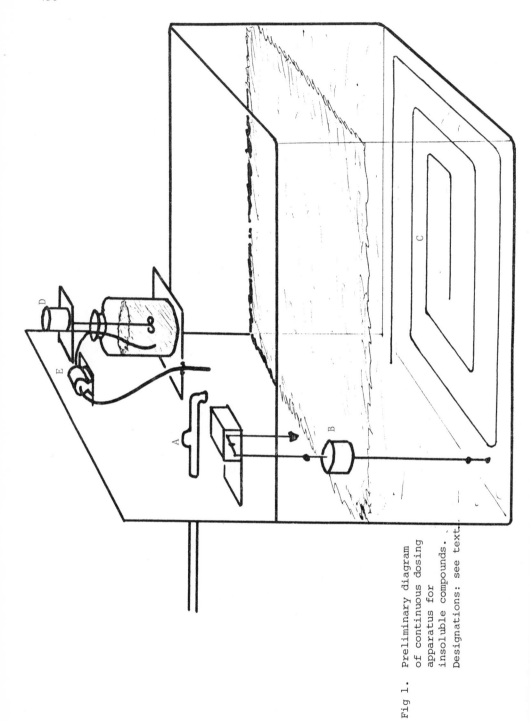

Fig 1. Preliminary diagram of continuous dosing apparatus for insoluble compounds. Designations: see text.

by activation of the stock solution mixer (D) followed by an injection of anthelmintic through the dosing pump (E). The length of time the dosing pump operates will vary according to the number of calves being treated.

Calves consume the liquid, and when the float reaches its lower point the system is filled with fresh water. The electrical appliances and stock solution would, in practice, be enclosed to exclude light and rain.

RESULTS AND DISCUSSION

Relationship between calf bodyweight and water intake (indoor experiment 1).

The results of this trial were analysed statistically and lines of best fit are shown on Figure 2. An interesting feature is the direct relationship between the degree of parasite control (Downey and O'Shea, 1977) and level of calf water intake. No significant relationship was found between calf weight and level of water intake for non-treated infected calves whereas this was the case in groups where levamisole treatment was most effective. The lower water intake in infected animals probably was associated with reduced feed consumption.

Factors affecting calf water intake under grazing conditions.

Figure 3 shows the changes observed in calf liveweight, water intake and rainfall for grazing experiment 1. The three main observations are: water intake is heavily influenced by degree of rainfall, levels of water intake rarely fall below 0.5 gallons per day and due to variability in the amount consumed it was difficult to administer a constant daily dose when anthelmintic was administered in the drinking water at fixed concentrations.

A statistical appraisal of the results obtained from grazing experiment 2 is shown in Table 1. In non-treated groups

TABLE 1

EQUATIONS RELATING CALF WATER INTAKE TO WEIGHT AND LEVEL OF RAINFALL. GRAZING EXPERIMENT 2.

Treatment	Equation	t_{Value}	r^2	sig.
Control	W.l = 13.93 − 0.379 wt + 0.00272 wt^2 − 0.0220 R	−1.8	0.80	NS
Low morantel	W.l = 4.05 − 0.125 wt + 0.00110 wt^2 − 0.0131 R	−1.6	0.82	*
High morantel	W.l = 7.71 − 0.233 wt + 0.00190 wt^2 − 0.0174 R	−2.0	0.88	**
Levamisole	W.l = 6.79 − 0.196 wt + 0.00155 wt^2 − 0.0141 R	−2.0	0.82	*
Conventional	W.l = 6.75 − 0.205 wt + 0.00170 wt^2 − 0.0116 R	−0.86	0.79	NS
Overall	W.l = 6.18 − 0.183 wt + 0.00150 wt^2 − 0.0145 R	−3.8	0.77	***

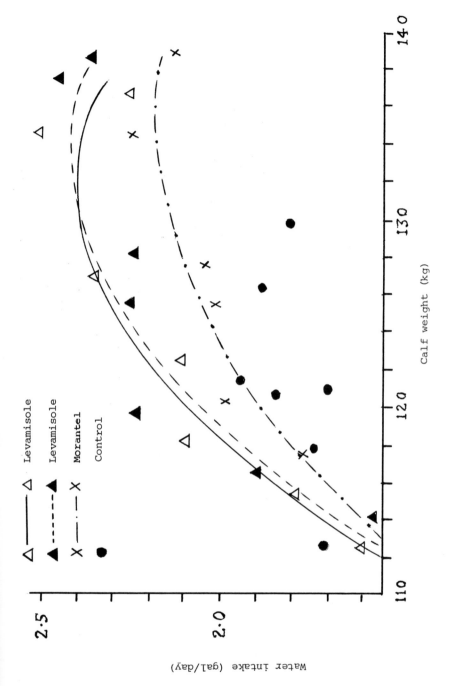

Fig 2.   Relationship between calf bodyweight and water intake under indoor feeding conditions.

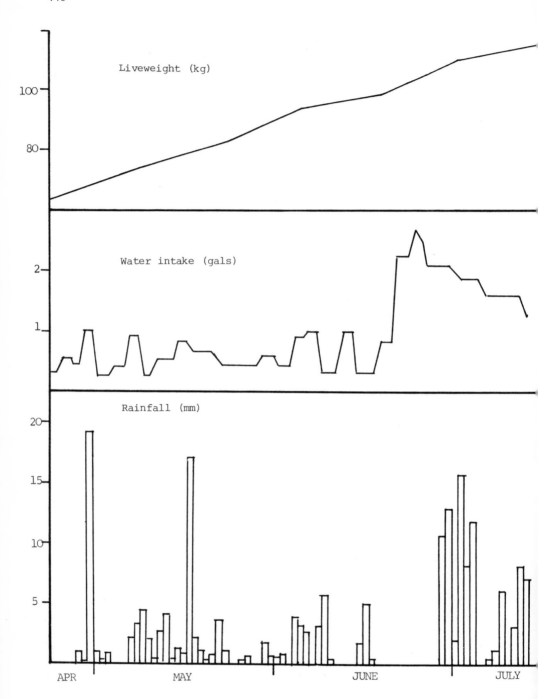

Fig 3. Calf liveweight, water intake and rainfall data for grazing experiment 1.

the relationship was not significant, tending to support the finding for indoor experiment 1 that water intake is severely depressed for animals bearing parasite burdens. The data suggests that the level of water intake may provide usefull supporting evidence on the severity of parasitic infection.

The overall results support the theory, mentioned earlier, that environmental weather conditions, by affecting the consumption of water, may lead to wide variations in amounts of anthelmintic acquired by an animal.

Individual calf water intake and palatability considerations.

The measurement of individual calf water intake in group grazing situations presents considerable difficulties (Wright et al. 1978). One approach is to observe visually the length of time each animal spends drinking. Such observations were carried out for the second indoor feeding trial. The results are shown in Table 2. These indicate that, even in conditions where medicated water was consumed within 50 minutes, with one possible exception, animals spent a reasonably constant period of time drinking. The variability encountered is probably unimportant if the prophylactic nature of this form of anthelmintic treatment is considered. Though individual water intake was not recorded, parasitological findings for individual animals indicate that calves were receiving reasonably uniform doses of anthelmintic.

In the series of grazing experiments (see Downey and O'Shea, 1980, these proceedings, Table 2, Experiment 2 - 4) in which anthelmintics were administered in the first 0.5 gallons of liquid consumed daily by calves, no evidence of unpalatability was found. Also group intake of anthelmintic was constantly at the dosage level intended.

Advantages of proposed system.

The main advantages of the proposed system are: the system is simple and does not need complicated calf pasture

TABLE 2

INDIVIDUAL CALF DRINKING BEHAVIOUR (INDOOR FEEDING EXPERIMENT 2).

Calf	Time spent drinking (seconds)					Total
	Day 1	Day 2	Day 3	Day 4	Day 5	
1	75	55	60	90	50	330
2	0	20	70	30	50	170
3	75	155	73	90	71	464
4	84	38	128	50	63	360
5	69	130	61	110	65	435
6	117	77	60	80	80	414
7	84	98	58	20	81	341
8	93	29	55	70	45	322
Mean time (minutes) taken by group to finish medicated water.	45	47	40	44	49	

management practices; a variety of anthelmintics may be used
including insoluble compounds, ensuring complete flexibility;
the automatic nature of the system is labour-saving and eliminates the upset to animals occasioned by conventional oral-
dosing; it may be used for other medication purposes in addition to anthelmintic administration.

REFERENCES

Downey, N.E., O'Shea, J. and Spillane, T.A., 1974. Preliminary observations
on the use of low-level medication in calves' drinking water as a
means of endoparasite control. Irish Veterinary Journal, 28,
221-222.

Downey, N.E. and O'Shea, J., 1977. Calf parasite control by means of
low-level anthelmintic administered via the drinking water.
Veterinary Record. 100, 265-266.

Wright, D.E., Towers, N.R., Hamilton, P.B. and Sinclair, D.P., 1978.
Intake of zinc sulphate in drinking water by grazing beef cattle.
N.Z. Journal of Agricultural Research. 21, 215-221.

GENERAL DISCUSSION

R.M. Jones *(UK)*

I would like to make a comment on the question of low level administration of anthelmintic and resistance. I think it is important that we differentiate between giving low level anthelmintics, which are larvacidal in their effect (killing larvae as they are ingested) and also adulticidal (killing adults in the intestine) from the system that Dr. Downey mentioned where an anthelmintic was used to control egg deposition. If one used an anthelmintic to control egg deposition then, obviously, this increases the chances of resistance to the drug developing since new generations of worms are produced in the presence of the anthelmintic. However, if you use low level anthelmintics in a parasiticidal manner you have the intent of killing the parasites just as effectively as you would with a single larger therapeutic dose.

N. Downey *(Ireland)*

Most of our dose levels would be helminthicidal. The one using phenothiazine, would certainly not be.

H. de Keyser *(Belgium)*

Has Dr. Downey experience with phenothiazine caused skin allergy in white animals, when long-term application is used?

N. Downey

No, we have no information on that. At low dosage levels it is unlikely this problem would arise.

J.-P. Raynaud *(France)*

Is it an advantage to use insoluble anthelmintics (the machine is more complicated) or could you limit yourself to soluble anthelmintics?

E.J.L. Soulsby

I did not necessarily mean a larvicidal effect but an effect against, the exsheathing mechanism; if the larvae does not exsheath it does not become parasitic. One might be able to inhibit exsheathment at substantially lower levels of drug than would be larvicidal. That would prevent completely the establishment of a parasite in the host.

R.M. Jones

In vitro one can go down to very low levels. One can get a paralysing effect at very low levels. An increase in concentration leads to a lethal effect.

E.J.L. Soulsby

That is with Morantel?

R.M. Jones

Yes.

J. Armour *(UK)*

I would like to ask either Dr. Downey or Dr. O'Shea, how do you insure adequate uptake of drug by each calf in the group. Have you done any estimations using labelled drug?

J. O'Shea *(Ireland)*

We believe that from the individual parasitic records that we can be reasonably sure that animals are receiving the correct dose. However, if we wanted to assess this, we could ensure each animal would go to his own trough and then we could measure intake.

J. Armour

How many troughs do you envisage having?

J. O'Shea

Only one, for the purposes of assessing individual variations.

J. Armour

Does stocking rate have any influence on the uptake? Some of my colleagues in the animal husbandry department have been looking at uptake of drug from feeding blocks. This seems to vary considerably in relation to the stocking rate. For example, in a small pen or paddock uptake is good, but once the grazing area is extended it does not work well at all.

J. O'Shea

The principle we used was that a calf would drink approximately half a gallon a day. We decided to put all the dose into that half gallon and give no further water until that half gallon had been consumed.

N. Downey

I would like to add to that comment. Drinking water is a different vehicle for drugs than the feed block. Cattle need to drink, and in our experiments, sometimes they have had to walk long distances to get to water.

F.H.M. Borgsteede *(The Netherlands)*

I have a question for Dr. Foldager. The system which is advocated in our country is the late turning out of calves after the first mowing of the pasture. Can you tell us the results of this late turning out?

J. Foldager *(Denmark)*

I can demonstrate that best with some results:

TABLE 1

DAILY GAINS IN EXPERIMENTS ON DATE OF TURN OUT IN CALVES AT PASTURE

Exp. No.	TRT		Gain in periods, g/day					
			Before date of paddock change (mid July)			After date of paddock change (mid July)		
			$-PC^A$	$+PC$	$+PGC^B$	$-PC$	$+PC$	$+PCG$
U10	N* (		759			162		
	< (		791	775	717	202	317	228
	L**		611	579		347	442	
U13	N		74	239		200	190	
	L		382	449		32	38	
U21	N		348	449		82	411	
	L		399	533		545	400	

A   Paddock change   * Normal date of turn out

B   Paddock change to grazed area   ** Late turn out

Two trials were conducted in dry years (U10 and U13) and one trial was conducted in a normal year (U21). The daily gains before the paddock change are much the same in all groups. However, in the second half of the season there is a tendency in normal years towards higher gains in those turned out late.

We get the same gain in the sub-groups turned out late, and either maintained or moved. The group which was turned out normally, in May, and then moved to a clean paddock in the middle of July, has the same weight gain as groups turned out late.

F.H.M. Borgsteede

What do you call late, under Danish circumstances?

J. Foldager

The middle of June.

P. Nansen *(Denmark)*

We have done some other experiments in support of this.
The effect of late turning out has been documented: a delay
of two weeks in turning out had an effect over the entire
season, both on the herbage contamination and on the performance
of the animal.

Our experiments indicate that late housing - especially
when the stocking rate is high and the grass production is
poor - may destroy all the efforts made during the season with
different management systems. In a few weeks one can eliminate
all effects of alternative grazing systems.

I would like to ask John Foldager a question that is
often put by Danish farmers. Is the effect you find after
moving animals to the aftermath in July - not just a question
of better grass, more succulent grass, being available? This
would explain the weight gains. But I think we may have some
figures on the grass production.

J. Foldager

Yes, we did mention grass production in one of the trials.
We had a first cutting and then moved calves onto the herbage
later. Here we had the lowest production according to all our
estimates.

D. Düwel *(FRG)*

I would like to go back to Professor Pouplard's
contribution concerning the treatment of lungworms. The data
did not correspond with Dr. Jørgensen's findings. Could I ask
Dr. Jørgensen for his comments on that?

R.J. Jørgensen *(Denmark)*

All I can do is to refer to my experimental results
which you can find under 'Prediction on outbreaks'.

L. Pouplard *(Belgium)*

Each year, in our country, the evolution of parasites is approximately the same. A good moment to treat is at 6 and 12 weeks.

R.J. Jørgensen

Perhaps I went through this experiment too quickly and maybe it should have been presented in the control section. However, it showed that at the time of an outbreak, the severity of the outbreak, was correlated with the time of turning out. These were the early turned out animals with the very high peak of larval output which occurred six weeks after they had been turning out. If you compare these with animals turned out six weeks afterwards you will see that with the first turned out animals it was in mid-June, and with the later turned out animals it was around the 1st July that there was a pathogenic peak in the pasture larvae.

J.-P. Raynaud *(France)*

In those countries where it is the practice to turn out late, do the farmers put animals out to graze the pasture early in the season or do they cut it only?

F.H.M. Borgsteede

They cut the pasture for silage.

J.-P. Raynaud

They never use the pasture for grazing animals?

F.H.M. Borgsteede

After the regrowth of the pasture they turn out the calves.

J.-P. Raynaud

It would have been possible to contaminate the young animals if they put adults or heifers out first.

N. Downey

We could limit ourselves to a soluble anthelmintic but
I think it is desirable to have this flexibility for insoluble
forms.

D. Barth *(FRG)*

Dr. Downey, what were the actual daily doses of the
various anthelmintics received by the animals?

N. Downey

With Morantel we reduced the dose to 1.7 mg/kg body
weight per day at one stage. With levamisole it is not quite
as good; we have to go to 3 mg/kg. With oxfendazole we have
used 1 mg. This is far higher than is needed and we are now
aiming at a 60% reduction on that dose at the moment and it
seems to be working. Diethylcarbamazine was used at 10 mg/kg.
Thiophenate did not seem to work all that well unless we went
to about 14%.

E.J.L. Soulsby *(UK)*

I would like to ask a question from the Chair. In
addition to all the effects which you have mentioned, I wonder
if low dosage has any effect on exsheathment and initial
migration of larvae?

R.M. Jones

We believe that the effect of Morantel, is against the
ingested third stage larvae. Doses as low as 0.25 mg/kg per
day, will effectively prevent the establishment of third stage
larvae; in fact it is larvicidal at that dose level. Slightly
high dose levels are also effective against established adult
infections over a period of time. Therefore, we are seeing
both effects - a larvicidal effect, preventing the third stage
larvae from actually invading the tissues, and also a
therapeutic effect against established infections.

F.H.M. Borgsteede

It is just done to avoid re-infection.

J. Armour

I would like to raise a point in relation to the treatment of bovine parasitic bronchitis. This relates to the reaction that occurs when animals, suffering from clinical parasitic bronchitis, are treated. Two very severe lesions occur following treatment, and which persist for some time after treatment. We have had clinical cases referred to us where animals were treated not only with fenbendazole, as was suggested in one publication, but also with levamisole - producing exactly the same lesions. These animals showed respiratory malfunction for some time after treatment.

E.J.L. Soulsby

I would like to bring the discussion back to the low level or continuous dosage schemes and the question of resistance of parasites to anthelmintic drugs. Despite the disclaimers made by the proponents of this method, resistance has not occurred in the past, but there is no guarantee that it will not occur in the future. Especially under a great degree of pressure, possibly continuous pressure, over several years. I wonder if anyone has any comments to make on this. It is known to occur with some anthelmintics of course, especially under continuous medication such as with phenothiazine. Do you wish to comment, Dr. Michel?

J.F. Michel (UK)

No, nothing further than the point which I have already made. If you recall I asked for comment from someone better educated than I.

J. Eckert (Switzerland)

If these long-acting devices come into use in Europe, we should be able to offer methods for monitoring the resistance

problem. I think this is a point which could be included in
future research. It would be necessary to improve the
application of methods for practical use, as the egg hatching
method is a rather complicated one which requires the isolation
of the pure strain.

E.J.L. Soulsby

It seems to me that almost all invertebrates, when they
are exposed to chemicals of some kind, eventually develop some
sort of resistance. It is well known in the field of arthropods
and insecticides.

R.M. Jones

I think you have to relate the risk of resistance
against the historical situation; in economic terms, resistance
has not yet become an economic problem. Resistance, as a
problem, is limited to a relatively small area in Australia.
Much of the resistance work, and most of the extrapolations
which are made from the data, are based on laboratory work.
The economic impact is very small in relation to the use of
anthelmintics in the production of livestock, but this does
not mean to say we should not be conscious of it and indeed,
as Professor Eckert said, there are methods for monitoring
resistance *in vitro*. We are concerned with this and do work
in this area in the laboratory. We are conscious of it, but
I do not think we should get the problem out of perspective
because, at the moment in an economic sense, it is not a serious
problem.

J. Euzeby *(France)*

I think we know very little about the development of
resistance to anthelmintics. Perhaps it is not the same
thing as the resistance of insects because, as you know, the
resistance of insects is not obvious because it exists prior
to treatment. When all susceptible strains have been wiped
out by insecticides, the ones which are resistant are revealed.
Therefore, where insects are concerned, resistance appears to

occur quicker when large doses - high doses - of insecticides are sprayed. There may be a comparison of course, but this has to be studied.

R.M. Jones

In terms of resistance to insects, we are talking about resistance factors which are huge, where you need to multiply the dose a hundred times to get the effect. There is no such problem here, at least for the present. When we have a situation which is described as resistance, the maximum increase in the effective dose required, in any of the literature, is about three times. If you relate that to insect situation it depends on your definition of resistance - increased tolerance. But high selection pressure is the way that insect resistance was developed.

SESSION 5

PROBLEMS ASSOCIATED WITH MODERN
ANIMAL HUSBANDRY PRACTICES
Chairman: H.J. Over

EPIDEMIOLOGY AND CONTROL OF GASTRO-INTESTINAL HELMINTHOSIS IN CATTLE INTENSIVE-BREEDING

J.A. Euzeby

Ecole Nationale Vétérinaire de Lyon,
Parasitologie et Maladies Parasitaires
Marcy l'Etoile, 69260, Charbonnières-les-Bains, France

ABSTRACT

The following report summarises the measures to be implemented to control helmintic infections in intensive cattle breeding units in order to reduce economic losses resulting from sub-clinical infections. The various systems of cattle-management are reviewed and various types of infections in these systems are considered. Control is then considered chiefly emphasising the measures to be taken in herds which alternate between housing and grazing periods. Finally, the necessity of integrated control is stressed and the economic benefits from implementing control are discussed.

P. Nansen, R.J. Jørgensen, E.J.L. Soulsby (eds), Epidemiology and Control of Nematodiasis in Cattle.
Copyright © 1981 ECSC, EEC, EAEC, Brussels – Luxembourg. All rights reserved.

THE ANIMALS AND THEIR PARASITES

The animals dealt with in the present report are:
1) <u>reproductive cattle and dairy-cows which alternate between housing and grazing periods</u> for several years until they are slaughtered after fattening (these animals are liable to infection by strongyles), 2) <u>dairy-cows in large specialised industrial dairy farms</u>, permanently housed (these cows, which are fed on concentrate and dry hay, do not risk any helmintic infection) and, 3) <u>cattle for fattening</u>.

All cows under study are reared from calves which are liable to acquire helminths directly from the cow. Thus *Toxocara vitulorum* and *Strongyloides papillosus* may either be transmitted before calving via placenta or more likely via colostrum from the first suckling and over the following 10 - 15 days. Once infected the cow may transmit *T. vitulorum* to its offspring at successive calvings without being re-exposed to infection. On the other hand, young calves can also acquire *S. papillosus* infection perorally or percutaneously.

Cattle for fattening may be bred in three major systems of husbandry.

The first is the penned veal-calf system which involves rearing in two ways:

Early-weaned calves are removed from their mothers at 5 - 6 days of age and kept isolated in small, grate-floored pens. They are fed on milk-substitutes from self-feeders, or,

Suckled-calves are penned with their mothers in straw-littered pens and supplied extra food.

Calves in both systems are slaughtered when 3 - 4 months old, weighing 150 - 180 kg (liveweight). Except for toxocariasis and strongyloidosis that they may have acquired from their mothers they do not risk many other helmintic infections. However, calves belonging to the suckle-reared group may be exposed to *S. papillosus* during their short life. In cases where the cows are infected with *Trichuris discolor* or *Bunostomum phlebotomum* the suckled calves may acquire these parasites as well.

The second system to be considered is that of young stock kept in feedlots for fattening until slaughtering when weighing 550 - 650 kg (liveweight) and at about 15 - 18 months of age(*). These animals may be dairy breeds or beef breeds. In both cases, calving takes place in winter-time. When the calves of dairy breeds are kept in nurseries up to an age of 3 months and after weaning and transfer to feedlots, these animals are not exposed to strongyles. Calves from beef breeds are kept on pastures and moved into feedlots when they are 7 - 8 months of age. During this time they become infected with strongyles (and tapeworms). In feedlots animals are usually kept on hard soil or on concrete covered with loose straw or accumulated bedding. They are no longer liable to infection with *T. vitulorum* or *S. papillosus*, having reached an age when they are no longer susceptible. Nevertheless they may harbour various species of helminths, especially *Trichuris discolor* and *Bunostomum phlebotomum*, which can readily develop in the microclimate of the soil and litter of the feedlot. Strongyles may be introduced into feedlots by animals removed from pasture and the strongyle eggs passed by these animals can develop in the humid straw-litter into L_3 in 8 - 10 days. Usually, cattle in feedlots do not become severely infected if the farm is well kept. However, calves of beef breeds which have experienced a few preceding months on pastures (e.g. in late autumn/early winter) may harbour hypobiotic L_4 of *Ostertagia ostertagi* and this may lead to clinical disease in late winter or early spring in the feedlot.

The third system of husbandry for cattle for fattening is the conventional grazing-cattle, kept as store bullocks and alternating between pasture and cattle housing over three grazing seasons and eventually being slaughtered when they are three years

---

* Instead of being kept in feedlots, young calves may be kept outdoors on pastures. In this type of management, which requires dehorning, strong fencing, epidymectomy, helminth infection may occur.

This may become a common practice in the future due to the high cost of farm buildings and concentrate. In Western Europe climatic features allow production of low-cost pasture ('green petrol!')

old and weighing 600 kg. These cattle belong either to beef
breeds or to dairy breeds and they may be divided into three
age-groups, namely, young animals up to 12 months old; animals
from 13 to 24 months of age, and oxen from 24 to 36 months of
age. All age groups are exposed to strongyles and, besides, the
first age group of calves may also be infected by tapeworms
(Moniezia spp), which, however, are not very harmful and thus not
mentioned further in this report.

As far as strongylosis is concerned calves reared for beef
from dairy breeds are often heavily infected because they may be
kept for several months after calving in small paddocks close
to the farms so as to be near their mothers and cared for by the
farmer; overcrowding in such paddocks favours larval uptake leading to heavy burdens of strongyles.

Whatever the type of breeding, calves are kept and moved
after very well defined periods. Thus, dairy breed animals, at
8 days of age, after completing absorption of colostrum, are trans
ferred to pens or nurseries and then on to feedlots. Or when they
are 3 - 4 months old (weaned lean-calves market animals) they are
then moved out to feedlots. The meat type breed calves may be
slaughtered at 7 to 8 months or retained with fattening on pasture
until they are between 18 and 30 months of age. The stay in
allotment centres is very short and does not allow cattle to be
infected by helminths although this period of stay in such centres
may give rise to infections by fungi (ring-worm) and mange or
lice.

On the individual farms, irrespective of type of breeding
practised, helmintic infections are transmitted in two ways:
vertically due to endemicity within the farm, and horizontally due
to transmission from contaminated to non-contaminated farms. The
control of vertical infection requires systematic regular treatments of animals and disinfection of the environment. The control
of horizontal infection can be accomplished by preventing infected
animals from entering non-contaminated farms, i.e. by quarantine
detection of infected animals and treatment of these animals.

One should, of course, always be on the lookout for sub-clinical infections.

CONTROL

Control measures must focus on: infected animals and the elimination of their helminths and the protection of the healthy ones and the environment. The environment should be decontaminated and used strategically so as to lower the risk of infection.

The control of prenatal and neonatal infections requires treatment of pregnant cows at about 4 - 5 weeks before and for 10 days after calving in order to control *T. vitulorum*. Treatment, a few days, say five or six, before calving and for ten consecutive days after calving will control *S. papillosus*. However, this kind of treatment is not easy to administer, indeed, as far as *T. vitulorum* is concerned in pregnant cows, it would necessitate the use of fenbendazole and administering it at 15 mg/kg bodyweight for 15 days. In the case of *S. papillosus*, the same drug or thiabendazole (100 mg/kg) can be used over 15 consecutive days. Control also requires the treatment of newborn calves from two days after birth and for ten consecutive days thereafter in order to control *T. vitulorum* and *S. papillosus*. In the case of ascaridosis, other treatments may be given at 3 weeks of age including fenbendazole (7.5 mg/kg), levamisole (5 mg/kg), thiabendazole (100 mg/kg) or morantel tartrate (5 mg/kg).

Cleaning and disinfection of contaminated premises, removal of old bedding and careful 'stream-washing' should be performed twice a week.

The control of helmintic infections in penned veal calves, kept by themselves in individual, grate-floored pens presents no infection problem provided the grate-floor is washed every day. On the other hand, before entering their pens the calves should be given the treatment mentioned above. With suckled calves, penned with their mothers, control requires the same methods as those already quoted for control of neonatal infections.

The control of helmintic infection in feedlots concerns the control of horizontal and vertical infection. In the former, before entering feedlots, all animals, whether they come from nurseries or from pasture, should be dewormed so as to prevent horizontal infection. Deworming should be carried out at least five days before entering the feedlot in order to ensure that all eggs are expelled before introduction into the lot. Moreover, young animals, having experienced an earlier grazing period in autumn, should be treated in early winter in order to prevent outbreaks of Type II ostertagiosis.

Control of vertical infection may be implemented by thorough removal of manure and bedding once a week. At the end of a feed-lot process, thorough cleaning, including 'stream-washing' with 2% sodium hydroxide is recommended.

The control of helmintic infections in conventionally grazing cattle, is obviously the most difficult to deal with. It requires means aimed at both animals and grassland.

The animals involved include reservoir animals; these are those which have experienced one or several grazing seasons which have allowed them to become infected. The most important animals are those belonging to the 12 - 18 months old group, after having experienced one grazing season during which time they were able to spread many eggs onto the pasture. Older animals acquire immunity and although they do ingest infective L_3, they do not pass as many eggs as animals of the 12 - 18 months group do and thus they may be considered as 'pasture-cleaners' rather than 'pasture-spoilers'.

Receptive animals are young calves, born in winter or early spring, and turned out to graze either immediately after weaning or even before completed weaning. They are fully susceptible to strongyle infection and their main source of infection is, as previously mentioned, the 12 - 18 month old group of animals.

With regard to grassland control, pastures become

contaminated when grazed by infected animals or when fertilised
with contaminated slurry.

The L_3 contamination of grassland is not of an even all-
year-round pattern but follows a pattern intimately linked to
climatic features in a given area and to intrinsic resistance
of the infective larvae themselves. The larvae not only survive
on grass or soil, but may also occur in the soil, even when
buried down to a depth of 10cm. In western-Europe, L_3 can overwinter so that pastures are contaminated from the very beginning
of the succeeding grazing season. However, as soon as the temperatures rise to $10^{\circ}C$ and higher, the over-wintered larvae regain
their activity. They soon deplete their energy reserves and die
about late March or early April. Clearly, pastures will become
contaminated again by eggs passed out by the infected stock, the
12 - 15 months old group being the main contributors. These eggs
accumulate on grass and soil and the rising temperature in spring
and early summer gradually accelerate hatching and development
into L_3 (minimum $10^{\circ}C$: optimum $22 - 25^{\circ}C$). This factor explains
why the numbers of L_3 on grass rises dramatically around late-
June and mid-July. This is, in fact, the period when young
cattle are most liable to infection by strongyles while they are
experiencing grazing for the first time. Strongyles at this
period may be of a 'fulminating type'. Subsequently, a certain
number of L_3 die from dryness and heat and the risk of infection
dwindles during the summer. Later, commencing around late-summer/
early autumn, as soon as rainfall occurs, another peak of L_3
occurs as well and this leads to another infection spell. Of
course, this general pattern may vary from country to country.

Based on these data the following control methods in grazing
herds are possible:

Offensive means of control involving animals

Among reservoir animals, for example, the group of 12 - 18
months old animals should be dewormed before being moved on pasture and an anthelmintic treatment has usually already been given
soon after their first grazing season, that is to say at a time

when the animals are 9 - 10 months cld and had been housed for
3 - 4 weeks. This will prevent subsequent Type II ostertagiasis
outbreaks. It might perhaps not seem necessary to treat again
at the end of the housing period before turning the animals out
in the spring, however, this second treatment is very useful because it is supplementary to the first treatment in reducing
pasture contamination in the early grazing season. Though modern
anthelmintics belonging to the benzimidazol compounds can have
ovicidal and larvicidal effects, it is recommended to treat cattle
while still housed so that the strongyle eggs are expelled in
cow-sheds and not on the pasture.

Though deworming is less necessary in the 24 - 30 months
old group, it is advisable to treat these animals in the same
manner as above. In any case, mother-cows which graze with new
born calves must be treated.

Control against infection in young calves that are experiencing their first grazing season is important. Such animals
are highly susceptible and liable to infection from the beginning
of the grazing season and throughout the whole grazing period.
Anthelmintic treatment of these animals can be carried out in
two ways: firstly, by discontinuous full-dose treatment 3 and 6
weeks after calves have been turned out to grze so as to rid them
of worms which have developed from over-wintering larvae. The
anthelmintics used should also inhibit the development of eggs
into L_3. Treatment in late June/early July at the time when the
first peak of L_3 occurs on grass (the optimal time will depend on
the climatic conditions of a given area) is advised and also at
the time of the autumn peak. Secondly, continuous low-level
treatment with anthelmintic drugs; though unable to kill the worm
it prevents egg laying. Thiodiphenylamine was the first anthelmintic used in this way and is still useful in sheep management,
however, more suitable anthelmintics are available for cattle such
as morantel tartrate (at 1.5 mg/kg) from two weeks before the star
of the grazing season until early or mid-July. This drug is now
being tested in the form of 'eight-week boluses' that are inserted
into the rumen where the active substance is continuously released

over 8 weeks. Levamisole, fenbendazole and oxfendazole are under study for the same purpose. If such procedures are effective they will perhaps reduce the necessity of moving herds to 'new' pastures in July.

Management to prevent contamination of pastures can be achieved by applying the medication regimens referred to above. Additionally, pasture-manuring using slurry from infected animals should be avoided unless this slurry has been decontaminated by biological means.

There are various methods of 'cleaning' contaminated grasslands. The effectiveness of chemical compounds is under debate. For example, calcium-cyanamide is quite effective against L_3 and it provides the pasture with Ca and N. However, it is also rather expensive and it makes grass grow too quickly. If used it should be spread in late winter/early spring to kill overwintering L_3 and before young receptive cattle are turned out to graze or at the time of the early summer L_3 rise, or at the end of the grazing season to prevent L_3 from overwintering. For biological control, the role of coprophilic beetles as 'cleaning' agents has been emphasised. However, in view of the ability of L_3 to penetrate deep into the soil, the role of these insects becomes doubtful. Further studies are necessary in this area.

Farm management practices are also important. For example, pasture may be improved by ploughing deep enough to prevent L_3 from migrating to the surface again. However, ploughing implies that pastures may not be available for grazing for two years and this is possible only on large farms. When used, it has other purposes than helminth control. Cutting grass should remove any L_3, which would die either in dry hay or in silage. The remaining larvae on the pasture will be exposed to sun and dryness. Cutting might take place in early spring to remove over-wintering L_3. Unfortunately only large farms can afford this practice. However, cutting should be carried out at the end of the grazing season on the grass tufts surrounding faecal pats. These grass tufts, which are a result of the selective grazing behaviour of the animals, are usually heavily contaminated with L_3.

Herd management is important. Pasture resting, if put into practice, should have a duration such as to exceed the longevity of L_3. Therefore its application depends upon the climate in a given area. It also depends upon the resistance of various species of L_3, which in summer is about 6 weeks for *Haemonchus* and *Trichostrongylus* spp. and up to 12 weeks or more for *Ostertagia* and *Nematodirus*. Therefore, the practice of returning calves in late summer to plots they had been removed from in early July is not always good and will definitely not work with *Ostertagia*. This practice may also lead to a high risk of a Type II infection. If associated with the application of calcium cyanamide the effectiveness of pasture-resting would be enhanced.

Alternate-grazing by cattle and sheep and, if possible, horses is an effective method of pasture management and depends on the fact that there is no transmission from cattle to sheep and vice versa for *Ostertagia, Nematodirus, Bunostomum* and only very few possibilities of cross-transmission for *Cooperia* and for *Trichostrongylus* spp. of the small intestine. On the contrary, the abomasal worms *Trichostrongylus axei* and *Haemonchus* spp. can be crosstransmitted between cattle and sheep. Nevertheless, wherever possible, alternate grazing between these animals is quite valuable because the non receptive animals remove a lot of L_3 without passing many eggs. However, alternate grazing usually is possible only in large farms because a suitable number of both sheep and cattle must be available. The optimal rate is about 35 cattle for 200 ewes at lambing.

Alternate grazing by young (receptive) and older (non receptive) cattle is a further approach in herd management. Animals more than 24 months of age usually have low faecal egg counts although they may ingest many L_3. They may therefore 'clean' the pastures. In the case of *O. ostertagi* infections, old cattle, alternating with young stock, may risk heavy infection, but this has not been reported and it should not prevent the use of the above principle. Alternate grazing with young and old stock might take place in early July; young

receptive calves being transferred to pastures until then
grazed by old cattle. It is not advisable to allow young
calves experiencing their first grazing season to graze after
animals of the 12 - 18 months old group. Mixed grazing might
be put into practice according to the same principles. For
practical reasons this method may be more acceptable to the
farmer.

Defensive measures designed to prevent the marked
uptake of L_3 by receptive calves, include the following: by
delaying the time of turning out, animals are not introduced
into the paddock before a high proportion of the overwintered
larvae has died out (i.e. about late March - April according
to the climate of a given area). In this way, calves may
only get slight, harmless (and possibly immunising) infection.

Mixed grazing with second-grazing season cattle (12 -
18 months old animals, see above) and even with mother-cows
should be avoided, at least from the time of the year when
climatic conditions allow a rapid L_3 development (i.e. early
July, and then later on, when the second peak of L_3 occurs,
i.e. late summer and autumn). The moving of young receptive
calves from contaminated pastures in early July to new or
less contaminated pastures will prevent 'fulminating infection'
of these calves. Rotational grazing, which is often difficult
to implement consists of grazing by calves ahead of the 12 -
18 months old group of cattle (leader-follower system) is
a useful defensive control measure.

An important aspect in control is the strengthening of
resistance of highly receptive animals. This may be achieved
by regular anthelmintic treatments given according to the
principles already mentioned and which will support resistance
in exposed animals. However, in some areas, animals grazing
for their second or even third season may be severely affected
by larval oesophagostomiosis. Such animals should be given
anthelmintic treatment at housing, or if housing is delayed,
first at the pasture and again at the time of housing.

Supplementary feeding will assist resistance if grass is sparse and of low quality. A supplementation with concentrate similarly will help animals to overcome helmintic infections. The artificial immunisation of young receptive cattle is not possible, so far, but development of immunity may be initiated by light infections acquired from pasture in spring. A possible influence of repeated anthelmintic treatments on the immunising process has not been clearly documented and it should not preclude the use of anthelmintics if and when necessary.

The selection of resistant strains of animals is a method of control under study in sheep but no precise information has so far been established on it in cattle.

OBSERVATIONS

Control must be determined according to the type of animals, the type of management and the epidemiology of infections. As far as epidemiology is concerned, this varies according to local climatic conditions. No control can be planned without perfect knowledge of epidemiological patterns. On grasslands, these patterns can be analysed first of all by detecting grass contamination and by the use of tracer animals.

Integrated control combines all defensive and offensive measures.

It is necessary to assess the economic benefits of control. One must be aware of the fact that besides clinical disease, sub-clinical infections often have important consequences for animal performance in that retarded growth may markedly reduce the farmer's profit. On the other hand, farmers have to balance cost of control with benefits provided through this control. Indices of economic profit, such as mean liveweight, may be misleading. The real index of economic benefit is based on an estimate of the net return from various antiparasitic schemes in comparison with that of a control group. The most profitable system is usually the one that would give an intermediate level of parasite control, while a scheme aimed at achieving the best control (at high cost) would be acceptable only when beef price is high.

DISCUSSION

J. Armour *(UK)*

I would like to congratulate Professor Euzeby on this unique presentation, which I enjoyed very much. I have one short question. If we buy in Charolais heifers from France, what advice do we give the farmers on how to treat them to prevent toxocariasis?

J. Euzeby *(France)*

This is the trouble. We have to treat them about six weeks before calving.

J. Armour

With what?

J. Euzeby

With a drug which can act upon larvae which are still encysted in the tissues. I take this from my experience with dogs and I am not sure whether the same effect would occur in heifers. I do not think there is any major risk. Perhaps Dr. Düwel can comment. Fenbendazole is active on encysted larvae in dogs, and perhaps it would be of use in cows?

D. Düwel *(FRG)*

That is right, but it needs treatment extending over 14 days.

J. Euzeby

Fourteen days in dogs, and four to six weeks in cows.
If the action is the same in cattle we have a good opportunity
to kill encysted larvae and migrating larvae during their
passage from the site of encystment to the mammary gland.

R.J. Jørgensen *(Denmark)*

I noticed that you distinguished between infected farms
and sound farms. This is the set-up which we are adopting
with infectious diseases. For instance, in our industrialised
pig production we have SPF farms. This approach is in contrast
to the management of parasitic diseases.

J. Euzeby

I should not have said 'sound' farms because there are
actually no real sound farms; I should have said 'less infected'.
If one is careful when moving animals from a well-known
infected farm to a 'sound farm, and if careful treatment for
sub-clinical infection is done before putting them onto the
sound farm, there is an opportunity to avoid a big infection
in the so-called 'sound' farm. Are you happy about that? You
don't look too happy!

THE IMPORTANCE OF STOCKING RATE TO THE UPTAKE
OF GASTROINTESTINAL NEMATODES BY GRAZING CALVES

[1]J.W. Hansen, [1]P. Nansen and [2]J. Foldager

[1]Institute of Veterinary Microbiology and Hygiene,
Royal Veterinary and Agricultural University,
13 Bülowsvej, DK-1870 Copenhagen V, Denmark.

[2]National Institute of Animal Science,
25 Rolighedsvej, DK-1958 Copenhagen V, Denmark.

ABSTRACT

The effect of three different stocking rates and two grazing methods (3 x 2 factorial experiment) on grass production, grass availability, grazing behaviour, herbage intake, larval infection and weight gain was studied in 36 female calves of the Red Danish Milk breed. The age and the weight at the start of the trial were 6.2 months and 170 kg, respectively.

Six paddocks, two by two of equal size (1.10, 0.70, and 0.57 ha) were established during spring on an old pasture grazed by yearling heifers the previous year. One paddock of each size was grazed by 12 calves from mid-May to mid-July. The other three paddocks were harvested. In mid-July 6 calves from each paddock were moved to the comparable harvested paddock, and the other 6 calves remained in the original paddock.

At increasing stocking rate the growth rate decreased. There was no significant difference in grass production potential, but the herbage availability was decreasing at increasing stocking rate, and simultaneously the grass intake decreased, despite an increased parasitic load as indicated by increasing serum pepsinogen at increasing stocking rate. This was correlated with scarcity of grass, forcing the animals to graze closer to the faecal pats (at high stocking rates).

These effects at increasing stocking rate were less pronounced in all three groups moved from the original to a harvested area in mid-July.

P. Nansen, R.J. Jørgensen, E.J.L. Soulsby (eds), Epidemiology and Control of Nematodiasis in Cattle.
Copyright © 1981 ECSC, EEC, EAEC, Brussels – Luxembourg. All rights reserved.

INTRODUCTION

Performance by animals on pasture depends on grass quantity and quality and the efficiency of utilisation of grass consumed. Parasitism and other disease problems may interfere with this.

A large number of experiments have been conducted in order to obtain maximum production from grassland. In 1956, McMeekan claimed that stocking rate rather than the grazing system held the key to grassland productivity, and a large number of experiments have since then indicated that under most practical conditions McMeekan was right. Thus Mott (1960), McMeekan and Walshe (1963), Holmes et al. (1966), Yiakomettis and Holmes (1972), Sørensen and Lykkeaa (1974) and others investigated and discussed the production per animal and the production per hectare seen in relation to stocking rate. However, in most experiments, mainly grass production and weight gain parameters were considered, while possible interfering mechanisms such as parasitism were apparently overlooked. This is surprising since grassland utilisation is inevitably linked with a potential risk of parasitism and it has been clearly documented that live weight gain may be strongly affected by internal parasites when animals are grazing at high stocking rates (Campbell and Field, 1960; Michel 1968; Sejrsen et al., 1975).

The interrelationship between parasitism and stocking rate may be explained as follows: when the stocking rate is increased, the grazing behaviour of cattle may be affected. The quantity of grass per animal is reduced, and the normal selective grazing cannot be maintained, e.g. the animals are forced to eat the grass tufts surrounding the faecal pats. This may lead to increased uptake of parasites, since the concentration of trichostrongylid larvae, for example, is usually considerably higher in the vicinity of the faecal pat.

The purpose of the present experiment was to analyse in detail the influence of stocking rate on trichostrongyle

infection, grazing behaviour, weight gain etc., of yearling
calves under Danish conditions.

MATERIALS AND METHODS

Experimental design

The effect of stocking rate and grazing method on trichostrongyle infection was studied in a 2 x 3 factorial experiment.
A permanent pasture, grazed by yearling calves the previous
year, was divided into six paddocks, two by two of 1.10, 0.70
and 0.57 ha, respectively.

All paddocks received the same amount of chemical fert-
iliser/ha prior to the grazing season. Paddocks 2A, 2B, and
2C were fertilised again after the cut for silage.

The paddocks were grazed according to the schedule in
Table 1. Three paddocks of different sizes were grazed from
mid-May to mid-July and the other three paddocks were harvested.
All paddocks were grazed from mid-July onwards. By this
procedure, the stocking rates were tested during continuous
grazing throughout the summer and paddock change in mid-July,
and simultaneously the stocking rates were reduced by 50%.
Under Danish conditions 2/3 of the grass production takes
place in the first half of the grazing season. Furthermore,
the herbage contamination with trichostrongyle larvae starts
to rise in late July.

Animals

Six groups of 6 female calves of the Red Danish Milk
breed were formed on the basis of age, weight and sires.
Calves within groups were randomly assigned to treatment combinations. The average age and weight of the calves at the
start of the experiment were 6.2 months and 170 kg, respectively.

TABLE 1

TREATMENT COMBINATIONS. USE OF PADDOCKS DURING THE GRAZING SEASON.

11th May – 15th May				
Paddock	Stocking rate	Grazing method	No. of animals	No. of animals/ha
1A	Low	moved and non-moved	12	12
1B	Medium	moved and non-moved	12	17
1C	High	moved and non-moved	12	21
2A		Cut for silage		
2B		Cut for silage		
2C		Cut for silage		

15th July – 15th September				
Stocking rate	Grazed by group	No. of animals	No. of animals/ha	Grazing method
Low	1A	6	6	non-moved
Medium	1B	6	8.5	non-moved
High	1C	6	10.5	non-moved
Low	2A	6	6	moved
Medium	2B	6	8.5	moved
High	2C	6	10.5	moved

Measurements: Grass

Grass production: the grass production potential was measured weekly. In each of the six paddocks a representative area was fenced off, and the grass was cut on a 20 m^2 area with a lawn mower. The production potential was calculated as tons of green herbage/ha/week.

Grass availability: herbage on offer was measured and calculated from 20 random recordings every week in each paddock with an electronic capacitance meter.

Grass tufts: the average size of the grass tufts surrounding the faecal pats was determined every week. Within each of the six paddocks, 3 circular areas with a radius of 5 m were selected. The area of all faecal pats and surrounding grass tufts in the test areas was recorded and then averaged.

Grass contamination with trichostrongylid larvae: every fortnight the larval herbage contamination was determined in each paddock 1) by analysing grass samples collected randomly following a w-shaped pattern, and 2) by analysing grass from the grass tufts surrounding faecal pats. Grass cut within 15 cm from the edge of the pats was designated Sample I, and grass from 15 cm to the outer rim of the tuft was designated Sample II.

Trichostrongylid larvae were isolated and quantitated according to Jørgensen (1975).

At the same intervals grass samples were randomly collected in each paddock and analysed for dry matter, crude protein, crude fibre and *in vitro* digestibility.

Meteorological observations

Precipitation as well as daily maximum and minimum temperatures were recorded at a meteorological unit situated nearby.

Animals

The animals were weighed at three-week intervals throughout the season. On the same occasions faecal samples and blood samples were taken.

Parasitological analyses on animals

Faecal egg counts were made according to a modified McMaster technique. Serum pepsinogen was determined using the method described by Ross et al. (1967).

Grazing behaviour

On three occasions, 27th - 28th June, 25th - 26th July, and 22nd - 23rd August, the behavioural activity (resting, eating, walking, etc.) of the animals in paddocks 1A, 2A, 1C and 2C was recorded every 5 minutes during a 24 h period.

Herbage intake

The herbage intake by the grazing animals was calculated from the chromiumoxide content in faeces. The determinations took place from the 1st - 15th September. Each calf received a chromiumoxide capsule per os at 9.00 am daily, and 24 h later faecal samples were collected.

RESULTS

Weight gain figures

The growth rate curves for the respective groups of calves are shown in Figure 1. Up to mid-summer the animals had comparable growth rates. However, from July and onwards the growth was affected both by stocking rate (P < 0.001) and grazing method (P < 0.001). The well known beneficial effect of moving animals to aftermath in mid-July was clearly demonstrated at all stocking rates, but the effect was larger at high than at low stocking rates (P < 0.01).

Average weight gain per animal and per ha are listed in Table 2.

Grass production potential, availability, grass tuft size and quality

The grass production potential calculated from the

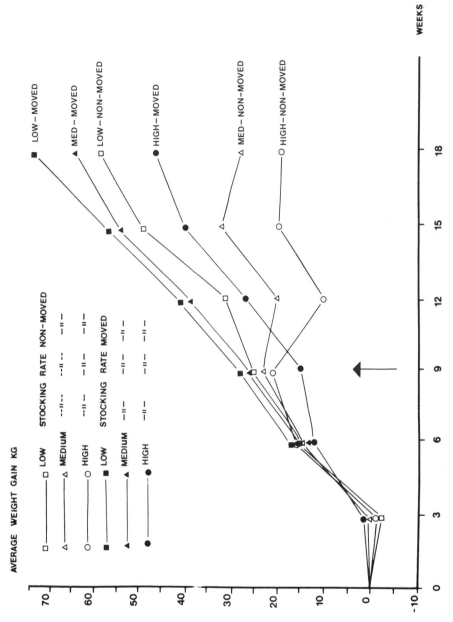

Fig. 1   Weight gain curves of the various groups of calves.

478

TABLE 2

EFFECT OF STOCKING RATE ON LIVE WEIGHT GAIN PER ANIMAL AND PER HA

	Stocking rate (cattle/ha) moved			Stocking rate (cattle/ha) non-moved		
	6	8.5	10.5	6	8.5	10.5
Live weight gain (kg)						
Per animal	72	63	46	58	28	19
relative	100	88	64	81	39	26
Per ha	394.2	541.5	494.6	371.5	240.7	204.3
relative	100	137	125	81	61	52

harvested amount of grass in the 20 m^2 plots was comparable in all six paddocks.

Grass availability, estimated with the electronic capaci-tance meter, exhibited a general seasonal trend. The amount of grass decreased from the time of turning out until July. In July there was a temporary increase which coincided with halving of stocking rates and high rainfall (see later). From mid-July to mid-September there was a linear decline in grass availability. Throughout the season there was a very clear influence of stocking rate. At the end of the season the foll-owing differences were observed. The herbage on offer per ha at low stocking rates was 2 - 3 t more than at medium stocking rates, which in turn had ½ - 1 t more per ha than at high stock-ing rates. On paddocks grazed throughout the season, grass availability was somewhat higher than in corresponding paddocks grazed only after mid-July.

Grass tuft sizes are shown in Table 3. It will be seen that the average size of grass tufts was not influenced by stocking rate in early summer. However, from July onwards marked differences were observed between low and high stocking rate paddocks. At the end of the season the average size of grass tufts in paddocks with high stocking rates was less than one half the size of tufts in paddocks with low stocking rates. These differences were observed in paddocks of both grazing methods.

Grass analysis: differences between the six paddocks in crude protein, crude fibre and *in vitro* digestibility were not significant.

Grazing behaviour and grass intake

The time spent grazing in three 24 h periods is presented in Table 4. In June and August the animals at high stocking rates spent considerably more time grazing than did animals at low stocking rates. However, in July the grazing times were

TABLE 3
AVERAGE SIZE IN M^2 OF GRASSTUFTS SURROUNDING FAECAL PATS.

		Stocking rate	8/6	22/6	6/7	20/7	4/8	17/8	2/9	15/9
						Dates of recordings				
Non-moved		Low	0.182	0.199	0.201	0.292	0.401	0.369	0.281	0.319
		Medium	0.162	0.235	0.228	0.204	0.187	0.220	0.193	0.235
		High	0.184	0.190	0.142	0.142	0.171	0.173	0.205	0.143
Moved		Low	-	-	-	-	-	0.553	0.292	0.434
		Medium	-	-	-	-	0.237	0.315	0.250	0.270
		High	-	-	-	-	0.290	0.265	0.182	0.150

TABLE 4

TOTAL GRAZING TIME DURING THREE 24-HOUR OBSERVATIONS OF GRAZING BEHAVIOUR

Stocking rate	Grazing time in minutes			
	Low non-moved	High	Low moved	High
Dates of registrations				
27 - 28/6	417	502	-	-
25 - 26/7	453	453	453	485
22 - 23/8	404	501	436	537

comparable. This latter observation took place shortly after mid-July when stocking rates in all paddocks were halved by 50%.

Herbage intake was determined in all animals and the results are presented in Table 5. The organic matter intake per animal and per 100 kg body weight was clearly influenced both by the stocking rate (P < 0.001) and by the grazing method (P < 0.001). The interaction was not significant. This is noteworthy in view of the slightly higher grass-availability in the permanently grazed paddocks. These features could evidently be related to differences in parasitic loads as indicated by differences in the serum pepsinogen levels.

Meteorological observations

The rainfall was well scattered throughout the season with July being above average.

Parasitological findings

Herbage contamination: the pasture larval contamination of the paddocks grazed throughout the season is shown in Figure 2. With the exception of paddock 1C there was a normal midsummer rise in herbage contamination. Most of the grazing season larval counts were roughly comparable, but in September larval counts were lowest at low stocking rate. The finding that

TABLE 5

HERBAGE INTAKE OF THE SIX GROUPS OF CALVES CALCULATED FROM THE *in vitro* DIGESTIBILITY AND THE CHROMIUMOXIDE INDICATOR IN FAECES (AFTER HØJLAND FREDERIKSEN ET AL., 1979).

Average values	Non-moved			Moved		
Stocking rate	Low	Medium	High	Low	Medium	High
Bodyweight 24/8 kg	218	2O2	189	227	224	21O
Faecal organic matter g/day	1.181	835	749	1.324	1.27O	1.142
O.M. intake/ animal/day kg	3.65	2.58	2.32	4.1O	3.94	3.54
O.M. intake/1OO kg bodyweight kg	1.67	1.28	1.23	1.80	1.76	1.69
Serum pepsinogen 24/8 units tyrosine/l	2.73	3.95	3.63	1.30	1.81	2.1O
Crude protein of O.M. in faeces %	26.2	31.5	3O.6	24.1	22.O	22.9

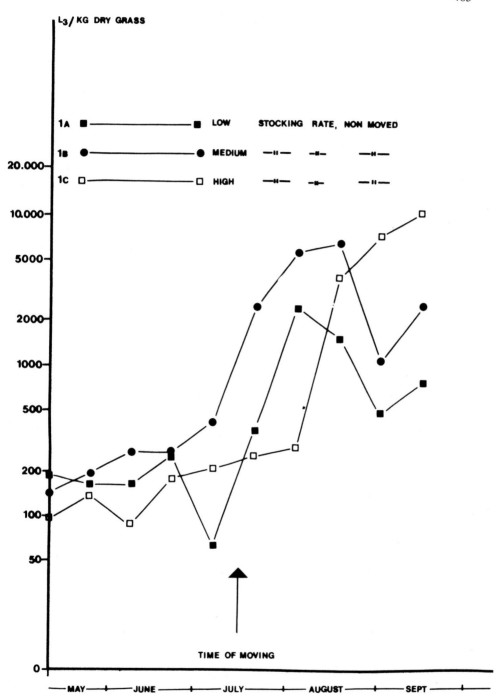

Fig. 2   Pasture contamination. Numbers of infective larvae (L_3) per kg dry herbage. Samples collected randomly in the paddocks grazed the entire season.

pasture larval counts were unexpectedly high in the paddocks grazed only after mid-July (Figure 3) may be related to the lower grass availability in these paddocks than in the permanently grazed paddocks.

The larval concentration on grass sampled close to the faecal pats was considerably higher than on grass sampled at random.

Figures 4 and 5 show larval counts from permanently grazed paddocks with low (1A) and high (1C) stocking rates, respectively. It will be seen that larval counts, particularly in Sample I, rose earlier and reached higher levels than larval counts in random samples.

While the number of L_3 larvae close to the pats is similar at the low and high stocking rates, marked differences can be seen in the random samples at the two stocking rates. The number of L_3 larvae on the 1C paddock is approximately 5 times higher than in the 1A paddock.

Examinations on animals

Faecal egg counts for the various groups of calves are presented in Figure 6. Eggs were demonstrated in faeces 3 weeks after turning out the animals, and during the following 5 - 6 weeks the faecal egg counts increased for most groups reaching a peak in July.

Average serum pepsinogen levels for the six groups of calves are presented in Figure 7. It appears that the levels were highest in the non-moved animals at medium or high stocking rates - especially towards the end of the grazing season.

Clinical observations

The animals grazing at high stocking rates (1C) developed diarrhoea during the first two weeks of July. The clinical condition improved considerably for the group which was moved

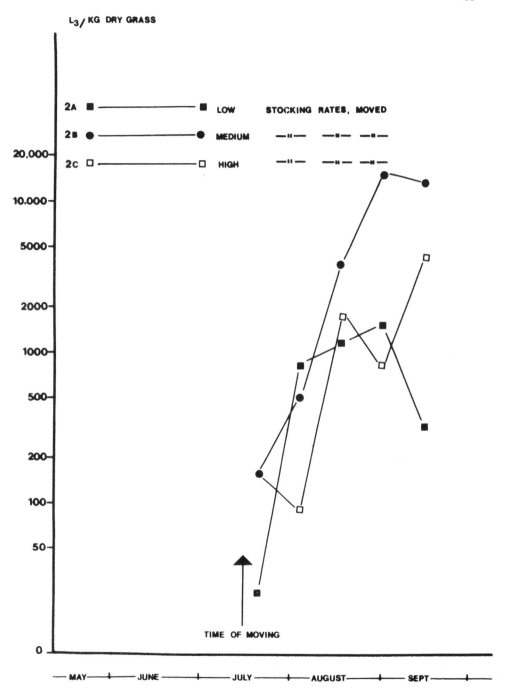

Fig. 3   Pasture contamination. Number of infective larvae (L₃) per kg dry herbage. Samples collected randomly in the paddocks grazed after 15th July only.

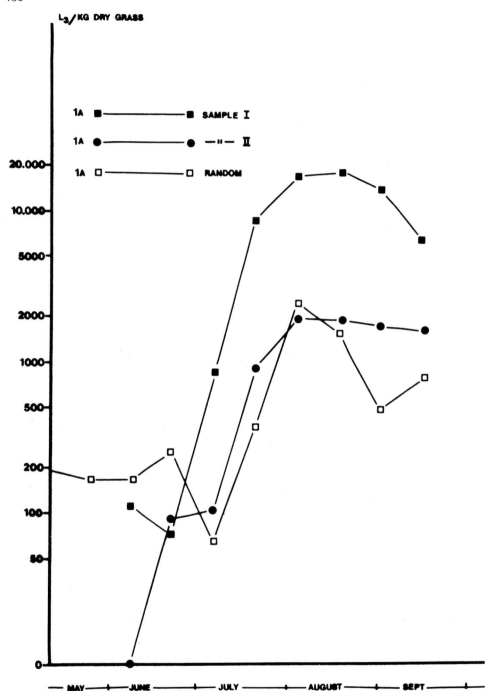

Fig. 4 Pasture contamination. Number of infective larvae (L$_3$) per kg dry herbage. Samples collected close to faecal pats and at random in paddock 1A (low stocking rate, non-moved).

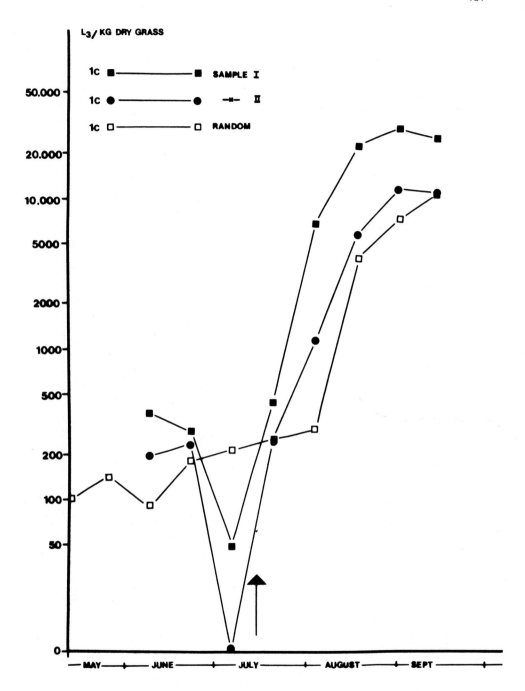

Fig. 5   Pasture contamination. Number of infective larvae (L_3) per kg dry
         herbage. Samples collected close to faecal pats and at random in
         paddock 1C (high stocking rate, non-moved).

488

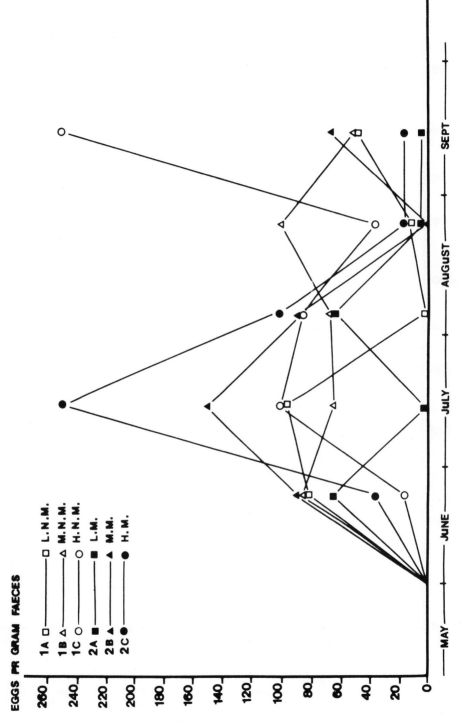

Fig. 6   Mean faecal egg counts for the various groups of calves.

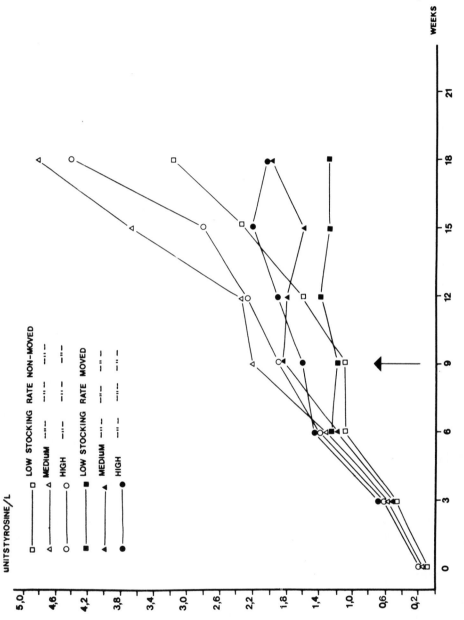

Fig. 7 Serum pepsinogen levels during the grazing season in the six groups of calves.

to clean pasture (2C) and then remained normal for the rest of the grazing season. The group grazing the same paddock showed some improvement shortly after moving half of the animals, but they developed diarrhoea again at the beginning of August. They were in a very poor condition at the time of stabling.

A few individuals in the other groups also developed clinical signs of ostertagiasis. Thus, two animals grazing 1B at medium stocking rate non-moved had to be taken out of the experiment during the last week of August.

DISCUSSION

The large differences between the three stocking rates in the output per animal and per ha, both within non-moved and moved groups, was apparently not due to differences in the herbage production potential per ha of the respective paddocks. The influence of stocking rate (Conway, 1963; Campbell, 1966) was cearly confirmed in our experiments. Throughout the season the herbage availability was significantly higher at low stocking rates than at medium and high stocking rates, in non-moved as well as in moved groups. While in many cases this results in a lower production per animal, the herbage utilisation may improve and lead to an increased output per ha (Evans and Bryan, 1973; Conway, 1975). At low stocking rates, where there is an abundance of feed, the animal may freely select its preferred grazing localities and grass species. However, at higher stocking rates the animals may not be able to practise selective grazing and they are forced to eat less acceptable herbage. The selective grazing of animals also concerns fouled herbage. This may be avoided when the grass is plentiful, but not when the stocking rate is increased (Marsh and Campling, 1970; Castle and MacDaid, 1972; Greenhaigh, 1975). In the present experiment this was assessed indirectly by quantitative measurements of a large number of grass tufts surrounding faecal pats. It was shown clearly in both permanently grazed paddocks and in paddocks grazed only after July that the size of grass tufts became significantly reduced when the stocking rate was increased.

The parasitological grass analyses are in accordance with those of many workers (Rose, 1970; Williams and Bilkowitch, 1973; Schultz, 1977). The trichostrongylid larval contamination of herbage increased faster and reached higher levels close to the faecal pats than elsewhere on the pasture. The very conspicuous finding that acquisition of infection by the grazing calves increased markedly with increasing stocking rates may be explained by the raised uptake of fouled herbage - with high larval contamination.

Moving the calves to clean pasture in midsummer reduced the parasite problem significantly, but it did not eliminate the effect of stocking rate. Moved animals grazing at high stocking rates also showed raised serum pepsinogen levels and lowered weight gain figures, compared with moved animals at lower stocking rates.

Decreased herbage intake at high stocking rates have been demonstrated by Hodgson et al. (1971). In the present experiment the non-moved animals ate less than those moved in mid-July. Furthermore, animals at medium and high stocking rates ate less than those at a low stocking rate (Højland Frederiksen et al., 1979). However, this cannot be explained by less herbage on offer since the permanently grazed areas had the same production potential as the clean pastures. Rather, the explanation may be that an increased stocking rate leads to an increased fouling of the pasture and changes in the grazing behaviour of the animals (Marsh and Campling, 1970). This was confirmed in this experiment as the animals spent more time grazing as they tried to avoid the contaminated grass (Table 4). The bite size of fouled herbage is also reduced. An increased worm burden towards the end of the grazing season may also influence the appetite of the animals resulting in a lower herbage intake.

The animals at medium and high stocking rates had a considerable worm burden as indicated by the raised serum pepsinogen values.

The results of this experiment indicate that the ever present problems of parasitism affect the animal production. At increased stocking rates the grass availability is decreased and the animals are forced to eat herbage close to the faecal pats. Hereby they acquire an increased wormburden as proven by increased serum pepsinogen levels and decreased herbage intake. However, under Danish conditions the adverse effects of increased stocking rates may be partly alleviated if the animals are moved before the mid-July rise in herbage contamination.

ACKNOWLEDGEMENT

The studies were part of a joint Nordic project (NKJ - No. 36) on gastrointestinal nematodes of cattle, supported in Denmark by the Danish Agricultural and Veterinary Research Council (Grant no. 533/8).

REFERENCES

Campbell, A.G., 1966. Grazed pasture parameters. I. Pasture dry matter
    production and availability in a stocking rate and grazing management
    experiment with dairy cows. J. Agric. Sci. Amb., 67, 199-210.

Campbell, A.J. and Field, A.C., 1960. Helminth infestation, a complicating
    factor in nutritional and grazing experiments. Proc. 8th International
    Grassld Congr., 715-718.

Castle, M.E. and MacDaid, E., 1972. The decomposition of cattle dung and
    its effect on pasture. J. Br. Grassld Soc., 27, 133-137.

Conway, A., 1963. Effect of grazing management on beef production. II.
    Comparison of three stocking rates under two systems of grazing.
    Irish J. Agric. Res., 2, 243-258.

Conway, A., 1973. The implications of grazing on land use. Occasional
    Symp. No.8, Br. Grassld Soc., 15-17.

Evans, T.R. and Bryan, W.W., 1973. Effects of soils, fertilisers, and
    stocking rates on pastures and beef production of the Wallum of
    south-eastern Queensland. 2. Live weight change and beef production.
    Aust. J. Experim. Agric. and Anim. Husbandry, 13, 530-536.

Greenhalgh, J.F.D., 1975. Factors limiting animal production from grazed
    pasture. J. Br. Grassld Soc., 30, 153-160.

Hodgson, J., Taylor, J.C. and Lonsdale, C.R., 1971. The relationship
    between intensity of grazing and the herbage consumption and growth
    of calves. J. Br. Grassld Soc., 26, 231-237.

Holmes, W., Jones, J.G.W. and Adeline, C., 1966. Feed intake of grazing
    cattle. IV. A study with milk cows of the influence of pasture
    restriction combined with supplementary feeding on production per
    animal and per acre. Anim. Prod., 8, 47-57.

Højland Frederiksen, J., Hansen, J.W., Sejrsen, K., Foldager, J., Agergaard, E.
    and Nansen, P., 1979. Løbetarmparasitter hos kalve på graes.
    Specialundersøgelse over graestilbud, fordøjelighed og optagelse af
    organisk stof. Statens Husdyrbrugsforsøg, Meddelelse Nr. 300.

Jørgensen, R.J., 1975. Isolation of infective *Dictyocaulus* larvae from
    herbage. Vet. Parasit., 1, 61-67.

Marsh, R. and Campling, R.C., 1970. Fouling of pastures by dung. Herb.
    Abstr., 40, 123-130.

McMeekan, C.P., 1956. Grazing management and animal production. Proc.
    7th Int. Grassld Congr., 146-154.

McMeekan, C.F. and Walshe, M.J., 1963. The interrelationships of grazing
method and stocking rate in the efficiency of pasture utilisation
by dairy cattle. J. Agric. Sci., 61, 147-163.

Michel, J.F., 1968. The control of stomach-worm infection in young cattle.
J. Br. Grassld Soc., 23, 163-173.

Mott, G.O., 1960. Grazing pressure and the measurement of pasture production.
Proc. 8th Int. Grassld Congr. Reading, 606-611.

Rose, J.H., 1970. Parasitic gastro-enteritis in cattle. Factors influencing
the time of the increase in the worm population of pastures. Res.
Vet. Sci., 11, 199-208.

Ross, J.G., Purcell, J.A., Dow, C. and Todd, J.R., 1967. Experimental
infection of calves with *Trichostrongylus axei*: the course of
development of infection and lesions in low level infections.
Res. Vet. Sci., 8, 201-206.

Schultz, A., 1977. Epidemiologiske studier over ostertagiose hos kalve.
Thesis, Copenhagen.

Sejrsen, K., Larsen, J.B., Klausen, S., Henriksen, Sv.Aa., Nansen, P.,
Jørgensen, R.J. and Ludvigsen, J., 1975. Løbetarmparasitter hos kalve
på graes. 29, Meddelelse, Statens Husdyrbrugsforsøg.

Sørensen, M. and Lykkeaa, J., 1974. Forskellig kvaelstofgødskning og
forskellig belaegning i forsøg med stude på graes. Meddelelse Nr. 12,
Statens Husdyrbrugsforsøg.

Williams, J.C. and Bilkovich, F.R., 1973. Distribution of *Ostertagia
ostertagi* infective larvae on pasture herbage. Am. J. Vet. Res.,
34, 1337-1344.

Yiakomettis, I.M. and Holmes, W., 1972. The effect of nitrogen and stocking
rate on the output of pasture grazed by beef cattle. J. Br. Grassld
Soc., 27, 283-291.

DISCUSSION

H.-J. Bürger *(FRG)*

How do you measure the amount of grass available?

J.W. Hansen *(Denmark)*

By an electronic capacitance meter, which is a mechanical device with a number of electrodes going down into the herbage and which measure electrical variances of resistance or conductivity. By this conductivity you can calculate the amount of herbage on the pasture at that particular time.

H.J. Over *(The Netherlands)*

It would be nice to have a demonstration.

J. Armour *(UK)*

Should you not be calculating the overall production per hectare, taking into account the stocking rate. Although the weight gains of the animals are different, the total yield per hectare might be more significant. I wondered if this, plus the possible effect of conservation, would have to be taken into account.

J.W. Hansen

One can calculate stocking rate either as the performance per animal i.e. the weight gain per animal, but also one can calculate it as the production per hectare. If you are a farmer, you like your animals to look good when they return from grazing and when they are sold. However, in the context of production, it is possible one may have to measure the production by the criterion of kilo of meat per hectare, for example.

J. Armour

What do your figures imply?

J.W. Hansen

You can have a higher production per hectare with a rather higher stocking rate and with a lower performance per animal. There is a point where there is an ideal situation from the point of production per hectare. It is very difficult to explain to the farmer that it does not matter that his animals do not look as well as they could but they may benefit from the increased production per hectare.

P. Nansen *(Denmark)*

Was the lowest performance per hectare on the highest stocking rate per hectare?

J.W. Hansen

I will have to ask John Foldager about that.

J. Foldager *(Denmark)*

Yes it was - however, the agronomist's point of view and the animal production man's point of view may be in conflict. The production per hectare and production per animal may differ and it is a question of pinpointing where the two coincide.

TRICHOSTRONGYLID NEMATODE INFECTIONS ASSOCIATED WITH THE HANDLING OF CATTLE SLURRY - A SURVEY OF DANISH STUDIES*

P. Nansen[1], Sv.Aa. Henriksen[2], R.J. Jørgensen[1] and J. Foldager[3]

[1]Institute of Veterinary Microbiology and Hygiene,
Royal Veterinary and Agricultural University,
Bülowsvej 13, DK-1870 Copenhagen V, Denmark.

[2]State Veterinary Serum Laboratory,
Bülowsvej 27, DK-1870 Copenhagen V, Denmark.

[3]National Institute of Animal Science,
Rolighedsvej 25, DK-1870 Copenhagen V, Denmark.

ABSTRACT

The application of cattle slurry to pastures may lead to raised herbage contamination with trichostrongyle larvae and subsequent parasitism in grazing animals. The liquid manure handling may lead to variable and unforeseeable epidemiological events, and even permanently housed animals may be exposed to infection. Precautions suggested for minimising the parasitological hazards are discussed, including the possible role of the biogas process in decontaminating slurry.

* The studies wre supported by a grant (No. 523/7/7) from the Danish Agricultural and Veterinary Research Council.

INTRODUCTION

Rationalisation of livestock production has implied that animal manures are now being handled as slurry rather than as solid manure. Low oxygen and low temperature in the slurry tanks (e.g. under winter conditions) are factors concerned with the more prolonged survival of nematode eggs or larvae in liquid than in solid manure (dung heaps).

This has been studied by workers, first in Sweden and Germany, and more recently in Ireland. The survival and persistence of microbial and helminth infective agents was the main topic in a CEC workshop held in Dublin in 1977 on animal effluents, and this workshop concluded that there was a relatively high survival rate of free-living stages of helminths in slurry tanks.

Analyses of the epidemiological consequences following application of slurry to grassland are few. For this reason we believe it relevant to summarise, at this workshop, experimental results and data from field situations.

Persson (1974a) in Sweden probably was the first to consider the risk of transmission of infective larvae to grass and subsequently to animals. He predicted that pastures fertilised with slurry during autumn, winter or early spring might be dangerous to calves turned out to graze the following spring. This has since been documented in reports from Ireland (Downey and Moore, 1977, 1979) and Denmark (Nansen and Jørgensen, 1977; Nansen et al., 1979).

SLURRY APPLICATION AND EPIDEMIOLOGY OF PARASITISM IN GRAZING CALVES

The application of slurry to pasture is almost certain to have varying and unforeseeable consequences. The severity of problems that will occur in the field will depend on a series of factors some of which are listed in Table 1.

TABLE 1

FACTORS INFLUENCING TRANSMISSION OF PARASITES VIA SLURRY

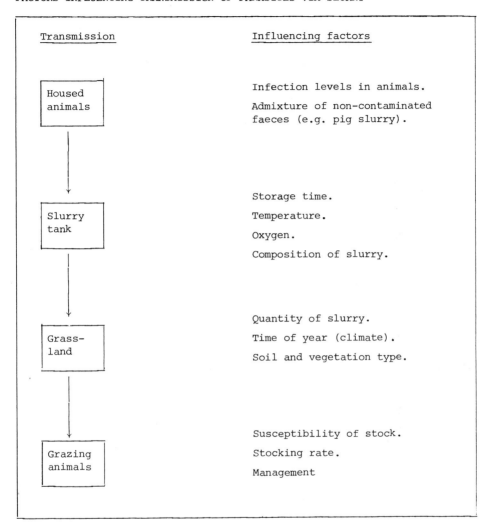

Transmission	Influencing factors
Housed animals	Infection levels in animals. Admixture of non-contaminated faeces (e.g. pig slurry).
Slurry tank	Storage time. Temperature. Oxygen. Composition of slurry.
Grass-land	Quantity of slurry. Time of year (climate). Soil and vegetation type.
Grazing animals	Susceptibility of stock. Stocking rate. Management

We have made experimental simulation of some situations that may occur in the field. The situations are presented in Table 2 with information on time of slurry application, herbage larval counts and acquisition of infection by the grazing stock. In all experiments slurry was spread on one half of a permanent paddock, the other half serving as a control area. The latter was given chemical fertilisers to promote comparable grass growth in the two areas. The quantity and composition of the fertiliser was calculated from the nutritive value of the liquid manure applied. The two paddocks were grazed by comparable groups of yearling calves which initially were parasite-free.

The data presented in Table 2 illustrates the variability in consequences of slurry application. In our experiments the extreme mid-summer drought of 1976 played a major role.

In an experiment conducted in 1978 we had the opportunity to study herbage larvae counts on a pasture which had not been grazed previously, but had been fertilised with slurry on several occasions; the latest in the beginning of April (1978), i.e. approximately 6 weeks before the introduction of parasite-free calves.

The L_3 contamination pattern of this paddock is presented in Figure 1 and is compared with the contamination of another permanently grazed paddock (grazed the year before by infected calves). In both paddocks the larval counts were extra-ordinarily low in May and June due to the unusual drought. However, coinciding with the rain in late June there was a rise in larval counts in the slurry-treated paddock - whereas with the non-slurry treated paddock this rise did not occur and there was a normal mid-July rise and a continuous increase over the rest of the season. In the slurry-treated paddock the larval curve showed a peculiar decline in early August. The calves grazing this field did not show clinical manifestations of trichostrongylosis and perhaps this is partly explicable by an anthelmintic treatment in July. The calves in the non-slurr

TABLE 2

THE EFFECT OF SLURRY APPLICATION ON INFECTION PARAMETERS AND PERFORMANCE. SUMMARY OF FIELD EXPERIMENTS

Experiment	Time of appl.	kg per m2	Trichostrongylids per kg — Eggs	Trichostrongylids per kg — Larvae	Herbage contamination**)	Date of introduction into field	Experimental calves**) — Infection parameters	Experimental calves**) — Weight gains	Special notes
A*)	March 1976	3.0	820	160	Significantly raised larval counts in May – June	May 17th	Mild clinical infection in early July – e.p.g. but not serum pepsinogen significantly raised	Significant weight gain reduction in May – July	Extreme drought in mid-summer. Anthelmintic treatment in mid-July
B*)	March 1976	2.0	–	270	Significantly raised larval counts in May – June	May 17th	Clinical infection of slurry-exposed calves in early July. In June – July significantly raised e.p.g. and serum pepsinogen	Significant weight gain reduction in May – July	Extreme drought in mid-summer. Anthelmintic treatment in mid-July
C*)	July 1st 1976		340	1110	No significant change	July 19th	No significant change	No significant change	Extreme drought at the time of slurry application
D	July 1st 1977	2.0	70	600	No significant change	July 23rd	No significant change	Significant weight gain reduction in July – Sept.	

*) Nansen et al., 1979.   **) The comments refer mainly to differences between slurry-exposed and non-exposed animals.

502

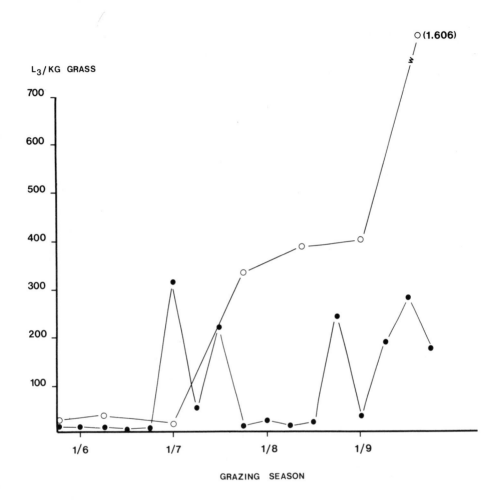

Fig. 1. Herbage larval counts (L_3/kg dried grass) in a slurry-
contaminated paddock not previously used for grazing (●-●)
and a normal permanent calf paddock (o-o). For details see
text.

503

treated paddock showed clinical signs of helminthiasis in late
summer. Thus it may be concluded that slurry application
in spring is responsible, at least partly, for the unusual
herbage larval fluctuation in the grazing season, but it is
not easy to deduce the underlying mechanisms .

The present example illustrates that the effects of
slurry is not only a question of raised herbage contamination,
but it may also be a question of a changed/displaced herbage
contamination pattern over the grazing season.

GRAZING BEHAVIOUR AND GRASS INTAKE IN SLURRY CONTAMINATED FIELDS

One of our experiments (Nansen et al., 1979) allowed us
to conclude that calves reject slurry-contaminated grass as
long as non-contaminated grass is available. We do not have
precise information about total grass intake by animals on
pastures which are widely contaminated with slurry, however,
the observation that slurry application may lead to weight gain
depressions in the absence of significant parasitism (Table 1)
suggests that slurry contamination of a paddock may lower the
grass intake by animals over a substantial period. In this
context it is relevant to mention the possible influence of
slurry contamination on the normal ability of cattle to avoid
herbage close to droppings where grass larval counts are usually
very high. The slurry may mask palatability differences and
thereby interfere with the selective grazing of cattle. This
is an area for closer study.

SLURRY APPLICATION AND PARASITISM IN PERMANENTLY HOUSED ANIMALS

We have received field reports indicating that slurry
application may also lead to parasitic problems in farms where
all animals are housed permanently. One outbreak of parasitism
was subjected to a detailed analysis (Nansen and Jørgensen,
1977) and the following points were noted: clinical ostertagiasis
occurred as early as June in housed calves and heifers and was

explicable on the basis of an efficient mechanical transmission
of the infection. Faeces were continuously transferred from
the stable to one big slurry tank. Slurry from this tank was
used during winter and at frequent intervals during summer for
fertilising grassland from which a cut was taken daily and fed
to the housed stock. In periods of low rainfall the area was
artificially irrigated. Larval counts of the herbage provided
a full explanation for the clinical outbreak. Ostertagiasis
with this type of history may lead to difficulties in diagnosis
and differential diagnosis at an early stage.

IMPLICATIONS AND CONTROL MEASURES

The results show that under certain circumstances
application of slurry to grassland may favour the propagation
of parasites and induce changes in the epidemiological patterns.
Our data on grazing calves in Denmark are in full agreement with
results reported by Downey and Moore (1977, 1979) in Ireland.
The data indicate that slurry application to pasture, in some
situations may significantly impair animal performance. The
situation posing most risk is perhaps the spring application
of slurry followed by grazing by susceptible calves. However,
it is important to emphasise that a number of unforeseeable
epidemiological changes may be expected, some of which may cause
production losses. In this context it should be emphasised that
impairment of production may be unnoticed since it will not
necessarily be accompanied by overt clinical signs.

It has become increasingly evident that precautions are
needed in the use of cattle slurry as a fertiliser. The
previously mentioned CEC workshop on animal effluents held in
Dublin 1977 suggested that minimum guidelines to minimise the
hazards are required. It was recommended that slurry should be
used on tillage crops wherever possible, but if there is no
practical alternative to spreading slurry on pasture the
fertilised area should preferably be used for conservation
(e.g. silage). However, where this is not possible a minimum

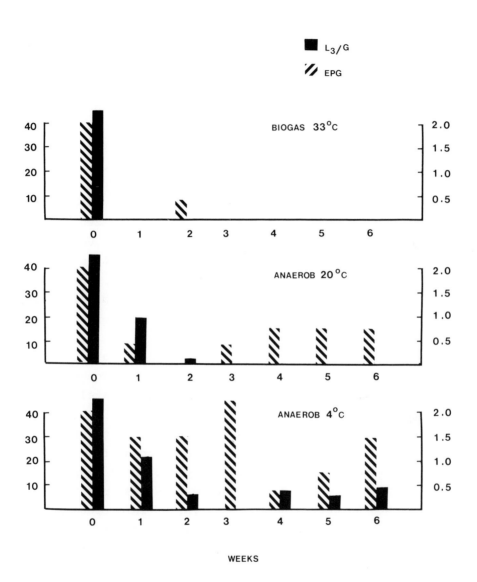

Fig. 2. Recoveries of viable trichostrongyle eggs and larvae under
          anaerobic storage (4°C and 20°C) and methanogenesis at 33°C.

506

storage time should be observed. Our data and those of
Persson (1974b) in Sweden suggest a storage time of 4 - 5 months
during winter and 2 months during summer, however, minimum
storage times, should definitely be determined with reference
to local climatic conditions.

Various methods of destroying parasite eggs and larvae
in slurry have been advanced (aerobic decomposition, addition
of lime or other chemicals, ionising radiation, etc.), but most
of them have practical and economical limitations.

Recommendations for grazing management were considered,
e.g. slurry contaminated pasture should not be grazed until
aftermath and then only by adult cattle or sheep. However, it
should be remembered that the recommendations discussed here
are made with reference to trichostrongyles only; there is a
lack of knowledge on the survival of many other parasites in
slurry.

The number of Danish dairy farms handling cattle manure
in the form of slurry has increased markedly in recent years,
the number now being almost 10 000 (i.e. approximately 10%Of
the total number of farms). It is estimated that the number
will double over the next decade. During the same period
the Ministry of Energy has estimated that biogas farm units
for the production of methane will be established in a high
proportion of these. As a consequence this has involved us
in experiments to determine the survival of infectious agents
(parasites, bacteria, viruses) during the production of methane,
Initial studies have shown a rapid destruction of trichostrongylid
eggs and larvae under both thermophilic and mesophilic anaerobic
fermentations (see Figure 2). The studies will be continued
and extended in an attempt to analyse the overall decontaminating
effect of the biogas-process.

REFERENCES

Downey, N.E. and Moore, J.F., 1977. Trichostrongylid contamination of pasture
    fertilised with cattle slurry. Vet. Rec. 101, 487-488.

Downey, N.E. and Moore, J.F., 1979. The possible role of animal manures in
    the dissemination of livestock parasites. CEC Workshop in Oldenburg
    1977.

Nansen, P. and Jørgensen, M., 1977. Øgede problemer med løbetarmstrongylider
    som følge af flydende gødingshåndtering i kvægbesætninger
    (Increased problems with trichostrongyle infections associated with
    liquid manure application in cattle farms). Dansk VetTidsskr,
    60, 249-254.

Nansen, P., Midtgaard, N., Jørgensen, M., Sejrsen, Kr. and Jørgensen, R.J.,
    1979. Trichostrongylid nematode infections in calves grazing slurry
    manured paddocks. Yearbook, Roy. Vet. Agr. Univ. Copenhagen 1979,
    53-71.

Persson, L., 1974a. Studies on the Occurrence of Parasite Eggs, Oocysts,
    and Larvae in Cattle Faeces and Manure, and of Larvae on Pasture
    where Manure has been Spread. Nord. Vet. -Med. 26, 151-164.

Persson, L., 1974b. Studies on the Survival of Eggs and Infective Larvae
    of *Ostertagia ostertagi* and *Cooperia oncophora* in Liquid Cattle
    Manure, Zbl. Vet. Med. B. 21, 311-317.

DISCUSSION

E.J.L. Soulsby *(UK)*

This is not a parasitological question, but how serious a problem is palatability of grass with excess application of slurry? It would seem to me to be rather objectionable to have all your food covered with a thin layer of faeces.

P. Nansen *(Denmark)*

I think it is a problem and it is recognised by the farmer. In these systems where you apply slurry to the field and you also use the field for animals, the farmers know that they cannot use the field for 3 or 4 weeks, depending on the rainfall, because the animals would not eat the grass. But if you feed animals in a stable they will eat the herbage - they have no alternative.

E.J.L. Soulsby

May I ask a supplemental question. Might some of the production results which you obtained be unrelated to parasitism but more related to palatability?

P. Nansen

Yes, that is what I wanted to say with these experiments where there is a poor correlation between weight gain and epidemiological parameters, but a close relationship to the application of slurry. There is one other point in connection with smell which I think is important. When the field is covered with slurry the palatability of herbage changes in the field and the selective grazing behaviour of the cattle is eliminated. Therefore, cattle eat more grass from the tufts of grass which, according to Jørgen Hansen, is more dangerous because that is where the larvae are more concentrated. The pasture could be more uniform in taste and this could have an adverse effect. That is something which we should look into.

J. Eckert *(Switzerland)*

What is the concentration of eggs in the slurry? Also,
what stage of development have they reached? Are eggs or
larvae present?

P. Nansen

We are not too sure about this because we have had problems
with the techniques initially. In the first experiments we had
third stage larval in the range of 200 - 300 larvae/kg slurry.

N. Downey *(Ireland)*

In one of our experiments the control pasture also
received slurry, but slurry which was not contaminated with
eggs. Nevertheless, there was a weight gain depression on the
pasture which had been contaminated with slurry. This has
bearing on the question of palatability.

H.J. Over *(The Netherlands)*

You mean it might work out as a repellent?

P. Nansen

There is one other aspect which we would like to
investigate. The conditions in the winter in the slurry tanks is
comparable with the environment from which after ingestion third
stage larvae become arrested in development in calves. Thus
larvae survive at 3 - 4°C over long periods, and it would be
interesting to know if this would have an effect on the
subsequent development of larvae when they are ingested in
the spring.

H.J. Over

One of the unforseeable epidemiological effects!

SESSION 6

OTHER ASPECTS OF NEMATODIASIS
Chairman: E.J.L. Soulsby

ACQUISITION OF IMMUNOLOGICAL COMPETENCE TO GASTRO-INTESTINAL TRICHOSTRONGYLES BY YOUNG RUMINANTS: EPIDEMIOLOGICAL SIGNIFICANCE

E.J.L. Soulsby, Gillian Monsell and Sheelagh Lloyd

Department of Clinical Veterinary Medicine,
University of Cambridge, Cambridge, UK

ABSTRACT

The acquisition of immune competence varies with the species of animal and with the kind of infection or antigen presented. The neonatal lamb fails to develop a significant protective immune response to helminth infections until it is several weeks or months of age. By this time, in the field, animals may have been subjected to a severe, even fatal, challenge from the herbage. Animals unable to mount a satisfactory immune response to control infection may be a major source of infection for other animals. There appears to be a sequential development of immunological competence in the lamb to various antigens and the differences in responsiveness to antigens of helminths on the part of lambs are discussed with reference to genetic variability of animals (responders and non-responders), maternally transferred antibody, colostral transfer of tolerogenic substances, suppressive factors in newborn serum, neonatal suppressor cells and induced suppressor cell formation.

P. Nansen, R.J. Jørgensen, E.J.L. Soulsby (eds), Epidemiology and Control of Nematodiasis in Cattle.
Copyright © 1981 ECSC, EEC, EAEC, Brussels – Luxembourg. All rights reserved.

INTRODUCTION

Parasitic gastro-enteritis of domestic ruminants is a disease syndrome which is most usually seen in young animals in their first grazing season. This may be due, in part, to greater susceptibility of young animals to the pathogenic effects of parasitic infection, but there is evidence that young animals are less able to mount an immune response which will reject an existing infection or prevent reinfection. This phenomenon is exemplified particularly by *Haemonchus contortus* and *Trichostrongylus* spp. infection in sheep, but the phenomenon is recognised in other species including neonatal rodents (e.g. rats infected with *Nippostrongylus brasiliensis*) and has been demonstrated in neonatal cattle infected with metacestodes of *Taenia saginata*. The derivative implications of these phenomena pose the following questions:

- does the young bovine respond promptly to infection with gastro-intestinal nematodes?

- does infection of the neonatal bovine compromise its ability to respond subsequently?

- does the immune response vary with physiological events, such as lactation, weaning, etc?

The present consideration will deal mainly with the failure of lambs to mount an effective immune response to gastrointestinal nematodes during the neonatal period. Of ruminants, the response of the lamb has been considered in the most detail, but there are indications that the lamb and the calf respond similarly to gastro-intestinal nematode infections.

OVINE NEONATAL RESPONSIVENESS TO NEMATODE INFECTIONS

The acquisition of immune competence varies with the species of animal and with the kind of infection or antigen presented: the foetal and neonatal lamb has been shown to respond immunologically by antibody and cell mediated responses to a range of unrelated antigens (Silverstein et al., 1963), but it fails to develop a significant protective immune response to helminth infections until it is several months of age. Thus lambs fail to develop immunity to *Haemonchus contortus* following vaccination with irradiated larvae when they are aged less than 6 months, whereas animals aged 9 months respond with a vigorous and effect- ive protective response (Urquhart et al., 1966). Similarly, results were obtained by Manton et al. (1952) also with *H. con- tortus*, who exposed lambs aged 3 to 4 months or 10 to 12 months to two doses of infective larvae followed by challenge 60 days later. The older animals showed highly significant reduction in worm burden while the younger ones did not. By this time, of course, in the field animals, these may have been subjected to a severe, even fatal, challenge from the herbage. Again, with *T. colubriformis* , strong immunity has been produced in sheep aged 6 months or more by vaccination (Mulligan et al., 1961; Gregg and Dineen, 1978) but lambs younger than 3 months respond poorly to an irradiated vaccine. Studies with repeated doses of normal larvae (e.g. Chiejina and Sewell, 1974) produced com- parable results in that lambs failed to become immune to *T. colu- briformis* when such immunisation was initiated in animals less than 3 months of age.

A comparable situation is seen in the field. For example, studies of a naturally infected flock of sheep demonstrated a continuous high mean faecal strongyle egg count which did not terminate until the lambs were about 6 months of age (Soulsby, 1966).

In contrast to the situation with *H. contortus* and *T. colu- briformis* lambs are capable of responding to *Nematodirus battus* at an earlier age. Provided the size of the primary infection is large enough (e.g. 60 000 larvae), lambs infected at 6 to 8 weeks of age reject the infection and by 12 weeks of age they are immune to reinfection (Ballantyne et al., 1978).

The inability of neonatal lambs to respond to helminth infections such as *H. contortus* is in contrast to their ability to be immunised successfully against bacterial and viral infections (Cole and Morris, 1973) and to the ready ability of both foetal and neonatal lams to respond to a range of non helminth antigens from mid-gestation onwards (Silverstein et al., 1963; Fahey and Morris, 1978). There appears to be a sequential development of immunological competence in the lamb to antigens such as Φx, ferritin, chicken red blood cells, etc., but the foetus does not respond to diphtheria toxoid, *Salmonella typhurium*, lipopolysaccharide or somatic antigens of this bacterium, though the lamb will respond to these latter antigens 80 - 140 days after birth despite foetal exposure to them (Fahey and Morris, 1978). Foetal lambs are also able to reject homografts and thus are capable of mounting a cell mediated immunity response (Silverstein et al., 1964).

Why then are there such differences in responsiveness to antigens of helminths on the part of lambs and what relationship might these have to responses of ruminants in general to gastro-intestinal nematodes?

POSSIBLE MECHANISMS OF UNRESPONSIVENESS

It is necessary, first, to define the unresponsiveness. The majority of studies have assessed this on the basis of resistance to a challenge infection. However, it should be noted that neonatal lambs are capable of responding immuno-logically by antibody production to infection with *H. contortus* (Varela-Diaz and Soulsby, 1972), such animals will undergo a self-cure reaction (Varela-Diaz, 1970) but this is in the absence of immunological protection against subsequent infection (Chen, 1972). Hence the immunological defect in the unresponsiveness to helminths in neonatal sheep at least to *H. contortus*, appears not to be a total lack of response, but that associated with resistance to reinfection. The immunological basis of this resistance to reinfection in sheep is not fully understood but if it is similar in basis to that of other hosts for the patho-genic trichostrongylus of domestic animals, then T lymphocyte dependent mechanisms, including cell-mediated immunity, probably play a significant role. Cell mediated immunity responses have

been demonstrated in sheep infected with *H. contortus* but such
responses are not acquired until the animal is several months
of age (Chen, 1972). Such results have been confirmed recently
in experiements which show that peripheral blood lymphocytes
of lambs infected with *H. cortortus* respond to antigen, *in vitro,*
at 19 weeks of age and not before (Monsell, Lloyd and Soulsby,
1980, unpublished results, Figure 1). During this period of
unresponsiveness of peripheral blood lymphocytes to specific
antigens, such cells respond to phytohaemagglutin throughout
the period of study. This is in contrast to the results of
Riffkin and Dobson (1979) who reported an absence of response
to PHA in lambs at birth, but this response developed during
the first 5 months in the absence of infection.

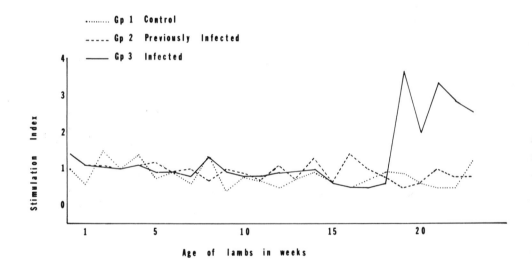

Fig. 1   Response of peripheral blood lymphocytes to specific antigen of lambs
variously infected with *Haemonchus contortus*. Three lambs in each
group.

Group 1: Control group; uninfected throughout experiment; Group 2:
Previously infected group; during weeks 1 - 7 given 50 infective
larvae (L3) of *H. contortus* per week; at week 8 given 2 000 L3.
Treated on week 18 with albendazole. Group 3: Infected group; given
2 000 L3 *H. contortus* on week 6; remained infected throughout the
experiment. Note marked response of lymphocytes to specific antigen
in all animals of this group at 19 weeks of age.

Genetic variability of animals

A further consideration is the innate ability of sheep to respond to immunisation. Dineen et al., (1978) have confirmed that there is a marked difference in the response of mature sheep and lambs to irradiated larvae of *T. colubriformis* but nevertheless lambs in these studies segregated into 'responders' and 'non-responders' in this work suggested that genetically determined factors play an important role in the responsiveness of lambs to vaccinations. In this respect Dineen and Windon (1980) have demonstrated that rams selected for responsiveness to vaccination with irradiated *T. colubriformis* larvae at an early age will permit the establishment of resistant generations of animals.

Genetic variation of susceptibility to infection by *T. colubriformis* in guinea pigs have been reported by Rothwell et al., (1978) and Wakelin (1975) has reported on the genetic control of the immune reponse to *Trichuris* in mice. The role of other genetically controlled factors (e.g. haemoglobin type) in immune responsiveness to intestinal nematodes has yet to be determined but may need to be taken into account when considering the ability of an animal to respond to infection. In this respect, Dineen and Windon (1980) were not able to show a relationship between haemoglobin-type and the responsiveness of lambs to vaccination with *T. colubriformis*.

A further point in the assessment of responsiveness is the interval allowed between immunisation and challenge. For example, Dineen et al. (1978) report that a higher proportion of responders were detected in lambs when the interval between immunisation and challenge was extended. These authors suggest that animals may be primed by vaccination but unable to mount an effective response until later.

Maternally tranferred antibody

A 'feed-back inhibition' of an active immune response by passively acquired colostral antibody may occur (Husband and Lascelles, 1975). However, Dineen et al. (1978) demonstrated

that there was no significant difference between colostrum fed
and colostrum deprived lambs vaccinated with irradiated *T. colubriformis* larvae. It was concluded that 'feed-back inhibition'
did not play a role in the difference between lambs and mature
sheep.

Colostral transfer of tolerogenic substances

The occurrence of tolerogenic substances in colostrum has
been reported by Auerbach and Clark (1975). Unresponsiveness to
sheep red blood cells was induced in mice suckled on mothers
injected with a high speed supernate of lysed cells. A role
for such a substance might occur in sheep undergoing the periparturient increase in worm burdens, possibly associated with
reactivation of previously hypobiotic larvae in the mucosa of
the digestive tract. Worm proteins (antigens) have been detected
in the serum of sheep infected with *H. contortus* (Stumberg, 1933),
however, it seems unlikely these could be a primary cause of
unresponsiveness since the phenomenon occurs in lambs born and
raised under worm free conditions. Furthermore, the fact that
no difference was noted in the responsiveness of colostrum fed
or colostrum deprived lambs to *T. colubriformis* (Dineen et al.,
1978) would also suggest that this is not a major factor in the
differential response. However, immunisation was attempted at
weaning in such studies when the effects of any tolerogenic substances might be minimal. Infection with gastro-intestinal
parasites before weaning might allow tolerising mechanisms to be
established which would then persist beyond weaning.

Suppressive soluble factors in newborn serum

Immune regulation of pregnancy by which the foetus sur-
vives has been discussed by Beer and Billingham (1978). A variety of non specific events accompany pregnancy of man (e.g.
increased production of adrenal corticosteroid, ovarian and
placental hormones, an involution of lymphoid tissue resulting
in temporary lymphocytopaenia, suppression of inflammation and
reduced lymphocyte responsiveness *in vitro*). In conjunction with
this is the evidence that pregnancy lowers maternal resistance

to a variety of infections and parasitic infections are examples of such. Particularly, there is a marked 'relaxation' of immunity in domestic ruminants to their gastro-intestinal nematodes which is maximised during the 'lactational rise' in egg output. There is no evidence that the periparturient lowering of the immune response of the dam is related to the subsequent neonatal unresponsiveness to helminth infections but the two in concert do provide a most effective mechanism for the transmission and maintenance of parasite species.

Recently, considerable attention has been directed to the role of alpha feto protein (AFP) in the suppression of cellular based immunity mechanisms which could hold maternal reactivity against foetal antigens in abeyance. AFP is a glycoprotein present in high concentrations in foetal plasma and amniotic fluid and may remain elevated in plasma for varying periods following birth. Tomasi (1978) has reported that AFP inhibits T cell mediated reactions in mice, though this might be through the induction of suppressor T cells and this would be consistent with the observation that new born animals (mice) have large numbers of suppressor T cells (Tomasi. 1978). AFP may also suppress proliferative responses. possibly through an effect on macrophages either via macrophage processing or macrophage-T-cell interactions (Tomasi. 1978).

Neonatal suppressor cells

Immunocompetent cells have been detected in the foetus of various species (e.g. man. mouse. sheep) and are capable of participating in both humoral and cell mediated reactions. However. in new born animals for the first few weeks after birth, thymic and splenic lymphocytes may be unresponsive to mitogenic stimulation and MLR. Further. new born human lymphocytes will inhibit PHA-induced transformation and suppress MLR, an effect mediated by T lymphocytes (Olding and Oldstone, 1976). Pavia and Stites (1979) have demonstrated similar cells in new born mice, such cells inhibiting responses of maternal (competent) cells to lipopolysaccharide and MLR. This effect persisted for the first two weeks of life of the mouse, was eliminated from cell populations by depletion of the T cells and was associated with a soluble factor released during culture. Pavia and Stites, (1979) suggest that murine new born suppressor cells belong to the Ly-1,2,3 subclass of lymphocytes and loss of suppressor activity is associated with repopulation of the spleen by Ly-1 and Ly-2,3 cells.

New born mice and humans lose their spontaneous suppressor cell activity within a few weeks after birth, but abnormal persistence might lead to lowered responses to specific antigens especially those concerned with B cells and immunoglobulin production since it is a IgM (Fc) binding sub-population of new born T lymphocytes which suppresses pokeweed mitogen induced differentiation of adult B lymphocytes (Haywood and Lydyard, 1978).

There is a paucity of information on the composition of the lymphocyte population of ruminants at birth and hence it is not possible to comment on whether, for example, the new born lamb possesses suppressor cells similar in function to the neonatal mouse or man. If they were to exist, then they could provide a base for consideration of neonatal unresponsiveness to helminth infections.

Induced suppressor cell formation

It has been known for several decades that orally administered antigen may suppress systemic immune responses. More recent studies (Ngan and Kind, 1978; Mattingly and Waksman, 1978) have shown that orally administered antigen induces antigen-specific suppressor cells in Peyer's Patches and mesenteric lymph nodes and these cells later are found in the spleen and thymus but not in Payer's Patches or mesenteric lymph nodes (Mattingly and Waksman, 1978). The cell responsible appears to be a long-lived, recirculating T_2 cell which may work in conjunction with a macrophage. The responses blocked included plaque forming and delayed type hypersensitivity responses to sheep red blood cells.

Induced suppressor cell formation is the likely explanation
for the induction of tolerance in neonatal mice with a T-dependent
antigen that is an obligate immunogen in adult mice (Etlinger
and Chiller, 1979$_a$). Etlinger and Chiller (1979$_b$) also reported
that this neonatal induced specific unresponsiveness was effective on T as well as on B cells. The unresponsive state could be
maintained on adoptive transfer of cells and persisted for up to
100 days in mice. Though unresponsiveness was observed to persist for so long this was not linked to suppressive factors
associated with serum or lymphnoid cells. This work is of
special interest since antigens normally highly immunogenic in
adult animals (e.g. aggregated human gammaglobulin) induce
unresponsiveness in a neonatal environment. Work needs to be
done to determine whether helminth antigens would have a similar
effect since mature animals' parasitic infections frequently are
obligate immunogens inducing strong immunity, whereas in the
neonate virtually complete failure of the immune response is the
situation.

The induction of specific immunological unresponsiveness
of lymphocytes by infection of sheep with *H. contortus* was reported
by Adams (1978). This work indicated that normal lymphocytes
from worm free sheep were stimulated mitogenically by antigen
prepared by the parasite antigen indicating a mitogenic component
for the antigen. However, lymphocytes from *H. contortus* infected
sheep were suppressed in their reactivity to specific antigen
but not to non specific phytomitogens. Termination of infection,
either naturally or by therapy, resulted in a return to reactivity
to antigen on the part of lymphocytes. Adams (1978) offers various explanations for these results, including a temporary withdrawal and sequestration of reactive cells from the circulation,
permanent dilution of clones of lymphocytes or blockade of potentially reactive cells by antibody or antigen. It has not been
possible to confirm the work of Adams (1978) and whereas the
lymphocytes of sheep may fail to respond to specific antigen
following infection, they do not show evidence of induced immune
unresponsiveness throughout the course of the infection (Monsell,
unpublished results).

CONCLUSION

Neonatal unresponsiveness to helminth infections is at present an enigma which contrasts with the strong response generated by adult animals. The duration of this unresponsiveness may be critical for the survival of the young animal. There is need, therefore, to understand this phenomenon further in the neonatal ruminant and to develop means whereby such neonates are rendered as responsive as their adult counterparts.

524

REFERENCES

Adams, D.B. 1978. The induction of selective immunological unresponsiveness
in cells of blood and lymphoid tissue during primary infection of
sheep with the abomasal nematode *Haemonchus contortus*. Aust. J. Exp.
Biol. Med. Sci., 56, 107-118

Auerbach, R. and Clark, S. 1975. Immunological tolerance: transmission from
mother to offspring. Science, 189, 811-813

Ballantyne, A.J., Sharpe, M.J. and Lee, D.L. 1978. Changes in the adenylate
energy charge of *Nippostrongylus brasiliensis* and *Nematodirus battus*
during the development of immunity to these nematodes in their hosts.
Parisitology, 76, 211-220

Beer, A.E. and Billingham, R.E. 1978. Immunoregulatory aspects of pregnancy.
Federation Proc., 37, 2374-2378

Burrells, C., Wells, P.W. and Sutherland, A.D. 1978. Reactivity of ovine
lymphocytes to phytohaemagglutinin and pokeweed mitogen during pregnancy and in the immediate post-parturient period. Clin. Exp. Immunol.
33, 410-415

Chen, P.C. 1972. Peripheral lymphoid cell responses of sheep to gastro-
intestinal parasitisms. Dissertation for the PhD degree. University
of Pennsylvania

Chen, P.C. and Soulsby, E.J.L. 1976. *Haemonchus contortus* infection in ewes.
Blastogenic responses of peripheral blood leucocytes to third stage
larval antigen. Int. J. Parasit., 6, 135-141

Chiejina, S.N. and Sewell, M.H.H. 1974. Experimental infections with *Trichostrongylus colubriformis* (Giles, 1892) Loos, 1905 in lambs: worm
burden, growth rate and host resistance resulting from prolonged
escalating infection. Parasitology, 69, 301-314

Cole, G.J. and Morris, B. 1973. The lymphoid apparatus of the sheep: its
growth, development and significance in immunologic reactions. Adv.
Vet. Sci. Comp. Med., 17, 225-263

Connan, R.M. 1976. Effect of lactation on the immune response to gastro-
intestinal nematodes. Vet. Rec., 99 476-477

Dineen, J.K., Gregg, P. and Lascelles, A.K. 1978. The response of lambs to
vaccination at weaning with irradiated *Trichostrongylus colubriformis*
larvae: segregation into "responders" and "non-responders". Int. J.
Parasit. 8, 59-63

Dineen, J.K. and Windon, R.G. 1980. The effect of sire selection on the response of lambs to vaccination with irradiated *Trichostrongylus colubriformis* larvae. Int. J. Parisit., 10, 189-196

Etlinger, H.M. and Chiller, J.M. 1979$_a$. Maturation of the lymphoid system. I. Induction of tolerance in neonates with a T-dependent antigen that is an obligate immunogen in adults. J. Immunol., 122, 2558-2563

Etlinger, H.M. and Chiller, J.M. 1979$_b$. Maturation of the lymphoid system. II. Characterization of the cellular levels of unresponsiveness induced in neonates by a T-dependent antigen that is an obligate immunogen in adults. J. Immunol., 122, 2564-2570

Fahey, K.T. and Morris, B. 1978. Humoral immune reponses in foetal sheep. Immunology, 35, 651-661

Gregg, P. and Dineen J.K. 1978. The response of sheep vaccinated with irradiated *Trichostrongylus colubriformis* larvae to impulse and sequential challenge with normal larvae. Vet. Parasit., 4, 49-53

Hayward, A.R. and Lydyard, P.M. 1978. Suppression of B lymphocyte differentiation by newborn T lymphocytes with an Fc receptor for IgM. Clin. Exp. Immunol., 34, 374-378

Husband, A.J. and Lascelles, A.K. 1975. Antibody responses to neonatal immunization in calves. Res. Vet. Sci., 18, 201-207

Manton, V.J.A., Peacock, R., Poynter, D., Silverman, P.H. and Terry, R.J. 1962. The influence of age and naturally acquired resistance to *Haemonchus contortus*. Res. Vet. Sci., 3, 308-313

Mattingly, J.M. and Waksman, B.H. 1978. Immunolgical suppression after oral administration of antigen. I. Specific suppressor cells formed in rat Peyer's Patches after oral administration of sheep erythrocytes and their systemic migration. J. Immunol., 121, 1878-1883

Mulligan, W., Gordon, H.McL., Stewart, D.F. and Wagland, B.M. 1961. The use of irradiated larvae as immunizing agents in *Haemonchus contortus* and *Trichostrongylus cubriformis* infection in sheep. Aust. J. Agric. Res., 12, 1175-1187

Ngan, J. and Kind, L.S. 1978. Suppressor T cells for IgE and IgG in Peyer's Patches of mice made tolerant by the oral administration of ovalbumin. J. Immunol., 120, 861-865

Olding, L.B. and Oldstone, M.B.A. 1976. Thymus-derived peripheral lymphocytes from human new borns inhibit division of the mothers lymphocytes. J. Immunol., 116, 682-686

526

Pavia, C.S. and Stites, D.P. 1979. Immunosuppressive activity of murine new born spleen cells. I. Selective inhibition of *in vitro* lymphocyte activation. Cell. Immunol., 42, 48-60

Riffkin, G.G. and Dobson, C. 1979. Predicting resistance of sheep to *Haemonchus contortus* infections. Vet. Parasit., 5, 365-378

Rothwell, T.L.N., LeJambre, L.F., Adams, D.B. and Love, R.J. 1978. *Trichostrongylus colubriformis* infection of guinea pigs: genetic basis for variation in susceptibility to infection among outbred animals. Parasitology, 76, 201-209

Silverstein, A.M., Uhr, J.W., Kraner, K.L. and Lukes, R.J. 1963. Fetal response to antigens stimulus. II. Antibody production by the fetal lamb. J. Exp. Med., 117, 799-812

Silverstein, A.M., Prendergast, R.A. and Kraner, K.L. 1964. Fetal response to antigenic stimulus. Pt. 4. The rejection of skin homografts by the fetal lamb. J. Exp. Med., 119, 955-964

Soulsby, E.J.L. 1966. The mechanisms of immunity to gastro-intestinal nematodes. In: Biology of Parasites (Ed. Soulsby E.J.L.), Academic Press, New York and London, pp 255-276

Stumberg, J.E. 1933. The detection of proteins of the nematode *Haemonchus contortus* in the sera of infected sheep and goats. Amer. J. Hyg., 18, 247-265

Tomasi, T.B. Jr. 1978. Suppressive factors in amniotic fluid and new born serum: Is α-fetoprotein involved? Cell. Immunol., 37, 459-460

Urquhart, G.M., Jarrett, W.F.H., Jennings, F.N., MacIntyre, W.I.M. and Mulligan, W. 1966. Immunity to *Haemonchus contortus* infection. Relationship between age and successful vaccination with irradiated larvae. Amer. J. Vet. Res., 27, 1645-1648

Varela-Diaz, V. 1960. The immunological response to gastro-intestinal parasites of sheep. Dissertation for the PhD degree. University of Pennsylvania

Varela-Diaz. V. and Soulsby, E.J.L. 1972. Immunoglobulin synthesis in sheep. IgG_2 deficiency in neonatal lambs. Res. Vet. Sci., 13, 99-100

Wakelin, D. 1975. Genetic control of immune response to parasites: Immunity to *Trichuris muris* in inbred and random-bred strains of mice. Parasitology, 71, 51-60

DISCUSSION

J. Eckert (Switzerland)

You demonstrate that there is quite a good cellular immune response in the sheep infected with Haemonchus. What is the relevance of this response with regard to the worm burdens? Is the worm burden retained or is it reduced or eliminated by this immune response,

E.J.L. Soulsby (UK)

No! The worm burden was maintained at a moderate level. The immune response in the animals under study did not result in the rejection of the worm burden.

J. Eckert

What is the significance of the finding that indicates an impairment of the effector arm of the immune response?

E.J.L. Soulsby

There are two mechanisms to consider. With Haemonchus there is the manifestation of resistance to a new infection, and then there is the elimination of the existing infection. These are probably two separate mechanisms. To assess the protective nature of the immune response it is necessary to challenge and assess worm burdens.

J. Armour (UK)

We have been doing much the same study with fluke infected animals and getting similar results. One comment is how relative is the lymphocyte transformation test to cell mediating immunity in ruminants?

E.J.L. Soulsby

Antigen induced lymphocyte responsiveness can be correlated with other parameters of cell mediative immunity, such as the production of macrophage inhibition factor (MAF). In the sheep

and in the bovine, the lymphocyte populations are not characterised fully. It is very difficult to measure T-cell populations,
and variations in these, simply because the techniques are not
available for measuring them. However, sheep and cattle are
sensitive, in a cell mediated immunity manner, to antigens such
as tuberculin. It is possible to measure and quantitate the
responses to these antigens by the techniques used in the present study.

J. Armour

What you are saying is that we should be looking for suppressor T-cells?

E.J.L. Soulsby

Yes.

J. Armour

You determined if alpha foetal protein plays a role in these
infections?

E.J.L. Soulsby

We suspect that it does play quite a role but we have not
looked at it in detail. It is a well-known suppressor in other
animals, for example, in mice and humans.

J. Armour

Has it been done in the ruminant?

E.J.L. Soulsby

Yes, I believe so. Work in Australia suggests it is associated with a reduction of responsiveness of peripheral blood
lymphocytes to phytomitogens.

J. Euzeby (France)

Does the sex of the animal have any influence on the unresponsiveness?

E.J.L. Soulsby

Not that we can determine. However, we work with females
rather than males, but in our work there is no real evidence
that the sex of the animal is important. There is some evidence
that the haemoglobin types do contribute to the responsiveness,
but it is a question of degree rather than absolute unresponsiveness and responsiveness.

PERFORMANCE OF RESISTANT AND NON-RESISTANT CALVES DURING REPEATED INFECTION WITH *Cooperia* spp. AND *Ostertagia* spp. AND MIXED SPECIES

A. Kloosterman and R. van den Brink

Department of Animal Husbandry, Agricultural University,
P.O. Box 338, Wageningen, The Netherlands

ABSTRACT

An experiment was carried out to examine the significance of resistance to Cooperia spp. for the weight gain performance of calves under conditions of severe re-infection with several species. Part of the variation in weight gains could be explained by variation in resistance. Resistant animals that showed a transient growth-depression after primary infection, ultimately performed better.

P. Nansen, R.J. Jørgensen, E.J.L. Soulsby (eds), Epidemiology and Control of Nematodiasis in Cattle.
Copyright © 1981 ECSC, EEC, EAEC, Brussels – Luxembourg. All rights reserved.

INTRODUCTION

Previous experiments have shown that when calves under uniform conditions of nutrition, age, sex and housing are inoculated with a single dose of 100 000 *Cooperia* spp. larvae, they show a marked variation in resistance, as measured by parasitological parameters and antibody titres. This variation is partly genetically determined (Albers, 1980; Kloosterman et al., 1978).

In these experiments there was an indication that the most resistant animals showed the greatest growth depression after primary infection. This is in agreement with the results of Riffkin and Dobson (1979) who worked with *Haemonchus contortus* infection in sheep and measured resistance by stimulation of lymphocytes with parasite-antigen. Because in earlier experiments only *Cooperia* spp. larvae were used and infections were rather short-lived, it could not be decided whether such resistance had any effect on the growth performance of calves under field conditions, i.e. continuous infections with several species during an entire grazing season.

It is possible that the growth depression of resistant animals is of short duration and that after prolonged, repeated infections resistant animals have ultimately some advantage. Therefore, the following experiment was carried out.

MATERIALS AND METHODS

Calves

Fifty-one calves, born within one week, were bought and reared at the University farm. At the age of 3 months the calves weighed approximately 95 kg and were on a ration of 2 kg concentrates/d and hay *ad libitum*. They remained on that diet for the further period indoors.

Parasites

Faeces of donor calves were mixed with wood shavings and cultured for 9 days at 27°C. The infective larvae were stored for 4 weeks at 4°C.

Cooperia spp. larvae consisted of approximately 70% *Cooperia onchophora* and 30% *C. surnabada*. *Ostertagia* spp. larvae were obtained from the Central Veterinary Institute, Department of Parasitology, at Lelystad. They consisted of 97% *O. ostertagi* and 3% *O. lyrata* (Borgsteede, personal communication).

Egg counts

Egg counts were done three times a week during the housing period, starting 15 days after primary infection. During the pasture period egg counts were performed once per week.

Antibody titres

Weekly serum samples were taken and antibodies were measured by the ELISA technique, using a saline extract of fourth stage larvae of *Cooperia* spp. Details of the method and the results obtained with extracts of adults, third stage larvae and fourth stage larvae of *Cooperia* spp. and *Ostertagia* spp. will be published elsewhere.

In the present paper the antibody titre against *Cooperia* L4, found at 5 weeks after primary infection, is used as a parameter for resistance.

Weight gains

The animals were weighed once a week. The daily gains during the various periods were calculated by taking the mean of three successive weighings at the start and at the end of the period in order to minimise the effects of weighing errors.

Experimental design

A primary infection with 100 000 *Cooperia* spp. larvae was given to determine the resistance of the calves. Twelve resistant

and 12 non-resistant animals were selected from the total of
51 animals on the basis of egg counts at days 17, 20, 22, 24
and 27 after infection. Egg output was the only measure for
resistance that could be used, because at that time antibody
titres were not yet available. Five of the remaining 27 animals
were chosen at random and used as controls. The animals were
treated twice with omnizole* on day 28 and 35 after primary
infection. The resistant and non-resistant calves were sub-
divided and infected every Monday, Wednesday and Friday with
larval numbers corresponding to daily doses of 25 000 *Cooperia*
spp., of 2 500 *Ostertagia* spp. or of 25 000 *Cooperia* spp. + 2 500
Ostertagia spp. according to the 2 x 3 factorial design given in
Table 1.

TABLE 1

THE EXPERIMENTAL DESIGN APPLIED DURING 7 WEEKS OF CONTINUOUS INFECTIONS.

Type of infection	*Cooperia* spp.	*Ostertagia* spp.	Mixed	Total
Number of resistant animals	4	4	4	12
Number of non-resistant animals	4	4	4	12
	8	8	8	24

For larval doses see text.

The course of the experiment

After 7 weeks of continuous infection, during which only
transient clinical signs such as diarrhoea, anorexia and depressed growth were observed in several animals, the calves
appeared to recover. To achieve more severe infections the
experimental calves, including the controls, were turned out
to pasture. They were grazed rotationally on 3 paddocks of

* A paste formulation of Thiabendazole, Merck Sharpe & Dohme Nederland B.V.,
Haarlem, The Netherlands.

about 1 ha each for 10 weeks. The pasture had carried no cattle
in the last two years. Ewes with lambs had been grazing on it
in the spring and the ewes had been treated with anthelmintic
at lambing time. The rotation of the calves was designed to
provoke auto-infection rather than to avoid it.

RESULTS

Egg counts

The criterion of selection of resistant and non-resistant
animals was by egg counts and it was not surprising that egg
counts differed between these groups after primary infection
(Figure 1). Mean peak egg counts of 1 200 and 8 000 epg were
reached by these groups respectively. After the first anthelmintic treatment, the egg output remained at 300 epg and after
a second treatment it decreased to a mean of 150 epg. Three
weeks after the start of continuous infections, egg counts rose
to a peak of 1 900 epg and 600 epg in non-resistant and resistant animals respectively. This difference was significant
(P < 0.05). The egg counts of the calves receiving mixed
infections were further analysed by means of larval differen-
tiations. Comparison of these results with the egg output of
pure infections of *Cooperia* spp. or *Ostertagia* spp. gave no
indication that the presence of one parasite species influenced
the fecundity of the other.

After being placed on pasture, the continuously infected
animals maintained the same level of egg output but the control
animals showed a significant increase in egg counts approximately
5 weeks after introduction onto pasture.

Antibody titres

At five weeks after primary infection, the antibody titre
against *Cooperia* L4 antigen differed significantly between
resistant and non-resistant animals (P < 0.05).

536

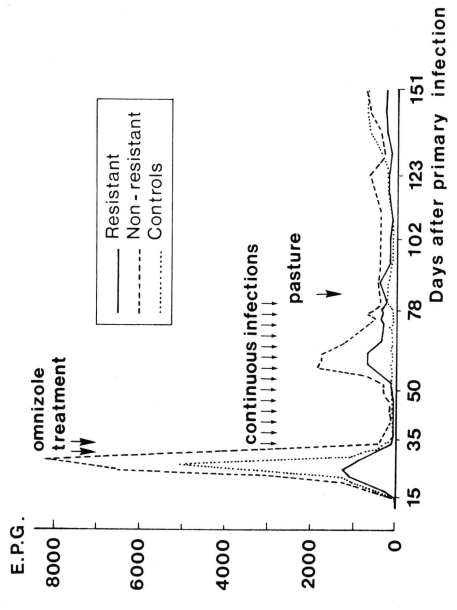

Fig. 1: The egg output of calves.

Weight gains

Table 2 shows the live weight gains of calves for the
various periods under study. Before infection (period 1) a
significant better weight gain (P < 0.05) was found in resistant
animals than in non-resistant and control animals. After infection (periods 2, 3 and 4) no significant differences between
resistant and non-resistant animals were found. The resistant
animals, however, maintained a slightly better weight gain
throughout the entire experimental period. The small growth
depression after primary infection was significantly larger
for resistant animals than for non-resistant and control animals.

During continuous infection the controls and the *Ostertagia*
spp. infected animals gained significantly better than calves
infected with *Cooperia* spp. and mixed species. At pasture the
weight gain was poor. Severe clinical signs were seen in several
animals.

As well as comparing the growth of the resistant and
non-resistant groups of animals it is possible also to examine
correlations between growth and resistance characteristics of
individual animals. This may be a more sensitive measure for
the relation between resistance and performance, especially
when the variation within groups is large. These correlations
are presented in Table 3. Two remarks should be made.
Firstly, during continuous infections (period 3) the control
and *Ostertagia* spp. infected animals had higher weight
gains than *Cooperia* spp. and mixed infected calves. At
pasture the controls, and to a lesser extent the *Ostertagia* spp.
infected animals, had the poorest gains. The effect of infection
on weight gain in period 3 had nothing to do with resistance
and was compensated in period 4. Therefore, it was decided to
take the total weight gain in periods 3 and 4 for correlation
between resistance and growth. Secondly, the resistance of
animals was measured by egg output and antibody response after
primary infection. Because these parameters were negatively
correlated (r = -0.44) a new, possibly more sensitive parameter

TABLE 2

THE DAILY GAIN (g/d) DURING VARIOUS PERIODS. STANDARD DEVIATIONS ARE GIVEN BETWEEN BRACKETS.

Resistance	Type of infection in period 3	Number of animals	Daily weight gain in period			
			1	2	3	4
Resistant	*Cooperia*	4	1092 (53)	1040 (161)	849 (110)	366 (178)
	Ostertagia	4	1045 (81)	972 (127)	967 (122)	612 (216)
	Mixed	4	1040 (81)	968 (99)	910 (206)	405 (210)
	Mean	12	1050 (70)	993 (124)	909 (147)	461 (215)
Non-resistant	*Cooperia*	4	929 (104)	1000 (142)	823 (152)	564 (39)
	Ostertagia	4	941 (142)	995 (72)	1010 (209)	286 (190)
	Mixed	4	963 (117)	930 (55)	796 (138)	360 (226)
	Mean	12	944 (112)	975 (94)	876 (182)	403 (198)
Control	Control	5	920 (153)	965 (88)	1069 (52)	344 (45)

Period 1 – 3 weeks before primary infection.
Period 2 – 3 weeks after primary infection (100 000 *Cooperia* sp.).
Period 3 – 7 weeks of continuous infections.
Period 4 – 10 weeks on pasture.

TABLE 3

COEFFICIENTS OF CORRELATION BETWEEN WEIGHT GAINS DURING VARIOUS PERIODS AND RESISTANCE CHARACTERISTICS OF 29 CALVES

	Weight gain in period			E	A	A/E
	1	2	3 + 4			
Weight gain period 1	—	0.25	0.20	-0.45**	0.32	0.43**
period 2		—	0.21	-0.12	-0.14	0.04
periods 3 + 4			—	-0.31	0.39*	0.40*
Egg counts after primary infection (E)				—	-0.44**	-0.76***
Antibodies after primary infection (A)					—	0.76***
'Resistance' (A/E)						—

* $p < 0.05$
** $p < 0.02$
*** $p < 0.01$

The periods referred to are described under Table 2.

was introduced by expressing resistance as:

$$\frac{\log_2 \text{ antibody titre after primary infection}}{\text{mean of } \sqrt{}\text{-transformed egg counts after primary infection}}$$

From Table 3 it can be seen that positive but non-significant correlations exist between weight gains in the successive periods.

A significant negative correlation was found between growth before infection and egg output after primary infection, while the correlation between pre-infection and growth and antibody titres after infection was positive but not significant.

After primary infection (period 2) these correlations have disappeared, and for antibodies the sign of the correlation coefficient has even changed. During continuous infections and on pasture, the correlation between weight gains and antibody response after primary infection is significantly positive.

DISCUSSION

The absence of an effect of 2 500 *Ostertagia* spp. larvae/d on weight gain is difficult to explain. There is no indication that a less pathogenic strain has been used (Borgsteede, personal communication).

If the primary dose of 100 000 *Cooperia* spp. actually had, in fact, some immunising effect, it is difficult to see why *Ostertagia* spp. would be more effective than *Cooperia* spp.

The good growth performance of infected calves during continuous infections (period 3) must be ascribed to the nutritional level. Similar experiences were obtained by Burden et al. (1978) and we agree with these authors that factors other than additive worm burdens are important for the expression of disease under field conditions.

The poor growth at pasture was partly due to the fact that calves had to learn to graze. But in the latter half of the pasture period, it was clear that auto-infection of calves had occurred. This could be concluded not only from the rise of egg counts in control animals, but also from their antibody titres. During continous infections these were maintained at the same level from 5 weeks after primary infection. The same was observed for anti-*Cooperia* L4 titres in *Ostertagia* spp. infected calves. About 6 weeks after introduction into pasture, the titres of control and *Ostertagia* spp. calves rose to the levels which *Cooperia* spp. and mixed infected animals had already reached during continuous infections.

With respect to the relation between resistance and growth performance, the following conclusions were drawn: resistance is positively related to weight gain before infection. It might be concluded that animals with a good potential for growth are also better able to mount an antibody response and to keep egg counts at a lower level than calves with a poorer growth potential. If animals with a good growth performance continue to grow better, regardless of the circumstances, the positive influence of resistance on weight gain at a later stage of the trial would be simply due to the fact that resistance is an attribute of fast growing animals. That this is not true can be concluded from two facts. Firstly, the growth depression after primary infection is greater for the resistant animals. Secondly, the correlations between growth in periods 3 + 4 and resistance are higher than those between growth in periods 3 + 4 and weight gain in the preceding periods.

The results found after primary infection are in good agreement with results of earlier experiments. Resistant animals show lower egg counts and higher antibody titres but, temporarily, have a greater growth depression than non-resistant animals.

Under continuous infections and on pasture there is a significant positive relation (r = 0.40) between resistance and growth performance.

It is concluded that resistance has a positive effect on weight gain under conditions of infection similar to those occurring in the field. This conclusion is in contrast with that of Riffkin and Dobson (1979). These authors considered only the weight gains after primary infections. We would have reached a similar conclusion if only a restricted period after primary infection had been considered.

It is therefore not justified to state, as Riffkin and Dobson (1979) do, that selection for high production has been into the direction of more susceptible animals. On the contrary, in view of the present results which indicate a positive relation between resistance and performance, it is quite possible that much unconscious selection towards resistance to nematodes has been exerted in the past.

It is doubtful whether deliberate selection for resistance against gastro-intestinal nematodes will be useful. A correlation between resistance and growth performance of r = 0.40 means that only 16% of the variation in growth can be explained by variation in resistance. Only a part of this is genetically determined. In cattle the generation interval is long and the number of offspring is relatively low. On the other hand, it is possible to measure the trait in the male animal, which can be used in large scale artificial insemination programmes.

Finally, it is possible that the parasites can adapt themselves much quicker to changes than man can breed for resistance in his animals.

REFERENCES

Albers, G.A.A., 1980. Genetic resistance to experimental *Cooperia oncophora* infections in calves. Thesis, Wageningen (in preparation).

Burden, D.J., Hughes, D.L., Hammet, N.C. and Collis, K.A., 1978. Concurrent daily infection of calves with *Fasciola hepatica* and *Ostertagia ostertagi*. Res. Vet. Sci., 25, 302-306.

Kloosterman, A., Albers, G.A.A. and van den Brink, R., 1978. Genetic variation among calves in resistance to nematode parasites. Vet. Parasit., 4, 353-368.

Riffkin, G.G. and Dobson, C., 1979. Predicting resistance of sheep to *Haemonchus contortus* infections. Vet. Parasit., 5, 365-378.

DISCUSSION

J. Eckert (*Switzerland*)

As I understand it, you took the measure of resistance
factor calculated from the antibody figure and the egg count
figures. At what time did you compare these two parameters?

A. Kloosterman (*The Netherlands*)

It was after primary infection. The antibody decreased
after primary infection, and the egg counts were the result of
the test infection with *Cooperia*.

J. Eckert

Yes, but I think that the time may be very important.
At what time was this comparison made? If you are comparing
the antibody figures immediately after infection, you may have
no antibody response and it may be some time before the egg
counts are high. What was the exact time used for calculating
this factor?

A. Kloosterman

The egg count was actually the square root transformation
of the egg count after primary infection. The antibody response
was the antibody titre against *Cooperia*, four weeks after this
primary infection. It is better than taking antibodies alone
or taking egg counts alone as a parameter of the system, because
they were always - in all our experiments - negatively correlated.
You cannot make a combination of these two independent parameters
for a system by dividing the antibodies by the egg output.

J. Armour (*UK*)

You use thiabendazole? I wonder if you have considered
the possible effect that thiabendazole has had on the situation,
since there is other work which shows that this increases the
susceptibility of animals to re-infection, certainly in an

experimental situation. I wonder if you would have got a
greater percentage difference between your two groups had you
used levamisole.

A. Kloosterman

I do not think so. If it has an effect on the immune
response or the resistance of the animals, I think it will be
the same for both types of animals.

F.H.M. Borgsteede *(The Netherlands)*

You have selected on the basis of resistance against
Cooperia and you have found some surprising results with respect
to the behaviour of the animals and their weight gain with
experimental infections of *Ostertagia* and *Cooperia*. You thought
that *Ostertagia* would be worse than *Cooperia* and the opposite was
the case. Could you speculate about the possibilities that
you have selected not for *Cooperia* but for *Ostertagia*?

A. Kloosterman

That is an interesting question. In past years we have
always worked with *Cooperia* calf models and we want to general-
ise the interesting results we get in genetical differences in
resistance against *Cooperia*.

R.M. Connan *(UK)*

There is an interesting correlation between the non-resistant group and the fact that animals were also growing better
initially. Results from Queensland, Australia, indicate that
the animals which were more resistant were also the ones which
were not growing. It was really a rather depressing finding.
One selects for resistance and one ends up with an animal which
does not grow well or breed well. I think your results are
encouraging.

INFECTIONS WITH *Cooperia oncophora* IN CALVES

Sv. Aa. Henriksen

State Veterinary Serum Laboratory,
Copenhagen, Denmark

ABSTRACT

Studies on monospecific infections with Cooperia oncophora *in calves have been initiated.*

Five calves, reared indoors, were each inoculated with 250 000 - 750 000 infective larvae. Mild and transient clinical signs were observed in two calves. Six calves were inoculated with 800 000 - 1 800 000 larvae. Three of these died from the infection. Slightly reduced weight gain presumably caused by cooperiosis was observed in a tracer calf turned out in August to graze a paddock contaminated with Cooperia *larvae. Immunity seemed to develop within 1½ - 2½ months following ingestion of 400 000 infective larvae, as judged by obvious resistance to challenge inoculation and simultaneous grazing in a contaminated paddock.*

A prepatent period of 16 - 19 days was recorded. In most calves there was no correlation between number of ingested larvae and faecal egg output. In two calves suffering fatal infections, EPG exceeded 10 000.

P. Nansen, R.J. Jørgensen, E.J.L. Soulsby (eds), Epidemiology and Control of Nematodiasis in Cattle.
Copyright © 1981 ECSC, EEC, EAEC, Brussels – Luxembourg. All rights reserved.

INTRODUCTION

In most countries of north-western Europe the dominant
bovine trichostrongylids are *Ostertagia ostertagi* and *Cooperia onco-*
phora. Most experimental and field studies on bovine trichostrongylid infections have been focused on *O. ostertagi*, whereas
C. oncophora has received little attention being considered a
relatively harmless nematode. Experimental monospecific infection
with *C. oncophora* in calves were initiated with special reference
to conditions in Denmark. Preliminary observations on faecal
egg output, pathogenicity and immunity are presented.

MATERIAL AND METHODS

Two experiments have been carried out, in which calves (Red
Danish Milkbreed) reared under worm-free conditions were inoculate
with infective larvae (L_3) of a Danish strain of *C. oncophora*. The
strain was isolated from a local field case and passaged through
donor calves. The larvae were extracted from faecal cultures
and stored at $15^{\circ}C$ for no longer than two weeks prior to inoculation.

Experiment 1: Eleven calves, 3 - 7 months of age, were dosed
with various numbers of L_3 as specified in Table 1. The calves
were kept indoors and offered a diet of pellets and hay.

Daily clinical examinations were made. In Table 1 clinical
signs of parasitism are graded by a simple scale (+++ indicates
fatal infection).

Examinations on faecal egg output were carried out daily, starting on Day 14 p.i. A modified McMaster technique was employed
(Henriksen and Aagaard, 1976). Data are given in Table 1.

Experiment 2: Four calves ($C_1 - C_4$), 4 - 5 months of age, were
turned out to graze in a parasite-free paddock (0.27 ha) on June
1st, 1979. During the first week the calves were dosed individually, each calf receiving 2 x 200 000 L_3.

From mid-July (cf. Fig 1 A) the calves were challenged fortnightly by inoculation with fairly massive larval doses (ranging
from 200 000 1 400 000 L$_3$). In mid-August a tracer calf (C$_5$,
not inoculated) was turned out to graze in the same paddock.

All calves were weighed at intervals of 2 - 3 weeks, and at the
same time faecal examinations and herbage larval counts were performed. Results from weighings are given in Figure 1 A. for C$_1$ -
C$_4$ (mean) and C$_5$, respectively. Data on faecal egg outputs and
herbage larval counts are given in Figure 1 B. Herbage larval
counts, determined by a modified Baermann technique (Henriksen,
unpublished) were made on samples collected close to faecal pats
and at a distance of >25 cm from them.

RESULTS

Experiment 1: As appears from Table 1, inoculation of five
calves with 250 000 - 720 000 L$_3$ caused no overt clinical signs,
although two calves were passing slightly soft faeces for 2 - 5
days. However, inoculations with 800 000 - 1 800 000 L$_3$ led to
fatal infection in three out of six calves.

In most calves a prepatent period of 16 - 19 days was noted. All
infected calves excreted eggs and peak counts were usually observed 3½ - 6 weeks p.i. There was no obvious correlation between
the number of larvae administered and faecal egg output (max. EPG
varied between 60 and 21 600). Faecal egg output from one calf
(No. 26), inoculated with 1 000 000 L$_3$, was recorded only during
a short period (40 - 42 days p.i.). Two calves suffering fatal
infections, but still alive 4 - 5 weeks p.i., were excreting
large numbers of eggs in the terminal stages (EPG >10 000).

Experiment 2: Clinical signs were observed neither in the four
experimentally infected and subsequently challenged calves nor
in the tracer calf. The mean weight gain of C$_1$ - C$_4$ was rather
constant during the last 3½ months of the experimental period.
The tracer calf had a lower rate of gain and during the last 3
weeks even a slight loss of weight.

Mean faecal egg counts from C_1 - C_4 did not exceed 50 except during the period from 3 - 7 weeks following the initial inoculations. During the rest of the experiment a low-level EPG was constantly recorded. In contrast, the tracer calf exhibited a rapid increase to a peak of 1 860 in September.

Herbage larval counts were negative until mid-July. During the remaining period *Cooperia* larvae were demonstrated constantly. The number of larvae observed in August-September indicated that a fairly moderate contamination of the paddock had been established

DISCUSSION

Cooperia oncophora is generally considered to be rather harmless to cattle, yet, more than 20 years ago, Morgan and Soulsby, (1956) pointed out that *C. oncophora* (together with *C. macmasteri*) might well be of importance in causing enteritis in cattle. Later, Herlich (1965), was able to produce severe enteritis and slight weight loss among a group of Jersey calves (5 - 8 months of age) by inoculating 1 500 000 - 3 000 000 L_3 of *C. oncophora*. No such effect was observed in calves receiving less than 1 500 000 L_3. In recent experiments by Borgsteede and Hendriks (1979) mild and transient diarrhoea and a slight weight gain depression was recorded in calves inoculated with 200 000 L_3 of *C. oncophora*. No signs whatsoever were observed in calves given only 20 000 L_3.

The present experiments would seem to suggest that *C. oncophora* is a parasite with fairly low or moderate pathogenicity: administration of 250 000 - 720 000 L_3 to parasite-free calves produced only clinical signs in a few animals, and the signs were mild and transient. Inoculation of 1 - 2 million larvae, however, resulted in fatal infection in most calves. In this connection one may admit that 1 - 2 million larvae represent extremely high dose levels. Nonetheless, under certain circumstances such numbers of larvae may be present in calf paddocks at the end of the grazing season (Henriksen, unpublished).

The slight weight gain depression in the tracer calf C_5 (not previously exposed to *C. oncophora*) in Experiment 2, could possibly be ascribed to the ingestion of *Cooperia* larvae from the paddock. Thus, Coop et al. (1979) found that dosing of parasite-free calves with *C. oncophora* reduced weight gains by 13.5% without producing obvious clinical signs. The calves in question were inoculated with 5 x 5 000 - 5 x 20 000 L_3 weekly during a 5 months period.

The fact that the permanently grazing calves of Experiment 2 maintained low egg excretion and satisfactory growth rates despite repeated high challenge inoculations and exposure to herbage infection, may suggest development of a strong resistance. This assumption is in agreement with observations by Herlich (1965$_b$), who found that calves given a single inoculation of 32 000 *C. oncophora* larvae developed a strong immunity against challenge inoculations.

A rapid build-up of resistance against intestinal nematodes (*C. oncophora* and *Nematodirus helvetianus*) has also been demonstrated by Smith and Archibald (1968) in calves grazing infected marsh-land pastures and according to Coop et al. (1979) resistance to *C. oncophora* can develop within 8 -'10 weeks.

A prepatent period of 16 - 19 days and peak egg outputs $3\frac{1}{2}$ - 6 weeks p.i. largely correspond with observations made by Isenstein (1963), Herlich (1965) and Coop et al. (1979). The obvious lack of correlation between larval dose size and faecal egg output, seems to be in accordance with many observations on trichostrongylid infections.

The extremely low egg output recorded for one calf (No. 26) may perhaps be viewed in the light of the experiments of Klooster-man et al. (1978) on genetic variations in resistance to *Cooperia* spp within a group of calves (Dutch Friesian).

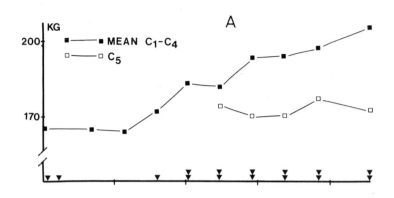

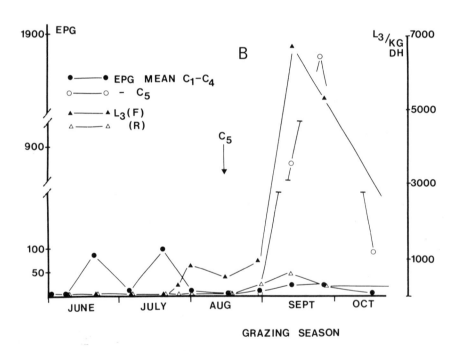

Fig. 1. A.   Weight curves. Each arrow indicates individual dosing of C_1 - C_4 with 200 000 L_3.

B.   Faecal egg outputs and herbage larval counts (DH: dry herbage). F: larval counts close to faecal pats. R: Larval counts at random places distant from faecal pats.

TABLE 1

CALVES ARTIFICIALLY INFECTED WITH *Cooperia oncophora*. DESIGN OF THE EXPERIMENTS AND RECORDING OF FAECAL EGG COUNTS

Calf No.	Total	Dosing scheme /period days	Clin. signs/ days p.i.	Days p.i.	Faecal egg output EPG Max/day p.i.
15	250 000	25 x 10 000 /25	-	20 - (56)*	2 430/38
16	250 000	25 x 10 000 /25	+/25 - 28	18 - 58	600/22
14	300 000	30 x 10 000 /30	-	17 - 44	1 650/27
17	420 000	14 x 30 000 /14	-	18 - (48)*	975/29
19	720 000	24 x 30 000 /31	+/45 - 47	18 - (49)*	2 970/39
24	800 000	8 x 100 000 /17	++/30 - 44	18 - 65	5 160/26
23	1 000 000	10 x 100 000 /22	++/29 - 44	19 - 62	1 200/25
26	1 000 000	10 x 100 000 /22	++/20 - 25	40 - 41	60/41
25	1 000 000	4 x 250 000 /8	+++/16 - (38)**	17 - (38)	(21 600/33)
22	1 200 000	12 x 100 000 /12	+++/26 - (38)**	16 - (38)	(10 200/37)
21	1 800 000	18 x 100 000 /18	+++/17 - (23)**	17 - (23)	(3 660/23)

*) Faecal egg output still manifest at slaughter.
**) Calves killed in extremis

CONCLUSIONS

The prepatent period is 16 - 19 days. There is usually lack of correlation between larval intake and faecal egg output.

Cooperia oncophora is a parasite of fairly low to moderate pathogenicity. However, by ingestion of 1 - 2 million infective larvae, fatal infections may be produced in susceptible calves.

Immunity seems to develop within 1½ - 2½ months following the ingestion of fairly large numbers of infective larvae.

REFERENCES

Borgsteede, F.H.M. and Hendriks, J. 1979. Experimental infections with *Cooperia oncophora* (Railliet, 1918) in calves. Results of single infections with two graded dose levels of larvae. Parasitology, 78, 331-342

Coop, R.L., Sykes, A.R. and Angus, K.W. 1979. The pathogenicity of daily intakes of *Cooperia oncophora* larvae in growing calves. Vet. Parasitol. 5, 261-269

Henriksen, Sv. Aa. and Aagaard, K. 1976. En enkel flotations- og McMaster metode. (A simple flotation and McMaster method). Nord. Vet.-Med., 28, 392-397

Herlich, H. 1965a. The effects of the intestinal worms, *Cooperia pectinata* and *Cooperia oncophora*, on experimentally infected calves. Am. J. Vet. Res., 26, 1032-1036

Herlich, H. 1965b. Immunity and cross immunity to *Cooperia oncophora* and *Cooperia pectinata* in calves and lambs. Am. J. Vet. Res., 26, 1037-1041

Isenstein, R.S. 1963. The life history of *Cooperia oncophora* (Railliet, 1898), Ransom, (1907), a nematode parasite of cattle. J. Parasitology, 49, 235-240

Kloosterman, A., Albers, G.A.A. and van den Brink, R. 1978. Genetic variation among calves in resistance to nematode parasites. Vet. Parasitol. 4, 353-368

Morgan, D.O. and Soulsby, E.J.L. 1956. New records of nematodes in British cattle. Vet. Rec., 68, 1029

Smith, H.J. and Archibald, R. McG. 1968. Experimental helminthiasis in parasite-free calves on marshland pastures. Can. Vet. J., 9, 46-55

ACKNOWLEDGEMENT

The author is grateful to Miss L. Hinz for skilful technical assistance. The study was supported by Grant No. 513-10026 from The Danish Agricultural and Veterinary Research Council.

DISCUSSION

E.J.L. Soulsby *(UK)*

Many years ago when I was at the University of Bristol, it seemed to me that *Cooperia oncophora* was a serious problem in young cattle in the south-west of England. Do any of the delegates from Britain have any comments on this?

J. Armour *(UK)*

In a study of the pathogenicity of *Cooperia oncophora*, Dr. Frank Jennings and I gave doses of up to a million without producing any clinical signs. This was a Scottish strain of *Cooperia oncophora*. A single dose of one million larvae produced a very mild softening of the faeces.

J. Eckert *(Switzerland)*

Did you see any evidence of self-cure reaction in these infections? Sometimes we have observed with artificial infections with *Cooperia punctata* that the egg counts drop very quickly after re-infection. This indicates that the wormburden had been eliminated rapidly. Did you observe a similar phenomenon with *Cooperia oncophora*?

Sv. Aa. Henriksen *(Denmark)*

In some instances there might have been such an effect, but our evidence is not strong.

R.J. Jørgensen *(Denmark)*

Could you just mention the most important lesions you found at postmortem in these infections?

Sv. Aa. Henriksen

There were marked pathological changes in the first part of the duodenum and the first part of the jejunum. There was necrosis and oedamatous changes in the mesenteric lymph nodes and mesentery.

EXPERIMENTS WITH MIXED INFECTIONS OF *Ostertagia ostertagi* AND *Fasciola hepatica* IN CALVES

H.J. Over, F.H.M. Borgsteede, Y.I.E.A. Wetzlar,
and J.N. v.d. Linden

Central Veterinary Institute, Department of Parasitology,
Edelhertweg 13, Lelystad, The Netherlands.

INTRODUCTION

An attempt was made in 1977 to simulate the Fascioliasis/ Ostertagiasis complex in young cattle (Reid et al., 1967). An experiment was designed that was assumed to be related to the conditions in the field. A comparable and parallel experiment was performed at Compton, the results of which were published by Burden et al. (1978). Their conclusions, in some respects, are inconsistent with the observations reported in this paper.

EXPERIMENTS

We assumed in the Netherlands, on fluke farms, that calves will ingest high numbers of *F. hepatica* metacercariae and third stage *O. ostertagia* larvae during the three months prior to stabling (i.e. August, September - October). Reid et al. (1967) and Urquhart and Armour (1973) have described pathological changes consisting of a reduced size of the liver and distended, thickened and calcified bile ducts occurring in animals in the winter following the original infection, this being a period of 100 days after infection. Consequently this trial was continued to the stage when chronic fasioliasis might be expected to occur for i.e. 4 months. The *F. hepatica* infection level was selected to ensure that chronic fascioliasis with consequent morbidity developed. The *O. ostertagi* infection level was selected for similar reasons. The design of the experiment is given in Table 1.

P. Nansen, R.J. Jørgensen, E.J.L. Soulsby (eds), Epidemiology and Control of Nematodiasis in Cattle.

TABLE 1

Group	Number of Animals	Daily dose days 1 - 100		Autopsy day	Mean weight gain %	Mean worm burden at autopsy			
						O. ostertagi		F. hepatica	
		Oo	Fh			ad.	EL4	ad.	juv.
1	3	5 000	–	217	139	4 730	14 670	–	–
2	3	–	100	217	167	–	–	144	168
3	3	5 000	100	131*, 148*, 217	122**	13 400**	14 400	297**	148
4	3	–	–	217	194	–	–	–	–

* Killed in extremis

** Surviving animal

At the start of the infection the male Friesian--
Holstein calves were 3 months of age. Prior to and over the
course of the trial they were kept under conditions which
precluded reinfection and they were fed a ration which would
produce an average weekly growth of 5 kg in normal animals.

RESULTS

Day 1 - 75; Phase I

Faecal egg output: Egg output of the *O. ostertagi* infected
animals showed the characteristic pattern. In group 1 it was
somewhat lower than in group 3. Populations of *F. hepatica* had
not reached the patent stage.

Serum enzymes: GLDH and γGt increased significantly in
groups 2 and 3 and pepsinogen in groups 1 and 3.

Haematology: During the first 10 weeks no differences
were observed in the red cell parameters between groups. The
mean number of leucocytes in the fluke infected groups rose
sharply from 2 weeks p.i., particularly the percentage of
eosinophils increased and the percentage of lymphocytes
decreased. In group 1 a slight increase in the percentage of
eosinophils was observed. Total protein in all infected groups
increased concomitantly with a change in the globulin/albumin
ratio.

Serology: Differences in the antibody titres in the
F. hepatica or *O. ostertagi* groups were not evident.

Weight gains: Only groups 1 and 3 showed a depression in
liveweight gain.

Day 75 - 150; Phase II

Faecal egg output: In this period in the *O. ostertagi* infected
animals (group 1) epg dropped. In group 3 animals the epg of
the surviving animal showed the same pattern but with the two

560

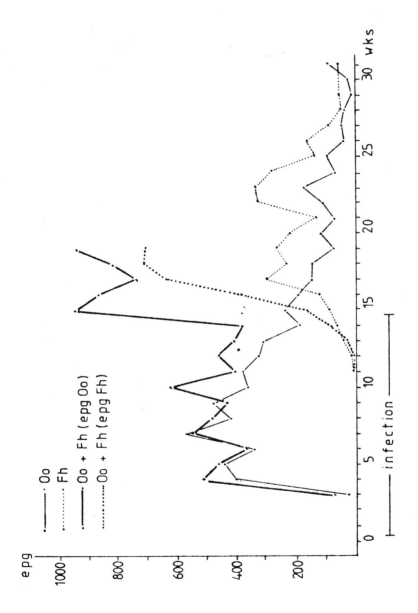

Fig. 1.

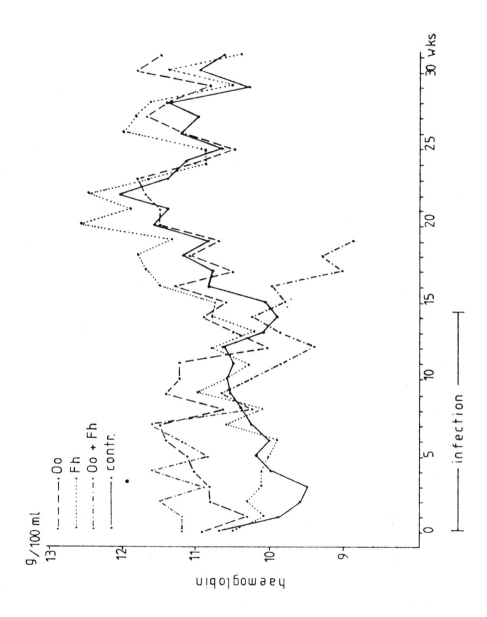

Fig. 2.

animals which succumbed to the infection, the egg output
continued to increase until the animals died. There were no
differences during the prepatent period in *F. hepatica* infected
animals between groups 2 and 3. Egg output was characteristic
and highest values were observed in animals that died (Figure 1).

Serum enzymes: There was no difference between groups for
GLD- and γGt-values or pepsinogen levels.

Haematology: During this period, differences between
group 3 and other groups were marked and two animals in group 3
had to be killed due to increasing anaemia (Figure 2). No
differences were noted between the other groups. In groups 2
and 3 leucocytosis was noticed particularly in the animal
killed first. On the other hand the second animal in this
group showed below normal leucocyte values.

Serology: Low titres against *F. hepatica* as well as against
O. ostertagi were obtained.

Weight gains: In this period group 1 resumed growth.
Group 2 showed a diminished growth rate and in group 3 only,
the surviving animal showed an increase in liveweight.

Day 150 - 217; Phase III

Faecal egg output: Egg output of both *O. ostertagi* and
F. hepatica infected animals decreased in all animals.

Serum enzymes: GLDH- and γGt-values dropped considerably,
similarly the pepsinogen values in group 1 fell.

Haematology: During this period there was an increasing
tendency for anaemia in the fluke infected animals. In group 1
values returned to normal. Leucocytosis was still apparent in
fluke infected animals but values in group 1 returned to normal.

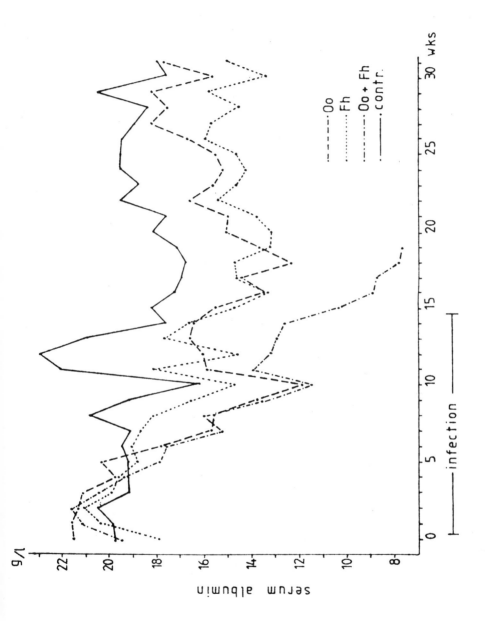

Fig. 3.

564

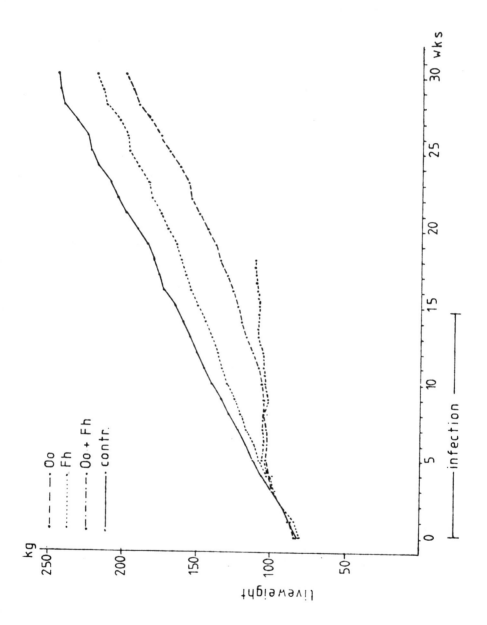

Fig. 4.

Total protein was normal as well as the globulin/albumin ratio in group 1 animals. In fluke infected animals, total protein continued to increase accompanied by hypoalbuminaemia particularly in the surviving animal in group 3.

Serology: Antibody titres over this period remained at a nearly constant level.

Weight gains: Liveweight increase in group 1 was higher than in group 2. The remaining animal in group 3 grew comparably to the fluke infected group.

DISCUSSION

In this experiment the differences between the development of disease in animals infected with *O. ostertagi* and *F. hepatica* were obvious. Both single species infected groups provided classical examples of the course of ostertagiasis and chronic fascioliasis respectively.

It is assumed that the clinical cases in the mixed infected group resulted from the combined action of the two parasite populations.

On the basis of worm counts and differential development there is some indication that in the mixed infected group the presence of adult worms was prolonged compared with the other groups. This resulted in an increased physiological change. The experiment indicated that a synergistic effect might occur between the two parasite infections, but even an additive effect in Fascioliasis/Ostertagiasis complex is sufficient reason for the course of the infection.

566

REFERENCES

Burden, D.J., Hughes, D.L., Hammet, N.C. and Collis, K.A., 1978. Con-
     current daily infection of calves with *Fasciola hepatica* and
     Ostertagi ostertagi. Res. Vet. Sci., 1978, 25, 302-306.
Reid, J.F.S., Armour, J., Jennings, F.W., Kirkpatrick, K.S. and Urquhart,
     G.M., 1967. The Fascioliasis/Ostertagiasis complex in young cattle:
     A guide to diagnosis and therapy. Vet. Rec., 80, 371-374.
Urquhart, G.M. and Armour, J. (ed)., 1973. Helminth Diseases of Cattle,
     Sheep and Horses in Europe, 98-100.

DISCUSSION

P. Nansen *(Denmark)*

The eosinophilia was of interest. There was no additive
effect in the double infection? We have seen this in the
Schistosoma and *Fasciola* double infections. There, the eosinophil
counts were lower in double infections than in single infections.

H.J. Over *(The Netherlands)*

Was that a combination of schistosomes and flukes?

P. Nansen

Yes. I have another question. We often find it hard to
interpret the faecal egg counts. Your double infected animals
are going rather poorly and probably have a reduced feed intake
as well. Do you think that the volume of faeces going out is very
limited, so that this might be responsible for the high egg counts?

H.J. Over

Yes. The fluke populations were rather comparable.
Animals dying at 16 - 20 weeks after infection had fluke burdens
that we did not think were of any great significance. Another
point of interest is that the portal lymph nodes in the two
animals that died (at approximately 17 weeks PI) were as in a
normal control animal, these animals had not responded.

J.F. Michel *(UK)*

The animals with *Ostertagia* alone showed the characteristic
egg count pattern. With addition of fluke infection you seemed
to break the normal restraints on egg output. It is a matter
of speculation as to what causes the restriction of egg output
of the entire population. I note you were giving 5 000
Ostertagia larvae a day and, in a proportion of the animals, I
would expect the egg count you obtained even without fluke
infection. It seems to me that it needed just a small extra
bit of infection to tip them over the edge.

H.J. Over

It is always difficult to have sufficient time and
animals. to produce a good solution with regard to that. If
there had been no effect we would have said, "Forget about
Fasciola/Ostertagia in this respect".

TOXOCARIASIS OF CATTLE IN BELGIUM

D. Thienpont and H. De Keyser
Janssen Pharmaceutica,
B-2340 Beerse, Belgium.

ABSTRACT

Toxocara vitulorum *infection in calves has been diagnosed in several European and in most subtropical and tropical countries. All breeds of cattle are susceptible to infection which is transmitted from cow to calf by the transmammary route. The infective larvae, present in the colostrum, develop directly to adult parasites in the calf. Clinical signs of disease depend on the wormburden and may cause severe enteritis and even death. In herds where toxocariasis is prevalent, a treatment with levamisole is indicated for the calf and the cow. The possibility of transmission to man to produce visceral larva migrans should be considered.*

P. Nansen, R.J. Jørgensen, E.J.L. Soulsby (eds), Epidemiology and Control of Nematodiasis in Cattle.
Copyright © 1981 ECSC, EEC, EAEC, Brussels – Luxembourg. All rights reserved.

INTRODUCTION

Some nematodes are able to undergo transmammary migration.
For example, Olsen and Lyons (1965) demonstrated the transmission of hookworm in fur seals via the milk. In cattle, the
nematode *Toxocara vitulorum* may become more widespread, because by
changing farming methods, suckling calves are exposed to this
nematode infection. The infection may pose a new zoonosis
problem since there are reasons to believe that *Toxocara*
vitulorum can be responsible for the condition of visceral larva
migrans in man.

PREVALENCE OF TOXOCARIASIS IN CATTLE

Though textbooks of parasitology consider this disease
a minor problem, it has been diagnosed in Western Europe in
Belgium, Germany and Italy and it also occurs in Hungary,
Yugoslavia, Rumania and USSR, where it is prevalent. Under
African and Asian cattle husbandry conditions the prevalence
of *T. vitulorum* in young calves is high to very high (Table 1).
Warren (1971) reported the parasite on a number of farms in
New South Wales in Australia and Thienpont (1977) has reported
the infection in cattle in Belgium.

TABLE 1

PREVALENCE OF *T. vitulorum* IN CATTLE

Country	Age	Animal Number	% infection
Yugoslavia	Calves	2 375	0 to 40
Yugoslavia	Calves	320	29
Egypt	Calves	2 261	66.7
	Young	962	4.1
	Adults	1 106	2.7
Tchad	Calves	163	18.4
Nigeria	Calves	91	89
Rwanda	Calves	420	22.8

Prevalence studies of the parasite are rare. Selim (1974) published data for 4 329 buffalo cattle, which showed that infection was high in young calves, but low in heifers or cows. From our own observations in Central-Africa (Rwanda and Burundi) the prevalence is probably under-estimated and the prevalence figure for Rwanda needs to be evaluated.

It is not known whether the calves from a first, a second or a later pregnancy are less or more sensitive to infection. Studies on acquired immunity in this infection would be very interesting.

Other animal species may be infected by adult *T. vitulorum*, these include the sheep (Macchioni, 1973; Matov and Vassilev, 1958) and goat (Vassilev, 1959). In Belgium, ascariasis of sheep is occasionally observed but it is due to *Ascaris suum* in the majority of cases.

SUSCEPTIBILITY OF CATTLE BREEDS

Various breeds of cattle and buffalo are susceptible to infection. For example it was observed in Ankole cattle in Rwanda (Thienpont unpublished data) it has been described in bison calves in Hungary (Tanyi and Kudrun, 1967; Tanyi and Danko, 1967). It is more common in buffalo than in cattle (Travassos and Lacombe, 1959) and Da Silva (1969) described the parasite in the water buffalo. Hasche et al. (1962) found the parasite in the USA in a Jersey calf and Enyenihi (1969a) and Troncy and Oumate (1973) found zebu cattle infected in Nigeria. In Belgium the infection has been observed only in Limousin cattle imported from France, where the disease is undiagnosed (Euzeby, 1963). The Limousin animals were imported as pregnant heifers and infection was detected in new-born calves. In Hungary, Nador (1975) reported that the disease was introduced by the importation of infected calves.

PATHOLOGY

Clinical signs have not been reported in adult animals except by Shoho (1970) who emphasises the extremely high eosinophilia, up to 70%. Pregnant animals become infected after ingestion of infective eggs containing a L_2 larva. Based on the life cycle, the major lesions are found in the intestinal wall, the lungs and the mammary gland of the pregnant cow.

In experimentally infected laboratory animals granulo-matous lesions caused by the presence of living larvae are found in the liver, the kidney, the lungs and the lymph nodes. In chickens, mice and guinea-pigs, the larvae are initially concentrated in the liver (Enyenihi, 1969b; Atallah et al., 1974) but later on they occur in the muscles (Warren, 1971).

These lesions are comparable to those associated with larvae of *T. canis*. Hence a clear relation exists between both parasites: thus they are pathogenic for the foetus or young animals, transmission occurs during the pregnancy, and parasites belonging to the same family and genus. Thus, one must expect that *T. vitulorum* may be pathogenic for man and farmers and veterinarians may be exposed to infection. The pathology in the calf has been described by Enyenihi (1969a) (Nigeria), Rai et al. (1971) (India) and by Thienpont et al. (1977) (Belgium).

The major pathology is observed in 2- to 3-month-old calves. Gastro-intestinal lesions are characterised by diarrhoea or steatorrhoea. Other signs are intestinal obstruction, colics, and evil smelling faeces. Toxemia with fever and allergic symptoms may occur. Anemia and poor weight gain are secondary effects.

Spontaneous worm explusion is observed frequently. Infection levels vary greatly. Selim and Tawfik (1966) found 70 to 500 worms pro calf. While Tanyi and Kudrun (1967) and Tanyi and Danko (1967) reported 572 worms in an animal.

Srivastava (1963) mentions 400 worms in the intestine. However, in older calves the worm burden decreases markedly and by the age of one year, most animals are negative as assessed by faecal examination.

LIFE CYCLE

The egg of *T. vitulorum* is similar to that of *T. canis* of dogs and *T. cati* of cats. The chitinous layer is typical for each species and specific identification is possible using the conventional light microscope.

Under optimal conditions the eggs become infective within 15 days and contain an L_2 larva. The embryonated egg is highly resistant to the common disinfectants and even to diluted sulphuric acid. The egg may remain viable for at least 2 years.

Ingestion of infective eggs by calves or young animals does not result in a patent infection. The larvae so acquired probably remains dormant in the parenchymatous organs, but in pregnant animals the larvae migrate from the intestine by a heart-lung-heart migration and are distributed all over the body as L_3 larvae. From eight months onwards they start to migrate again and reach the placenta and from there the amniotic fluid. Oral ingestion of larvae by the foetus permits the larvae to reach the stomach and afterwards the intestine, where they grow to adult worms after the birth of the calf (Mozgovoi and Shikhov, 1971; Mozgovoi et al., 1975).

However, the major number of larvae migrate to the mammary gland. Prior to birth the larvae accumulate in the colostrum and after birth are found in the secreted milk (Warren, 1971). Shoho (1970) showed that two types of larvae can be found in milk; on day 4 after parturition a larva with a dorsally bent tail and on day 11 after parturition the larvae have a straight tail. The transmammary migration of course is not specific for *T. vitulorum*; it has been described for *T. canis* in dogs, *Strongyloides ransomi* in pigs and *Uncinaria lucasi* in fur seals (Figure 2).

574

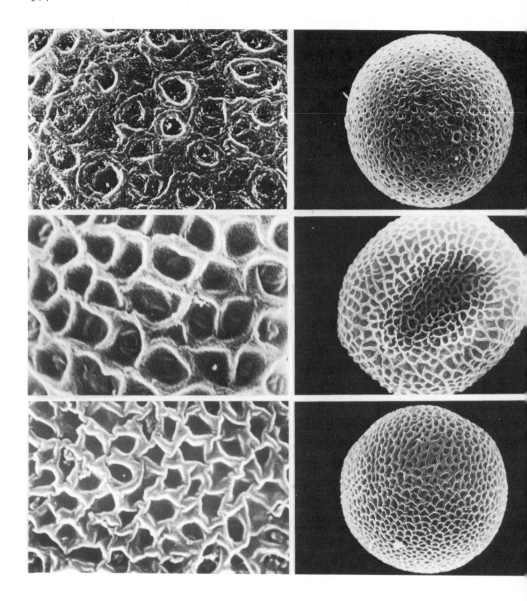

Fig. 1. Scanning microscopy of

a and b: *T. vitulorum*

c and d: *T. canis*

e and f: *T. cati*

General view (x 1 250) and close-up of cuticle (x 5 000).

Warren (1971) was able to prevent infection by
foster feeding of a new-born calf derived from an artifically
infected cow on a normal cow, but reciprocally, he produced
infection in a calf born of a normal cow, but foster fed on an
infected cow.

The L_3 larvae reach the intestine of the suckling calf,
here they rapidly moult to L_4 and L_5 and become adult male or
female worms. The egg production capability is enormous and
may reach 8×10^6 eggs daily per female worm. Egg-counts as
a result may be very high and epg of 100 000 or more are not
rare. The life span of the adult worms is short. Natural
expulsion starts as early as 37 to 38 days after birth. The
epg counts of young cattle are usually low but information on
the number of worms at post-mortem or in slaughter-houses are
not available.

MODE OF INFECTION

The life cycle of *T. vitulorum* is quite distinct from
that of the other common nematodes of cattle. The method of
rearing of calves under European conditions is different to
that followed by African and Asian cattle breeding systems, but
when transmission from cow to calf becomes optimal as in
suckling calves during the first days of birth. Then it is
probable the parasite will become more prevalent. The
economical aspects of beef production favour the suckling
of calves and because of this infection with *T. vitulorum* may
constitute a problem for this type of livestock farming. Oral
amniotic infection of the foetus is probably of minor
importance.

TREATMENT

So long as the exact life cycle was unknown, the
chemotherapy perforce is limited to the patent stage of
infection. Infections are found in the early weeks after
birth, when bacterial or viral infections are common, but an

576

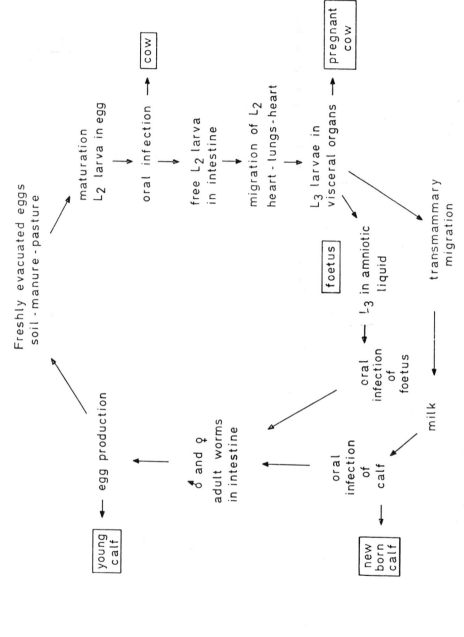

Fig. 2. Life cycle of *T. vitulorum*.

accurate diagnosis of *T. vitulorum* can be made only by copro-
logical examination.

Different treatments have been proposed. It is important
in case of bovine toxocariasis that a systemic anthelmintic
should be used and administered to the calf as well as to the
cow. The following have been suggested: Neguvon or Rametin
(Stamp, 1968), Haloxon (Ikeme, 1970), Piperazine (Tripathi,
1967; Tanyi and Kudrun, 1967; Tanyi and Danko, 1967),
Morantel (Troncy and Oumate, 1973), Fenbendazole (Gautam et
al., 1976). Levamisole was used by Shikhov (1971) and
Thienpont et al. (1977).

ACKNOWLEDGEMENT

This investigation was supported by a grant from the
'Instituut tot Aanmoediging van het Wetenschappelijk Onderzoek
in Nijverheid en Landbouw' (IWONL).

578

REFERENCES

Atallah, O.A., Mossalem, I. and Abdel-Rahman, M.S., 1974. Visceral larva
   migrans of *Neoascaris vitulorum* in laboratory animals. Acta Veter-
   inaria Acadamiae Scientiarum Hungaricae, 24, 207-220.
Burger, H.J., 1973. Helminth diseases of cattle, sheep and horses in
   Europe. Eds. G.M. Urquhart and J. Armour. Editor MacLehose.
Chauhan, P.P.S. and Pande, B.P., 1972. Migratory behaviour and histo-
   pathology of *Neoascaris vitulorum* larvae in Albino mice. Indian
   Journal of Experimental Biology, 10, 193-200.
Chauhan, P.P.S., Agrawal, R.D. and Ahluwalia, S.S., 1974. A note on the
   presence of *Strongyloides papillosus* and *Neoascaris vitulorum* in the
   milk of buffaloes. Current Science, 43, 486-487.
Chauhan, P.P.S., Bhattia, B.B., Arora, G.S. and Agrawal, R.D., 1977. A note
   on migratory behaviour of *Neoascaris vitulorum* larvae in Albino rat
   and chicken; a histological study. Indian Journal of Animal Sciences,
   44, 801-804.
Cvetkovic, L. and Nevenic, V., 1960. Epizootiology of *Neoascaris vitulorum*
   in calves. Acta Veterinaria, 10, 49-59.
Doughty, F.R., 1972. *Toxocara vitulorum* infection in calves in Northern
   New South Wales. Australian Veterinary Journal, 48, 62-63.
El-Sherry, M.I. and Tawfik, M.A.A., 1975. The pathology of experimental
   infestation of *Neoascaris vitulorum* in guinea-pigs. Assiut Veterinary
   Medical Journal 1, 47-59.
Enyenihi, U.K., 1969a. Studies on the epizootiology of *Neoascaris vitulorum*
   in Nigeria. Journal of Helminthology, 43, 3-10.
Enyenihi, U.K., 1969b. Pathogenicity of *Neoascaris vitulorum* infections in
   calves. Bulletin Epizootic Diseases in Africa, 17, 171-178.
Enyenihi, U.K., 1971. Migration of *Neoascaris vitulorum* larvae in guinea-
   pigs and calves. Nigerian Journal of Science, 4, 59-65.
Euzeby, J., 1963. Les maladies vermineuses des animaux domestiques. Tome 1,
   Fasc 2, Ed. Vigot Frères, Paris.
Gautam, O.P., Bansal, S.R. and Dey-Hazra, A. 1976. Field trials with fen-
   bendazole against *Neoascaris vitulorum* in buffalo calves. Indian
   Veterinary Journal, 53, 965-966.
Gautam, O.P., Malik, P.D. and Singh, D.K., 1976. *Neoascaris vitulorum* larvae
   in the colostrum milk of buffaloes. Current Science, 45, 350.

Hasche, M.R., Bilkovich, F.R., Todd, A.C. and Schwartz, B., 1962. *Neoascaris vitulorum* (Goeze, 1782) in a Wisconsin dairy calf. Journal of Parasitology, 48, 557.

Ikeme, M.M., 1970. *Strongyloides papillosus* and *Neoascaris vitulorum* naturally acquired mixed infections of calves in the plateau area of Northern Nigeria and the treatment given. Bulletin Epizootic Diseases in Africa, 18, 339-345.

Lamina, J., 1971. Neue Erkentnisse über den Kälberspulwurm, *Toxocara vitulorum* (syn. *Neoascaris vitulorum*, Goeze, 1782). Deutsche Tierärztliche Wochenschrift, 78, 181-182.

Levi, I. and Vaupotic, A., 1967. Veterinaria Saraj., 16, 255-258. Helminthological Abstracts, No. 722, p. 103 (1968).

Macchioni, G., 1973. Experimental microascariasis in lambs infected with embryonated eggs of *Neoascaris vitulorum* (Goeze 1782, Travassos, 1927). Annali della Facolta di Medicina Veterinaria di Pisa, 25, 274-285.

Mia, S., Dewan, J.L., Uddin, M. and Chowdhury, M.U.A., 1975. The route of infection of buffalo calves by *Toxocara (Neoascaris) vitulorum*. Tropical Animal Health and Production, 7, 153-156.

Mossalam, I., Hamza, S.M. and El-Abdin, Y.Z., 1974. Studies on blood of guinea-pigs experimentally infected with *Neoascaris vitulorum*. Journal of the Egyptian Veterinary Association, 34, 73-78.

Mozgovoi, A.A. and Shakhmatova, V.I., 1969. Study on the life cycle of *Neoascaris vitulorum* (Ascaridata: Anisakidae) of ruminants. Trudy Gel' Mint, 20, 97-101.

Mozgovoi, A.A. and Shikhov, R.M., 1971. *Neoascaris vitulorum* in ruminants. Veterinariya, Moscow, 48, 59-61.

Mozgovoi, A.A., Shakhmatova, V.I. and Shikhov, R.M., 1974. Helminthological Abstracts, No. 3731, p. 822.

Mozgovoi, A.A., Shakhmatova, V.I. and Shikhov, R.M., 1975. Helminthological Abstracts, No. 2128, p. 421.

Nador, A., 1975. Data on the *Neoascaris* infection of bought-in calves. Magyar Allatorvosok Lapja, 30, 345-346.

Orekhov, U.K., 1963. Occurrence of *Neoascaris* infection in the Tyumen region. Veterinariya, 40, 48.

Rae, P., Joshi, B.P. and Vihan, V.S., 1971. Clinical studies on ascariasis in buffalo calves. Oryssa Veterinary Journal, 6, 117-119.

Selim, M.K. and Tawfik, M.A.A., 1966. Incidence of *Ascaris vitulorum* in Egyptian buffaloes during the late autumn and early winter in United Arab Republic. Indian Veterinary Journal, 43, 965-968.

580

Shikhov, R.M., 1971. Nilverm against neoascariasis in calves and buffalo calves, Veterinariya, Moscow, 48, 58-59.

Shoho, C., 1970. Finding of the nematode larvae in fresh cow milk during the post-parturial period. Journal of Parasitology, 56, 318.

Srivastava, S.C., 1963. *Neoascaris vitulorum* (Goeze 1782) Travassos 1907, in intestinal perforation with its localisation in liver of buffalo calves. Indian Veterinary Journal, 40, 758-762.

Stampa, S., 1968. The efficacy of Neguvon and Rametin against *Neoascaris vitulorum* (Goeze 1782). Journal of the South African Veterinary Medical Association, 39, 57-59.

Stone, W.M. and Smith, F.W., 1973. Infection of mammalian hosts by milk borne nematode larvae. Experimental Parasitology, 34, 306.

Tanyi, J. and Kudrun, E., 1967. Magyar Allatorvosok Lapja, 22, 332. Helminthological Abstracts, 37, p. 294 (1968).

Tanyi, J. and Danko, G., 1967. Ibid. 22, 333. Helminthological Abstracts, 37, p. 222 (1968).

Thienpont, D., Vanparijs, O., Denollin, S. and Vermeiren, G., 1977. Toxocariasis in calves, Recent diagnosis and treatment. Tijdschrift voor Diergeneeskunde, 102, 1123-1128.

Tongson, M.S., 1971. *Neoascaris vitulorum* in milk of Murrah buffalo. Philippine Journal of Veterinary Medicine, 10, 60-63.

Travassos, L. and Lacombe, D., 1959. Excursão cientifica à cidade de Belem, Atas da Sociedade de Biologia do Rio de Janeiro, 3, 9-10.

Troncy, P.M. and Oumate, O., 1973. Treatment of Chad zebu cattle with morantel tartrate. II. Effect on nematodes of suckling calves. Revue d'Elevage et de Médecine Vétérinaire des Pays Tropicaux, 26, 199-202.

Vegad, J.L., 1970. Ascariasis in calves. Oryssa Veterinary Journal, 5, 171.

Vercruysse, J., 1980. Les nématodes gastro-intestinaux du veau en R.C.A. Revue d'Elebage et de Médecine Vétérinaire des Pays Tropicaux, 33, (in press).

Warren, E.G. and Needham, D.J., 1969. On the presence of *Neoascaris vitulorum* in calves in New South Wales. Australian Veterinary Journal, 45, 22-23.

Warren, E.G., 1969. Nematode larvae in milk. Ibid., 45, 388.

Warren, E.G., 1970. Studies on the morphology and taxonomy of the genera *Toxocara* Stiles, 1905 and *Neoascaris* Travassos, 1927. Zoologischer Anzeiger, 185, 383-442.

Warren, E.G., 1971. Observations on the migration and development of
Toxocara vitulorum in natural and experimental hosts. International
Journal for Parasitology, 1, 85-99.

DISCUSSION

J. Euzeby *(France)*

I am ashamed to see that France is spreading toxocariasis
all over Europe, all the more so since we have known about these
infections for quite some time. However, there is a special
symptom of infection: it is the smell of acetone which is produced by calves with the infection. When they enter a cowshed
you can recognise if there is one with toxocariasis.

T. O'Nuallain *(Ireland)*

I confirm that *Toxocara vitulorum* has been imported into Ireland in Charolais calves. We have established that the parasite
can survive in a herd to the third generation.

J. Eckert *(Switzerland)*

Could we have more information on the prevalence or incid-
ence. I have the impression that *Toxocara* is now a real problem.
How many cases have you diagnosed and what is the prevalence in
France?

H. de Keyser *(Belgium)*

In some beef cattle concerns in Belgium they are finding
this infection more and more. There are now more farms practi-
sing beef production similar to that of France or the USA, with
suckling calves the whole year round. We did not have these
problems when the farms had a mixed beef/milk production. This
is a problem which has become more prevalent with changes in
management.

J. Eckert

What do you mean by 'more'? Hundreds of farms?

H. de Keyser

No, until now it is just a few farms.

J. Eckert

How many cases?

H. de Keyser

There are ten farms up to the present.

STUDIES ON NEMATODES IN CATTLE PERFORMED AT UNIVERSITY OF BOLOGNA. A SURVEY WITH SPECIAL EMPHASIS ON *Strongyloides papillosus*

G. Canestri-Trotti

Università Degli Studi di Bologna
Istituto di Malattie Infettive, Profilassi e Polizia Veterinaria
Via S. Giacomo, 9/2
40126 Bologna, Italy

INTRODUCTION

Since its establishment in 1966, our institute, 'Istituto Malattie Infettive, Profilassi e Polizia Veterinaria, has based its activity mainly on the epidemiology, control and socio-economic impact of animal diseases. Information about the incidence of nematode infections in Italy was scarce at that time. Since then, the Institute received a special grant from the Ministry of Health (General Direction of Veterinary Services) to study helminth infections in animals. The first series of investigations (Borelli and Tassi, 1969; Delfino and Tassi, 1969) revealed a high incidence (17 - 47%) of *Strongyloides papillosus* in calves. A research programme on this parasite was initiated. The parasite seems adapted to traditional as well as some types of industrial cattle farming which have become important for Italy.

EXPERIMENTAL STRONGYLOIDOSIS

After a preliminary study (Mantovani et al. 1969) on the natural history and pathogenesis of *S. papillosus* infection, Restani and Borelli (1971) conducted experimental infections in calves. These studies revealed a prepatent period of 10 - 12 days and a patent period of approximately 3½ months. It was shown, furthermore, that the number of eggs in the faeces does not directly reflect the number of adults in the intestine and that only a small proportion of the larvae given to the animal become established as adult worms. Reinfection trials gave strong evidence that a significant resistance to reinfection could be acquired. Finally, studies on infective larvae showed survival times of not more than 20 days under optimal conditions.

P. Nansen, R.J. Jørgensen, E.J.L. Soulsby (eds), Epidemiology and Control of Nematodiasis in Cattle.

EXPERIMENTAL PRODUCTION STUDIES

Possible production losses caused by the infection were analysed by Restani et al. (1971). Eleven calves were experimentally infected with 20 000 larvae of *Strongyloides papillosus* and seventeen uninfected calves served as controls. Table 1 summarises the data on the EPG and the number of adult parasites found in the intestines of the infected calves at slaughter. The data show that the experimental infection with *S. Papillosus* had roughly comparable characteristics in all infected calves, with the exception of calf no. 375. At slaughter this calf still had a high number of eggs in faeces and adult parasites in the intestine. This apparent uniformity helps to evaluate the economic aspects of data in that valid average data can be provided. Table 2 shows the production and dressing-out data recorded in infected and control animals as well as the corresponding values of Student's t-test. An analysis of these data shows the following:

The mean daily weight gain of both groups was comparable and normal for this type of animal production. Over the entire experimental period the infected calves had daily weight gains slightly lower than those of the control animals: 1 119 and 1 145 g respectively. This difference was not statistically significant. Before infection (from the 1st to the 40th experimental day) the average weight gains were virtually the same (controls 681 g; infected 680 g); during the prepatent period of the infection (from the 41st to the 52nd day) the weight gains were higher in the infected group (controls 681 g; infected 716 g); whereas during the patent period (from 53rd to 125th day) the infected animals had a daily gain lower than that of the controls (controls 1 475 g; infected 1 426 g). All recorded differences, however, were not statistically significant.

Feed conversion was identical in both groups of animals (1.42), this value corresponding to a 70.3% milk efficiency. The control group consumed more milk (+ 36 g/day/head).

The final body weights, the slaughterhouse weights, the dead weights, the dressing-out percentages, were higher in

the control group, though the differences were not statistically significant when compared with the infected calves.

The weight of gastro-intestinal contents was higher in control animals than in infected animals (controls 11.59 kg;
infected 8.99 kg); this difference is statistically significant (P <0.05).

The differences between the average weights of the primary
offals (gullet, trachea, lungs, heart, liver and spleen)
was statistically significant (controls 8.05 kg; infected
9.21 kg; P <0.01). Also significant (P <0.01) was the difference between the weights of the empty gastro-intestinal
tracts (controls 12.34 kg; infected 14.32 kg).

The survey indicates that the higher body weight of controls
at the end of the trial (186.80 kg in comparison to 183.29 kg)
was mainly due to the high weight of the gastro-intestinal contents (controls 11.59 kg; infected 8.99 kg). In fact, the differences in the empty body weights were fairly low in the two
groups (controls 169.17 kg; infected 168.28 kg). The control
calves, however, had a dead weight (106.18 kg) higher than that
of the infected animals (103.45 kg), this being due to the fact
that the 'fifth quarter' (head, shanks and feet, skin, primary
offals, stomach and intestines) of the infected animals was
larger than in controls (50.53 kg compared with 47.32 kg). Thus,
there is a slight difference between the dressing-out percentages
in the two groups, but such a difference becomes more apparent
when the net dressing-out percentage is considered (carcase/empty
body) although there is still no statistically significant difference. The dressing-out percentage is largely influenced by
the contents of the gastro-intestinal tracts while the net dressing-out percentage (carcase/empty body) depends upon the 'fifth
quarter'.

In these investigations a fairly uniform infection was
obtained which led to reduced meat production without being
accompanied by overt clinical symptoms. The decrease was less
marked when comparing the weight gains of the two groups, but a

significant difference was noticed when comparing the weight of the carcases. Here the higher weight of the controls could be explained by lower weight of the so-called 'fifth quarter'. If one considers that the net profit of each animal was about 10 000 Lire under the market conditions prevailing at that time, it appears that the infected animals (taking into consideration both the feeding costs and the different selling conditions) had a lower profit (about 15% for the body weight and about 25% for the dead weight.

OTHER STUDIES ON STRONGYLOIDOSIS

Later, Mantovani et al. (1972) and Mantovani et al. (1974) demonstrated that the infective larvae of *S. papillosus* were capable of not only introducing *Sphaerophorus necrophorus* into the subcutaneous tissues of rabbit and sheep, but also of carrying the organism to the lungs of the rabbit, where a synergetic action between the organisms was exerted. Restani and Borrelli (1968) evaluated the efficacy of Thiabendazole in experimental infection with this nematode in calves and later (1971) the efficacy of Cambendazole.

SURVEY OF DISTRIBUTION OF GASTRO-INTESTINAL STRONGYLOSIS

A survey on cattle, sheep, goats, horses and swine in Italy was carried out by Tassi and Widenhorn (1972). Out of 4 522 cattle examined (belonging to 383 farms) 1 429 were positive (31.6%). Out of 7 224 sheep examined (belonging to 505 farms) 5 498 were positive (76.1%). Of 364 goats examined (belonging to 60 farms) 333 were positive (91.4%). Of 1 661 horses, 1 246 were positive (75.0%). Of 7 635 reproduction pigs examined (belonging to 503 farms) 3 185 were positive (41.7%). Of 1 727 fattening pigs examined (belonging to 233 farms) 250 were positive (14.4%).

The helminthological research of the Institute was then mainly devoted to sheep management, which represents an emerging problem in our country due to its economic implications in some regions, furthermore, to the study of economic problems associated

TABLE 1

RESULTS OF EPG AND DETERMINATION OF ADULT BURDENS IN 11 CALVES EXPERIMENTALLY INFECTED WITH 20 000 LARVAE OF *Strongyloides papillosus* ON JANUARY 21, 1971, AND SLAUGHTERED AFTER 12 WEEKS

| Calf no. | EPG Daily data | | | | | | EPG Weekly averages | | | | | | | | | | Total no. of adult parasites |
	29/1	30/1	31/1	1/2	2/2	3/2	4/2-10/2	11/2-17/2	18/2-24/2	25/2-3/3	4/3-10/3	11/3-17/3	18/3-24/3	25/3-31/3	1/4-7/4	8/4-14/4	
375	0	0	0	0	100	80	60	4550	10360	8680	10080	9070	5870	5030	1870	1160	855
370	0	0	0	140	–	600	600	4640	2510	1510	790	310	110	10	10	0	0
365	0	0	0	0	0	80	160	2270	1250	1070	500	470	70	20	0	0	3
341	0	0	0	100	740	320	1110	3340	5510	4180	1720	400	80	30	0	0	0
451	0	0	0	40	720	40	90	2470	860	1040	230	40	0	10	0	0	0
369	0	0	0	140	–	920	280	5150	3170	1280	430	90	30	40	10	10	0
254	0	0	0	20	480	1360	920	5850	7870	2680	3570	1440	470	30	40	10	0
345	0	0	0	180	1340	1560	940	5780	6150	5040	2670	1900	400	220	50	30	1
374	0	0	0	0	–	280	610	5930	5140	4700	3780	1090	120	30	60	0	2
338	0	0	0	20	180	200	1390	3030	4330	4130	2740	2660	590	550	190	50	0
411	0	0	0	20	560	–	160	4390	6330	3120	2500	640	190	160	0	20	20

(–) Faecal samples not collected

with these and other parasitic diseases such as fascioliasis and, finally, to the practical implementation of data both via veterinary and political channels. These activities formed the basis for a very recent enactment of a special law against parasitic diseases in Emilia-Romagna, which is one of the regions where the Institute carries out much of its activity.

TABLE 2

RESULTS OF THE WEIGHT GAINS, FEED CONSUMPTIONS, FEED EFFICIENCY AND SLAUGHTER-HOUSE PARAMETERS (MEAN VALUES)

	Controls	Infected	t (**)
No. of calves	17	11	–
Trial length, gg,	125	125	–
Initial body weight, kg,	43.65	43.36	0.400
Final body weight, kg,	186.80	183.29	1.029
Feed consumption/day/head, g,	1629	1593	–
Daily weight gain from 1^O to 40°, g,	681	680	0.039
" " " " 41° to 52° , g,	681	716	0.745
" " " " 53° to 125°, g,	1475	1426	1.643
" " " " 1^O to 125°, g,	1145	1119	0.957
Feed efficiency	1.42	1.42	–
Slaughterhouse live weight, kg,	180.76	177.27	1.030
Weight of head with skin, kg,	9.48	9.05	1.790
Weight of shanks and feet with skin, kg,	4.58	4.50	0.694
Weight of skin, kg,	12.87	13.45	1.517
Weight of primary offals,*, kg,	8.05	9.21	5.379
Weight of empty stomachs and intestines, kg,	12.34	14.32	3.273
Weight of gastro-intestinal contents, kg,	11.59	8.99	2.365
Dead weight, kg,	106.18	103.45	0.945
Net live weight, kg,	169.17	168.28	0.262
Dressing-out percentages, (Carcase/body weight, %,	58.72	58.34	0.479
Net dressing-out percentage, (Carcase, empty body weight,%,	62.74	61.41	1.541

* Gullet, trachea, lungs, heart, liver and spleen
** t Values:for =P 0.05; t = 2.056; for P = 0.01; t = 2.779

589

REFERENCES

Borrelli, D. and Tassi, P., 1969. Ricerche sulla presenza di uova di
   Strongyloides sp. nelle feci di bovini della pianura padana. Atti
   Soc. ital. Buiatria, 1, 410-415.

Delfino, F. and Tassi, P., 1969. Indagini sulla diffusione di *Strongyloides*
   papillosus in bovini di razza piemontese e suoi ibridi in una area
   della provincia di Cuneo. Atti Soc. ital. Buiatria, 1, 399-409.

Mantovani, A., Restani, R. and Borrelli, D., 1969. Storia naturale e
   patogenesi della infestazione da *Strongyloides papillosus* nel bovino.
   Atti Convegno Strongilosi Gastrointestinali Bovini Piemonte, 93-105.

Mantovani, A., Restani, R., Ricci-Bitti, G., Sanguinetti, V. and Biavati, S.,
   1974. Sulla trasmissione di *Sphaerophorus necrophorus* tramite larve
   di *Strongyloides papillosus* nella pecora. Vet. ital., 25, 122-132.

Mantovani, A., Togoe, I., Canestri-Trotti, G., Ricci-Bitti, G. and
   Gualandi, L., 1972. Sulla trasmissione di *Sphaerophorus necrophorus*
   tramite larve di *Strongyloides papillosus* nel coniglio.
   Parassitologia, 14, 149-162.

Restani, R. and Borrelli, D., 1968. Ricerche sulla attività del tiabendazolo
   nella infestazione sperimentale da *Strongyloides papillosus* dei
   vitelli. Atti Soc. ital. Sci. vet., 22, 722-725.

Restani, R. and Borrelli, D., 1971a. Osservazioni sulla infestazione
   sperimentale del vitello con *Strongyloides papillosus*. Parassitologia,
   13, 315-319.

Restani, R. and Borrelli, D., 1971b. Ricerche sull'attività del cambendazolo
   nella infestazione sperimentale da *Strongyloides papillosus* dei
   vitelli. Vet. ital., 22, 140-147.

Restani, R., Canestri-Trotti, G., Manfredini, M. and Romiti, R., 1971.
   Ricerche zooeconomiche sull'infestazione sperimentale da *Strongyloides*
   papillosus in vitelli da latte. Vet. ital., 22, 342-358.

Tassi, P. and Widenhorn, O., 1972. Indagine orientativa sulla distribuzione
   della strongilosi gastro-intestinale in allevamenti di bovini, ovini,
   caprini, equini e suini in Italia. Parassitologia, 14, 381-398.

DISCUSSION

J. Armour *(UK)*

Is the transmission of *Strongyloides* infection from the mother to the calf in the milk?

G. Canestri-Trotti *(Italy)*

We have not studied this problem.

J. Armour

When you first saw the infections in the field in calves, were they in very young calves?

G. Canestri-Trotti

Yes, in the very young calves. We infected the animals experimentally with 20 000 larvae of *Strongyloides papillosus*.

R.M. Jones *(UK)*

What is the basis of your incidence data? Was it based on worm counts or egg counts?

G. Canestri-Trotti

Egg counts, using the McMaster technique.

E.J.L. Soulsby *(UK)*

Is the infection seasonal?

G. Canestri-Trotti

We have not studied this aspect. In our region the animals are always at pasture and therefore the differences may not be so marked.

J. Eckert *(Switzerland)*

Can you give any information on the age groups? You reported that about 75% of sheep are infected with *Strongyloides* and nearly 100% of the goats. Were these animals of all age groups? What was the average age? Is this a strongyloidosis or a strongylosis?

G. Canestri-Trotti

It is strongylosis.

J. Eckert

Then my question is not valid. I thought this was strongyloidosis.

G. Canestri-Trotti

No. It was a mixed infection of gastro-intestinal strongyles.

PROPOSALS AND RECOMMENDATIONS

MADE BY WORKING GROUPS

Co-ordinators:
Peter Nansen and Rolf Jess Jørgensen

INTRODUCTION

J.F. Michel

The hazard of loss from helminthiasis is one of a number of constraints on agricultural innovation and hence there must be a close relationship between agricultural development and research in veterinary helminthology. Studies of the helminthological impact of new husbandry practices, after these are in general use, is far too late and ways should be found of fostering closer collaboration between agronomists and veterinary helminthologists.

Besides the effects of new systems of management, other changes also demand investigation. Thus, hosts, and therefore their parasites, may be moved from one region to another and parasite populations respond to changes in their environment. In particular they respond to the control measures directed against them by changes in their biological characteristics, their host tolerance or their resistance to anthelmintics.

It is evident that the large body of existing knowledge on the epidemiology and control of nematode infections in cattle is not making the practical impact that it might. The control measures that are available are only partially implemented; more attention should be devoted to translating epidemiological knowledge into realistic and workable recommendations, to studying the helminthological and agricultural consequences of their adoption and to developing lines of communication with farmers and their advisers.

Over the past few years, it has been considered that the epidemiology and control of the nematode infections of cattle were thoroughly understood and that points of detail only needed to be filled in. While such detailed work is still needed and epidemiological patterns have still to be worked

out in some parts of the EEC, it has been an important feature
of this workshop that a number of new developments have been
presented which bear directly on the epidemiology and control
of cattle parasites.

Nematode infections are an important cause of impaired
production. Deaths and losses associated with overt clinical
disease are of much less importance than those of reduced
production performance of apparently normal animals. The
incidence and severity of infections are closely related to
the methods of grazing management that are employed. Some
grazing systems contain a hazard of damage due to nematodes,
others do not. An adequate understanding of the epidemiology
of nematode infections is an essential prerequisite for the
design of control measures. These consist largely of the
selection of systems of management in which damaging infections
cannot arise.

The intensification of methods of production does not, of
itself, necessarily increase the severity of nematode infections
but the economic significance of such production losses that do
occur due to worm infection is far greater in intensive systems.
The real importance of nematode infections is that they
represent an obstacle to the development and adoption of more
efficient and more cost-effective methods of production.

The costs attributable to nematode infections of cattle
in the EEC are of three kinds: 1) losses due to impaired production; in present conditions of management these are estimated
at £75M annually in young cattle and, if recent studies in the
Netherlands and Belgium are confirmed, further losses of £400M
in milking cows should be added; 2) the cost of misdirected or
ineffective control measures, on the basis of recent studies
in the UK, is likely to exceed £15M annually: 3) losses
resulting from the use of practices less efficient than those
that might be used, were it not for the hazard of helminthiasis;
such are difficult to estimate, but almost certainly exceed
those listed under 1) and 2) above.

The capitalised benefit of reducing these losses by half seems to be not less than £800M. It could exceed £3000M. The support of properly directed research, development and extension work on the nematodes of cattle would thus be an excellent investment.

The following four working groups, dealing respectively with epidemiology, immunology, pathophysiology and anthelmintics, present recommendations which identify a number of areas where research is considered to be necessary.

*

PATHOPHYSIOLOGICAL STUDIES ON NEMATODE INFECTION IN ADULT ANIMALS

Chairman: J. Armour

Throughout Europe a large number of dairy cows are infected with gastro-intestinal worms. There is experimental evidence to show that infection with such worms can affect milk production. Some field evidence is available to indicate that worms in adult cows may be of practical economic significance.

To date there is no information on how such worms exert their effect and we believe this to be an area worthy of further study, preferably in collaboration with other workers (e.g. dairy scientists).

The following research areas are of particular relevance to these problems:

- Pathological changes following infections of young cattle and dairy cows, particularly the effect of continuous larval challenge.
- The effects on digestion and absorption associated with infection.

- The effects of helminth infection on milk production.
- The effects of helminth infections on reproductive performance.

*

EPIDEMIOLOGY AND CONTROL OF NEMATODES
Chairmen: H.J. Over and R. Connan

ECOLOGY

Studies should be made of the role of the soil in the ecology of larvae. For example, do larvae actively move into and out of the soil or are they dependent on other agencies? What effect does slurry have on the ability of the soil to serve as a reservoir for larvae?

These studies must be carried out in the diverse situations represented by the different regions of the European Community. They should embrace the differences of management, of soil structure and of vegetation types which these include.

Larvae in the soil are part of the overall larval pool. Every encouragement should be given to the development of methods and techniques for their study.

EPIDEMIOLOGY

(a) Gastro-intestinal nematodes

There is a considerable body of knowledge available on the epidemiology of ostertagiasis. However, there is a need for the continuous monitoring of the effect on parasite epidemiology of changes in farm practices and of the control methods employed. The behaviour of parasites may be modified by control pressures and these may differ in various regions.

There is need to re-examine other gastro-intestinal trichostrongylids in the light of knowledge of *Ostertagia*.

(b) *Dictyocaulus viviparus*

Pasture infection levels can change swiftly necessitating frequent sampling. The acquisition of knowledge of the epidemiology of *D. viviparus* has fallen behind that of *Ostertagia*. It still remains, for instance, to define the origins of natural infection and the particular determinants of disease. This should be a fruitful field for the collaboration of many laboratories in the different areas of the community.

CONTROL

There are problems associated with the application of control methods. Helminths are a major constraint on animal production and therefore parasitologists should have an input into the planning and development of new practices. Recommendations must be integrated into methods of management. This requires teamwork with agronomists, nutritionists and others and their recommendations may be subordinate to other factors in the development of efficient production methods. These will vary locally to suit differences of climate, social background, etc.

The disposal of slurry (animal waste) and of sewage sludge (human) presents special problems. Further study of these problems is recommended, aimed at finding safe and useful methods for disposal.

*

RESEARCH NEEDS IN IMMUNOLOGY

Chairman: E.J.L. Soulsby

The immune response probably plays an important role in the epidemiology of parasitic infections in cattle. There is a need to couple immunological and epidemiological studies to assess the influence of the immune status on parasite populations in animals, transmission rates, etc. However, there is still much basic information required on the immuno-logical system of the bovine, and basic studies of immune mechanisms and the epidemiological significance must go hand in hand.

Studies on the ontogeny of the immune response in calves to gastro-intestinal nematodes are necessary; they should include antibody and cell mediated responses, and character-isation of lymphocyte functions, to both abomasal (e.g. *Ostertagia*) and intestinal (e.g. *Cooperia*) parasites, with particular reference to the marked variability of calves to such infections.

Induced immunosuppression to other infections (parasitic and otherwise) has been noted in a number of parasitic diseases; it may be a feature of infection in animals of all ages or be associated more specifically with infections at an early age. There is no information on this phenomenon in gastro-intestinal parasitism in the bovine and work is necessary to investigate this aspect.

Periparturient relaxation of the immune response is a well-known phenomenon in various experimental parasitic infections. There is some evidence that it does occur in the bovine but there is need to study the phenomenon in the cow in greater detail.

Because of the general importance of *Ostertagia* in cattle and the paucity of knowledge about the immune response to this parasite, there is a major need to study the factors which govern the initiation and maintenance of immunity to it in cattle.

Various approaches to immunisation need investigation. These might include the use of less pathogenic strains of parasites from different geographical areas, attenuated infective stages, immunogens produced by *in vitro* techniques, and materials derived from the immune response (e.g. transfer factor).

Because of the major expense of immunological work in cattle with parasitic infections, there is need to search for more satisfactory *in vitro* correlates which would satisfactorily evaluate the immune status of an animal or a herd.

Research would be greatly assisted by the establishment of a register of species and strains of parasites of cattle, together with a system for the identification of isolates.

*

ANTHELMINTICS

Chairman: J. Eckert

In the past decade new anthelmintics, highly active against a broad spectrum of nematode species and developmental stages, have been introduced. Their application has contributed to the effective control of nematodiasis in cattle under various epidemiological conditions. However, further improvement is necessary in order to obtain optimal productivity in cattle farming. Therefore, the group defined the following research needs.

The evaluation is needed of new methods for the application of anthelmintics, such as long acting devices, continuous dosing, slow release preparations, etc.. There are

some indications that the use of such methods may improve
the effectiveness of nematode control in grazing animals.

The development of practical testing procedures to
monitor drug sensitivity is recommended.

Studies in the USA and some other countries indicate
that anthelmintic treatment of cows at parturition may be
beneficial for milk production. However, published results
are equivocal. A study of the economic and parasitological
effects and of the optimal timing of anthelmintic treatment
of cows should be undertaken.

Integrated control programmes, based on improved
epidemiological knowledge, pasture rotation and strategic
treatments require further evaluation under various agricultural and epidemiological conditions.

Immunity plays an important role in the protection of
cattle against diseases caused by nematodes. The influence
of anthelmintic treatments on the immune status of cattle
requires further clarification.

A working group attended by representatives from Denmark,
the Federal Republic of Germany, Great Britain and Switzerland
recommended the preparation of international guidelines for
the efficacy evaluation of anthelmintics.

Such draft guidelines have been prepared in the USA.
The aim of these guidelines is to standardise the evaluation
procedures and to make the results comparable. This could
reduce costs, manpower and experimental animals.

*

LIST OF PARTICIPANTS

J. ARMOUR
Wellcome Laboratory for Experimental Parasitology
University of Glasgow
Veterinary School
Bearsden Road
Bearsden, Glasgow G6I 1QH
UK

D. BARTH
Sharp and Dohme GmbH
Kathrinenhof
Walchenseestrasse 8-12
D-8201 Lauterbach
FRG

F.H.M. BORGSTEEDE
Centraal Diergeneeskundig Instituut
Afdeling Parasitologie
Edelhertweg 13
NL-8219 PH Lelystad
The Netherlands

H.-J. BÜRGER
Institut für Parasitologie
der Tierärztlichen Hochschule
Bünteweg 17
D-3000 Hannover 71
FRG

G. CANESTRI-TROTTI
Universita degli studi di Bologna
Instituto di malattie infettive, profilassi
e polizia veterinaria
Via S. Giacomo 9/2
I-40126 Bologna
Italy

R.M. CONNAN
Veterinary School
Department of Animal Pathology
Madingley Road
Cambridge CB3 OES
UK

N.E. DOWNEY
The Agricultural Institute
Dunsinea Research Centre
Castleknock
Co. Dublin
Ireland

D. DÜWEL
Hoechst AG
Helminthologie
Postfach 800320
D-6230 Frankfurt/Main 80
FRG

J. ECKERT
Institut für Parasitologie
Universität Zürich
CH-8057 Zürich
Switzerland

604

J. EUZEBY	Ecole Vétérinaire de Lyon F-69260 Charbonnieres-les-Bains France
J. FOLDAGER	National Institute of Animal Science 25 Rolighedsvej DK-1958 Copenhagen V Denmark
J.W. HANSEN	Institute of Veterinary Microbiology and Hygiene Royal Veterinary and Agricultural University 13 Bülowsvej DK-1870 Copenhagen V Denmark
O. HELLE	Institut for indremedisin I Norges Veterinaerhøgskole Boks 8146 Oslo Dep. Oslo 1 Norway
SV. AA. HENRIKSEN	State Veterinary Serum Laboratory 27 Bülowsvej DK-1870 Copenhagen V Denmark
F. INDERBITZIN	Institut für Parasitologie Universität Zürich CH-8057 Zürich Switzerland
D.E. JACOBS	The Royal Veterinary College Hawkshead House Hawkshead Lane North Mimms Hatfield, Herts AL9 7TA UK
J. JANSEN	Instituut voor Veterinaire Parasitologie en Parasitaire Ziekten 'De Uithof' Yalelaan 7 NL-3584 CL Utrecht The Netherlands
R.M. JONES	Pfizer Limited Central Research Sandwich, Kent CT13 9NJ UK
R.J. JØRGENSEN	Institute of Veterinary Microbiology and Hygiene Royal Veterinary and Agricultural University 13 Bülowsvej DK-1870 Copenhagen V Denmark

H. DE KEYSER	Janssen Pharmaceutica B-2340 Beerse Belgium
A. KLOOSTERMAN	Vakgrope Veehouderij van de Landbouwhogeschool Postbus 338 NL-6700 AH Wageningen The Netherlands
G. LUFFAU	Institut National de la Recherche Agronomique Station de Recherches de Virologie et d'Immunologie Route de Thiverval F-78850 Thiverval-Grignon France
J.F. MICHEL	Central Veterinary Laboratory Weybridge Surrey UK
P. NANSEN	Institute of Veterinary Microbiology and Hygiene Royal Veterinary and Agricultural University 13 Bülowsvej DK-1870 Copenhagen V Denmark
O. NILSSON	AB Svensk Laboratorietjanst Box 9003 S-291 09 Kristianstad Sweden
T. Ó NUALLÁIN	Department of Veterinary Parasitology Veterinary College Dublin 4 Ireland
J. O'SHEA	The Agricultural Institute Dunsinea Castleknock Co. Dublin Ireland
H.J. OVER	Centraal Diergeneeskundig Instituut Afdeling Parasitologie Edelhertweg 13 NL-8219 PH Lelystad The Netherlands
L. POUPLARD	Faculté de Médecine Vétérinaire 45 rue des Vétérinaires B-1070 Brussels Belgium
J.-P. RAYNAUD	Laboratoire Pfizer F-37400 Amboise France

606

E.J.L. SOULSBY

Veterinary School
Department of Animal Pathology
Madingley Road
Cambridge CB3 OES
UK

R.J. THOMAS

School of Agriculture
University of Newcastle upon Tyne
Newcastle upon Tyne
UK

G.M. URQUHART

Wellcome Laboratory for Experimental Parasitology
University of Glasgow
Veterinary School
Bearsden Road
Bearsden, Glasgow G6I 1QH
UK

E. VIGLIANI

Instituto zooprofilattico
Via Bologna 148
I-10154 Torino
Italy

RECORDING PERSONNEL

GILLIAN J. COOKES

S.E.W. HALLAM

Janssen Services
14 The Quay
Lower Thames Street
London EC3R 6BU
UK

Manuscript was prepared by:

Janssen Services, 14 The Quay, Lower Thames Street, London EC3 6BU, UK.